Forms for the Therapist

Forms for the Therapist

ALLAN G. HEDBERG

Amsterdam • Boston • Heidelberg • London • New York • Oxford
Paris • San Diego • San Francisco • Singapore • Sydney • Tokyo

Academic Press is an imprint of Elsevier

http://booksite.academicpress.com/Hedberg/forms/

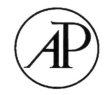

Academic Press is an imprint of Elsevier
32 Jamestown Road, London NW1 7BY, UK
30 Corporate Drive, Suite 400, Burlington, MA 01803, USA
525 B Street, Suite 1800, San Diego, CA 92101-4495, USA

First edition 2010

Notice
No responsibility is assumed by the publisher for any injury and/or damage to persons
or property as a matter of products liability, negligence or otherwise, or from any use or
operation of any methods, products, instructions or ideas contained in the material herein.
Because of rapid advances in the medical sciences, in particular, independent verification of
diagnoses and drug dosages should be made

British Library Cataloguing-in-Publication Data
A catalogue record for this book is available from the British Library

Library of Congress Cataloging-in-Publication Data
A catalog record for this book is available from the Library of Congress

ISBN : 978-0-12-374933-8

For information on all Academic Press publications
visit our website at www.elsevierdirect.com

Typeset by MPS Limited, a Macmillan Company, Chennai, India
www.macmillansolutions.com

Printed and bound by CPI Group (UK) Ltd, Croydon, CR0 4YY
Transferred to digital print 2012

Working together to grow
libraries in developing countries

www.elsevier.com | www.bookaid.org | www.sabre.org

ELSEVIER   BOOK AID International   Sabre Foundation

CONTENTS

Part I Starting and Managing Your Clinical Practice   1

Chapter 1
FORMS FOR SETTING UP AND DEFINING YOUR PRACTICE   3

Chapter 2
FORMS RELATED TO FEES

Chapter 3
HIPAA/PATIENT PRIVACY FORMS

Chapter 4
GENERAL INFORMATIONAL HANDOUTS FOR PATIENTS

Chapter 5
FORMS RELATED TO REFERRAL AND CONSULTING SERVICES

Chapter 10
TERMINATION OF TREATMENT/PRACTICE FORMS

Chapter 11
FORMS FOR SESSION NOTES

Chapter 12
CLINICAL ERRORS, BAD HABITS, ETHICAL COMPLAINTS, AND LAW SUITS

Part III Forms, Exercises, and Information for Treating Specific Disorders

Chapter 22
SUICIDAL BEHAVIOR   275

Chapter 23
PAIN MANAGEMENT AND COPING WITH MEDICAL DISORDERS   281

Chapter 24
ANGER AND VIOLENT BEHAVIOR   299

Part IV Skill Building Strategies and Tools for Personal Growth and Life Improvement   313

Chapter 25
STRATEGIES AND TOOLS FOR PERSONAL GROWTH AND HEALTH
AWARENESS   315

Chapter 26
COMMUNICATION TIPS AND EXERCISES

Chapter 27
EATING AND EXERCISE LOGS

Chapter 28
CULTURAL DIVERSITY APPRECIATION EXERCISES

Chapter 29
CONFLICT RESOLUTION AND PROBLEM SOLVING

Chapter 34
DEALING WITH GERIATRIC PATIENTS

Chapter 35
COUPLES THERAPY AND RELATIONSHIP ASSESSMENT AND EXERCISES

The website with electronic forms from this book can be found at:
http://booksite.academicpress.com/Hedberg/forms/

LIST OF ICONS

	FORM TYPE LEGEND
	Information for the Therapist
	Assessment Tools
	Patient Homework or Assignment Outside Therapy
	Information for the Patient
	Exercises to be Performed in Therapy
	Forms to be Completed by Therapist or Patient
	Sample Forms and Templates

LIST OF FORMS BY TYPE

INFORMATION FOR THE THERAPIST

Eating and Exercise

Cultural Diversity Appreciation

Dealing with Crisis

Serving Children and Their Families

Dealing with Geriatric Patients

Couples Therapy and Relationships

ASSESSMENT TOOLS

Organizing Your Charts and Evaluations

General Assessments: Intake, Brief, Comprehensive, and More

Specific Tests and Scales

Risk, Competency, Health, and Neuropsychology

Anxiety and Stress Relief

Addictive Behavior

Pain Management and Coping with Medical Disorders

Anger and Violent Behavior

Communication Tips and Exercises

Serving Children and Their Families

Dealing with Geriatric Patients

Couples Therapy and Relationships

PATIENT HOMEWORK OR ASSIGNMENT OUTSIDE THERAPY

Related to Patient Services

Anxiety and Stress Relief

Depression and Self-Esteem

Insomnia/Sleep Therapy

Addictive Behavior

Pain Management and Coping with Medical Disorders

Anger and Violent Behavior

Strategies and Tools for Personal Growth and Health Awareness

Communication

Eating and Exercise

INFORMATION FOR THE PATIENT

Related to Fees

Couples Therapy and Relationships

EXERCISES TO BE PERFORMED IN THERAPY

General Assessments: Intake, Brief, Comprehensive, and More

Anxiety and Stress Relief

Insomnia/Sleep Therapy

Anger and Violent Behavior

Strategies and Tools for Personal Growth and Health Awareness

Communication

Conflict Resolution and Problem Solving

Serving Children and Their Families

FORMS TO BE COMPLETED BY THERAPIST OR PATIENT

Fitness for Duty and Workers' Compensation

Related to Patient Services

Related to Therapist's Professional Activities

Managing an Office Staff

Termination of Treatment/Practice Forms

Forms for Session Notes

General Assessments: Intake, Brief, Comprehensive, and More

SAMPLES FORMS AND TEMPLATES

Fitness for Duty/Workers' Compensation Forms

Forms Related to Patient Services

Managing an Office Staff

Termination of Treatment/Practice Forms

Serving Children and Their Families

CONTRIBUTORS

Laura S. Brown
Seattle, Washington 98103, USA

Lowell M. Campbell
Shakopee, Minnesota 55379, USA

Yosef Geshuri
Porterville, California 93257, USA

Marty Harris
Vanguard University of Southern California, Costa Mesa,
California 92626, USA

Allan G. Hedberg
Fresno, California 93710, USA

Sharon L. Johnson
Fresno, California 93710, USA

Michael Kesselman
Fresno, California 93710, USA

D.H. Mapson
Fresno, California 93729, USA

David Modders
Ocala, Florida 34480-6187, USA

Duane Oswald
Avante Health, Fresno, California 93720, USA

Michael Regier
Fresno, California 93710, USA

Paul W. Schenk
Tucker, Georgia 30084, USA

Bradley A. Schuyler
Fresno, California 93710, USA

Norman M. Shulman
Lubbock, Texas 79446, USA

Joy D. Staley
Yakima, Washington 98908, USA

Sandra S. Valenzuela
Fresno, California 93710, USA

Steven Younker
Yakima, Washington 98908, USA

ABOUT THE EDITOR

Allan G. Hedberg, PhD has had a distinguished career in clinical psychology for over 40 years. Since his graduation from Queen's University, Kingston, Ontario, Canada, in 1969, he has engaged in the teaching of psychology, training of young professionals, writing on a variety of psychological topics, speaking on psychological issues to a wide variety of audiences, and applying psychological principles to various workplace and community problems through his consulting practice. In addition, he has maintained an active, community-based private practice, providing therapy to a host of individuals experiencing "problems in living" in troubled times.

Dr Hedberg has also served on many boards and committees. In so doing, his training and experience in psychology has been drawn upon to encourage these organizations to be committed to their mission and be intentionally purpose-driven.

Most importantly, he and his wife, Bernice, have reared three children, all of whom have married and assumed their own independent places of leadership in their individual spheres of influence.

PREFACE

My wife and I collect antiques. We have specialized in primitives. We started in 1960, during our honeymoon. We have collected ever since. One old antique dealer said to us, "Just collect, no matter what! The value is in how many of any item you have and the uniqueness of the collection." He further said, "Get your kids started young too. Help them collect whatever they are interested in even though it will change over time." So we did just that. We learned history through our stuff.

Professionally, I also collected stuff. I have had as many as six filing cabinets full of reprints, forms, lecture material, old lecture notes, articles that might be of help some day, and illustration material for a lecture or article I might write some day. The files were originally set up based on the Dewey Decimal System used to catalogue books. A little obsessive compulsiveness helps when you collect.

I also have three filing cabinets full of Psychological Testing materials and tests. I have collected tests over the years from many sources. I even have three kits of the original Wechsler. I still have my original Binet I used in graduate school at Queen's University. Paper and pencil tests are categorized by area of usage and purpose. Reprints and articles on test validity, reliability, utilization, false negatives and false positive, and relevant research are all intermingled in and among the various tests. Survey forms, tests, questionnaires, and checklists are all included in my file drawers of "Testing Supplies."

You never know when you will want to put some kind of number to an observation or behavior pattern. Just be ready to do so.

To my young colleagues, I say, "Collect." It does not matter what it is, as the value is in the range of professional materials collected and filed for ready access. Collect tests and forms. They will come in handy along the way of your professional career. Enjoy collecting. Look for new items for possible use. Look for things that may be helpful to you when you face an unexpected challenge in your practice.

This book, *Forms for the Therapist*, was written for you. It is designed to help you start, or add to, your own collection of forms for your clinical use. The forms contained in the book are there for you to reproduce and utilize freely. You will be a better clinician and a better scientist as you systematize your practice and approach with your patients. Start now. Use the forms. Learn to design your own. Share them. Modify them. Make forms part of your practice. You and your patients will be better for it!

All of the forms herein may be photocopied (or downloaded via the website) for individual use by therapists with patients. However they may not be posted elsewhere, distributed to anyone other than an individual patient, or used as teaching material in courses without prior permission by Elsevier.

This isn't meant to be a comprehensive book of all the forms one might need to have in starting, running, or growing a practice. They are simply the best of what we found on a number of common topics, to provide a start or continuation of the collection of forms you already have. We encourage clinicians to share best practices, and if you have a form you've found particularly helpful, I would be pleased to see it for a future edition of this book.

ACKNOWLEDGMENTS

To complete any work, it takes the diligent assistance of many others. Particular appreciation is expressed to:

Gina Beery, a very choice secretary and receptionist, who balanced the daily demands of the practice, making sure her duties as receptionist were not overlooked, while eagerly assisting me in many ways to produce this manuscript in a timely manner.

Kathy Hamlin, a faithful typist, who maintained a cheerful attitude despite her extra load. Kathy worked long hours, typing and correcting many pages, to assure that the book was readable, accurate, and completed on time.

Bernice Hedberg, my First Class wife of 50 years, who worked with me late into the evening to see that a chapter was completed before midnight! She helped me balance the extra writing, the demands of the practice, family life, and social relationships in a healthy manner. She is a dear wife with a living faith.

Nikki Levy, Barbara Makinster, Elaine Leek and Caroline Jones of Elsevier Publishing who shepherded the writing process, providing their wisdom and direction to help design and organize a useful book to meet the needs of the active professional therapist. They make a great team for any author to learn from and develop improved writing skills. As a result of their efforts to bring this book to the professional community, therapists will not have to reinvent the "Wheel of Forms and Documents" on their own as they establish a new practice or grow and mature their existing practices.

All the contributors who unselfishly offered forms and documents out of their own practices to share with the readers and users of this book. All of them saw value in this book and wanted to be part of it. It was important to them to share in the meaning and satisfaction of "passing it on."

And, lastly, any significant project becomes accomplished as a result of the efforts of a support team helping and being a source of encouragement. I thank my family members and friends that served in this capacity with me over the past year, as they have also done before on other projects I have undertaken.

Part I

Starting and Managing Your Clinical Practice

One of the exciting benefits of years of professional training, personal and professional development, work experience, and additional clinical experience, is the starting of a clinical practice. For some, it is joining an affiliation of therapists but having responsibility for their own practice. For others, it is a solo, independent practice venture. And for others, it is the establishment of some type of corporate entity.

Starting a practice is starting a small business. It is the time when the therapist feels ready to plant roots deep within the soil of the community and serve those in the community. While there is no rule of thumb as to when a person is ready to start their own practice, it is generally considered wisdom to hold off on such a decision until the therapist has had a few years of experience in some type of structured employment situation.

Starting a practice is an entrepreneurial effort and enterprise. Long office hours, community networking, building professional relationships, on-call availability, and establishing name recognition are all required, often without billable time opportunity.

Starting a practice is a journey. It is a journey with potholes that need to be avoided. Also, the journey has the opportunity for the joy of success, but success needs to be created and honed. Being well-prepared and having the tools necessary to create the success will make the journey a satisfying experience.

The forms, checklists, guidelines, information sheets, and templates in Part I will aid the therapist in starting the practice and growing it in a timely and orderly manner. The forms included in this Part will also help manage the practice successfully. It is vital that all patients and clients of the practice be well served to their satisfaction and that their personal growth is experienced fully.

Chapter 1

Forms for Setting Up and Defining Your Practice

Chapter Contents

Establishing a viable and successful practice needs to be properly planned and systematically developed. No longer can one begin a practice with shoestring financing or a shoebox accounting system. It takes a well-planned and carefully implemented sequence of steps to begin a small business of counseling. Likewise a small business usually grows and expands into a substantial business or practice of counseling. Over time, the practice becomes rooted in the community and is defined by the therapist's personality, lifestyle, and the office practice patterns. Eventually, a reputation is established and the practice follows suit.

This chapter provides the office forms, guidelines, exercises, and procedures for establishing a practice and growing it over time. While the process of starting a small business is complex, the forms in this chapter provide the guidelines for the therapist to utilize and follow.

EXAMPLE PROFESSIONAL RESUME (WEB VERSION)

| HOME | ABOUT | SERVICES | PUBLICATIONS | RESOURCES | CONTACT |

PROFESSIONAL SERVICES OF DR_____

- Lectures and workshops
- Consulting services
- Expert testimony
- Psychotherapy practice

PHOTO

Lectures and Workshops

_____ is available to offer lectures and workshops to professional and general audiences. Most of the following workshops can be presented to accommodate time slots varying from 1 hour to 2 days. Her usual fee for a workshop is _____ plus travel expenses. Feel free to contact her to discuss the needs and interests of your organization.

Topics on which Dr _____ is currently available to offer workshops include:

- Cultural competence in trauma treatment
- Assessment and treatment of trauma
- Trauma and memory
- Forensic issues for psychotherapists
- Integrating diversity into psychotherapy and assessment
- Developing multicultural competence
- Feminist therapy theory and practice
- Psychological assessment and diagnosis
- DSM-IV and beyond
- Self-care for therapists and vicarious traumatization
- Reality TV

A complete list of Dr _____'s workshop presentations can be found in her CV. Dr _____ is always interested in working with your group to develop new presentation topics within her broad general areas of expertise that are tailored to your group's specific needs.

Consulting Services

Dr _____ is available to consult with therapists about:

- Trauma treatment: Countertransference issues with trauma survivors, including vicarious traumatization; treatment planning; developing containment and self-soothing skills in severely dissociative trauma survivors; risk management with trauma clients
- Psychological testing: Dr _____ offers objective personality assessment for your clients with the MMPI-2, Personality Assessment Inventory, Trauma Symptom Inventory, and other similar tests. She is also available to consult with you on testing administered by other psychologists
- Diagnostic dilemmas: Assistance with differential diagnosis of complex cases, including questions of malingering
- Forensic issues: Preparing therapists and/or their clients for dealing with the legal system; consulting with attorneys on mental health aspects of civil and criminal cases related to trauma, dissociation, abuse, victimization, discrimination, and harassment

Consultation is available either on a one-time or on-going basis, by appointment. Current fees for consultation are $_____ /hour.

Forensic Expert Testimony

Dr _____ is available to attorneys to serve as an expert witness and consultant in legal matters involving questions of trauma, dissociation, abuse, victimization, discrimination, and harassment. Expert witness services include:

- Psychological assessment of plaintiffs in civil matters or defendants in criminal matters
- Review of records
- Deposition planning
- Research
- Report writing
- Expert testimony

If you are an attorney, please contact Dr _____ directly to discuss your case and her fees. Download forensic contract

Parties to civil or criminal cases, please arrange for your attorney to contact Dr _____, as she cannot deal directly with any party to a case.

Dr _____'s expert testimony has been referred to by the US 9th Circuit Court in the cases of:

- _____ v. US (sexual misconduct by therapists and nature of transference)
- _____ v. _____ (cross-gender body searches of women prison inmate by male correction officers)
- _____ v. _____ (service in the military by a lesbian)

Psychotherapy Practice

Dr_____'s psychotherapy practice is closed to new clients at this time. However, openings may occur unpredictably, so please contact her. Her current fee for psychotherapy is $_____ /session.

PROFESSIONAL PRACTICE PROFILE

MY CORE VALUES:

The core values of this practice shall be ...

1.

2.

3.

4.

5.

MY PROFESSIONAL MISSION STATEMENT:

The mission of this practice shall be ...

MY PROFESSIONAL VISION FOR MY PRACTICE:

The vision for this practice shall be ...

MY PLAN BY WHICH I WILL ASSESS MY SUCCESS:

Signature: _____ Date: _____

VISION IMPLEMENTATION PLANNER

MY VISION (5 YEARS): _____

MY MISSION (PURPOSE): _____

MY STRATEGY TO ACHIEVE MY VISION

Start Date	Support Person to Help	Primary Actions to Realize Vision	Secondary Actions to Realize Vision
		I will try	I will try
		I will try	I will try
		I will try	I will try
		I will try	I will try

COMMENTS:

STRATEGIC PLANNING WORKSHEET

Use this form to organize your thoughts and analysis when participating in a vision rising, strategic planning session or program development planning session. It can also be helpful if used in regular staff meetings when program development or planning is being discussed.

Developmental Areas	Goals and Objectives	Strategy	Issues: Time, Cost, Staff, Environment, Impact, Volunteers

PROFESSIONAL WILL AND INSTRUCTIONS

My legal and professional name(s):

My legal and professional practice address(es):

My chosen or preferred Executor:

My chosen or preferred successor Executor:

Location of my offices over past 10–15 years:

Names of hospitals in which I practiced and may have records:

Instructions for contacting my clients/patients (present and past):

Any special care to be extended to any particular clients/patients:

How to provide for continuity of care:

Location of files, keys, legal and professional documents, instructions, appointment book, e-mails, storage unit, filing cabinets, computer files, and contracts, etc:

Family member to assist in the execution of this Will:

Professional colleagues (two) to assist in the execution of this Will:

(1)

(2)

Directions for handling any and all records of clients/patients:

People/patients to be notified of my death, funeral/memorial, and future care:

Notify my attorney, CPA, billing service, secretarial service, insurance carriers, answering service, practice consultants, etc.

Notification plans for newspaper, BOP, insurance company, liability insurance company, professional associations:

Location of financial records, billing records, ARs, and bills outstanding:

All my writings and articles/publications shall be handled by the following family members:

_____, _____, and/or _____.

SPECIAL INSTRUCTIONS:

- Follow APA Code of Ethics, HIPAA and the APA Record Keeping Guidelines.
- Sell each client's/patient's files at market value to therapist taking over a case.
- Follow state and federal laws as they apply.
- Coordinate with the execution of my personal Will.
- Bill my estate for time and costs in executing these instructions.
- All professional and client materials and documents must be processed by the Professional Executor.
- Other ...

Signature: _____

Date: _____

E-mail address: _____

Access Pin Code: _____ Password: _____

Witness: _____

Date: _____

Witness: _____

Date: _____

Locations of this executed form:

People given a copy of this form:

CODICIL TO PERSONAL OR PROFESSIONAL WILL
Percentage of Adjusted Gross Estate

_____

"I hereby amend my said Last Will and Testament, dated _____, by adding a new Item as follows:

ITEM

In accordance with my appreciation of the graduate school I attended and/or the professional associations with which I have been associated and have benefited, I hereby give, devise, and bequeath _____ percent (__ %) of my adjusted gross estate to the _____ for scholarships and/or its general uses and purposes, provided said charitable organization is in existence at the time of my death and is an organization organized and operated exclusively for religious, charitable, scientific, literary, or educational purposes described in Sections 170 (c)and 2055 of the Internal Revenue Code of 1986, as amended; otherwise, if said organization is not in existence or does not so qualify, then to such charitable organization or charitable organizations so qualifying as my Executor shall determine. Except as herein modified, I hereby remake, republish and redeclare my Last Will and Testament, as heretofore amended."

Signature: _____   Date: _____

Witness: _____   Date: _____

Witness: _____   Date: _____

Witness: _____   Date: _____

PROFESSIONAL PROFILE DOCUMENTS NEEDED

The following documents are needed by every professional and should be readily available upon request by any patient, insurance company, attorney, Court, contractor, vendor, or social agency with whom business is conducted.

Generally, copies of these documents are kept in the office and sent to whomever upon a proper request.

- Professional resume (Curriculum vitae)
- Brief personal and professional biographical narrative (1 page)
- Fee schedule (Patients)
- Fee schedule (Forensic, Speaking, and Consulting)
- Professional license
- Proof of liability insurance
- Annual continuing education record of courses
- Listing of contracted Managed Care insurance companies
- Listing of Court hearing and depositions attended/testified
- Website that profiles the professional practice
- Listing of consulting contracts

BUSINESS DEVELOPMENT AND PROFESSIONAL RELATIONSHIPS

The following actions can be powerful in helping you build a practice in your community. Working closely with other professionals in the community can greatly assist you in serving your patients and meeting their needs.

1. Do you keep good contact and rapport with the doctors, lawyers, and agencies that are giving you referrals or that could be a source of referral in the future?
   - Send Christmas cards to their office. (No business cards here!)
   - Send "thank you" cards for each referral with business cards.
   - Call the secretary and arrange a time for you to drop by to meet and thank the referring professional in person.
   - As more referrals come in, call and invite that professional for lunch.

2. Do you learn about other counselors in your area who have different specialties than you?
   - They can become great business allies, so build strong relationships.
   - Ask for their brochure and business cards for you to have in your office.
   - Make referrals to them, as appropriate.
   - Arrange informal luncheons with your local group of professionals every few months.
   - If one of them is noticed in the local newspaper for some achievement, send them a copy and a brief congratulatory note.

3. Do you collaborate with social workers, nurses, teachers, and agency directors, etc. as to the needs of your community?
   - What workshops could you present that would meet a need?
   - What social support services could you offer?
   - What sub-group of people in your community are in need of some type of service?

ACTION PLAN: Circle the items above that you need to start doing or do better.

MAKING A BUSINESS PLAN

The Drucker Foundation created an assessment tool to help organizations develop a workable and strategic business plan as they consider their future. The following five questions, from this assessment tool, will guide you as you think through your future directions as a practice. While the questions were designed for a general business, they very well can be adapted to help focus the future of a practice in mental health.

WHAT IS OUR BUSINESS OR MISSION? (THERAPY/COUNSELING)

- What am I trying to achieve?
- What specific results am I seeking?
- What are my major strengths? What are my weaknesses?
- Does my mission need to be revisited?

WHO IS OUR CUSTOMER? (PATIENTS/CLIENTS)

- Who are my *primary* customers?
- Who are my *supporting* customers?
- Have my customers changed over time?
- Should I change my customer base?

WHAT DOES THE CUSTOMER CONSIDER VALUE? (HEALTH/WELFARE)

- What do my *primary* customers consider value?
- What do my *supporting* customers consider value?
- How well am I providing what my customers consider value?
- How can I use what my customers consider value to become more effective?
- What additional information do I need?

WHAT HAVE BEEN OUR RESULTS? (BEHAVIOR CHANGE)

- How do I define results for my organization?
- To what extent have I achieved these results?
- How well am I using my resources?

WHAT IS OUR PLAN? (TREATMENT/CARE PLAN)

- What have I learned and what do I recommend?
- Where should I focus my efforts?
- What, if anything, should I do differently?
- What is my plan to achieve results for the practice?

Cont.

WHAT IS THE PLAN FOR OFFICE SET UP? (OFFICE STRUCTURE)

- Is there a need for my service in a particular target area of the community?
- Does my savings account have sufficient funds to cover costs for at least a year?
- Am I ready to keep all the necessary records of income, expenses, capital costs, etc.?
- Am I properly structured to do business as a small business person?
- Should I set up a website to use for my business advantage?

INTENTIONAL STRATEGIC PLANNING

Strategic planning is best done when it is intentional. Essentially, strategic planning is decision making that originates with a well-defined vision. In brief, key leaders know how to create a vision, and they know how to make visionary decisions. As it has been said, "Write a vision, and make it plain upon the slate." That's where leadership all begins

The following decisive guidelines as set forth by Dr John Haggai can be helpful to any professional starting a practice, company or organization.

THE 12 STEPS FOR VISIONARY DECISION MAKING

1. Decide to define your vision for your professional practice, business, or company.
2. Decide to achieve what it is you are aiming to accomplish.
3. Decide to prove loving and caring for others works.
4. Decide to be humble and right in your work and practice style.
5. Decide to live without moral and ethical compromise.
6. Decide to persuade others and win.
7. Decide to invest your funds and efforts fearlessly.
8. Decide to profit from the impossible.
9. Decide to work so you will go further faster.
10. Decide to be there at the end.
11. Decide to lead by pacing yourself and with effortless grace.
12. Decide to thrive on ambiguity.

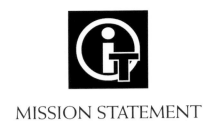

MISSION STATEMENT

WHO NEEDS A MISSION STATEMENT?

An agency or professional practice's purpose is only as good as its vision of itself. Once a vision has been determined, the vision must be expressed in terms of a Mission Statement. A Mission Statement sets the tone for the practice and provides it with focus. It lays out what the practice stands for and gives the staff something to live up to. It provides an attitudinal and behavioral challenge, i.e., a mission.

A Mission Statement provides the common vision for the total practice. An effective Mission Statement defines the fundamental, unique purpose that sets a practice apart from other practices and identifies the scope of the practice's operations. It describes the nature and concept of the practice's future and forms the foundation for strategic and operational plans. The Mission Statement helps to ensure the practice's consistency by aiding in obtaining understanding and support. It is not "buy in," as it does not have to be sold. It is a fulminate for "join in."

The actual statement generally will contain an umbrella statement of 15–30 words that identifies the conceptual nature of the service in which the practice is engaged. It should not include anything the practice is not willing to back up with action. It provides the foundation for priorities, tactics, strategies, and plans. It specifies the fundamental reason why a practice exists. At least once a year, the practice should make a formal review of its Mission Statement.

WHAT ARE THE COMPONENTS OF A MISSION STATEMENT?

A broad definition of an association's Mission Statement includes: (a) purpose; (b) strategy; (c) set of values; and (d) standards and behaviors. A Mission Statement may be the most visible and public part of a strategic plan. As such, it is comprehensive in its coverage of broad concerns to the practice. Guidelines for crafting an effective Mission Statement include:

1. Identification of the practice's desired public image and self-concept with a commitment to survival. Who are your customers? Clients?
2. Evokes a deep emotional attachment, connecting with the therapist's compelling professional/personal interests. Therapists have a strong and active passion about it. People become involved "on purpose!"
3. Specifies the key elements in the practice's philosophy. It makes the practice different from every other practice. It delineates what is unique about the practice. It sets the practice above and it states what is value added.
4. None of the Mission Statement's terms should be subject to interpretation. It should have no qualifiers or value modifiers (words such as "motherhood," "creative," or "excellent") because members can argue that meaning.
5. Identification of core scientific principles and principal services.

A good Mission Statement is to capture the vision and catalyze the collective energies of the members in a way that generates unprecedented synergy, momentum, innovation, and clarity.

OFFICE SET UP AND MARKETING NEEDS

The following products and marketing support services are needed early in the start up of a practice. These marketing products are available from any local marketing company or marketing consultant. It is best to contract with a marketing firm that caters to professional practices. It is also best to align with a local marketing firm that knows the local market in your field of practice. Of course, if the therapist is a marketing expert, these services can be self designed and utilized at a great saving.

LOGO AND IDENTITY CREATION

- Logo
- Letterhead
- Envelopes
- Mailing labels
- Business cards
- Newsletter format and design
- Signage for building and door

WEB AND MEDIA

- E-mail sign up
- E-newsletter
- Web hosting and design
- Blog setup

BROCHURES AND HANDOUTS

- Flyers and handouts on selected topics
- Brochures
- Announcements
- Give-away gifts

MARKETING SUPPORT SERVICES

- Direct mail
- Rental of mailing lists
- Photo shots for the media
- Professional resume design
- Purchasing power for durable supplies
- Purchasing co-ops

LETTER OF INTRODUCTION TO THE COMMUNITY

When a professional moves into a new community and initiates independent practice or affiliates with an existing practice or group, a letter of introduction is typically sent to potential referral sources. The letter may then be followed up by a phone call or an invitation to have lunch together so a working relationship can be established. This initial introduction to the professional community is vital to a positive and quick start in service delivery. Essentially, this is a business letter, not an informal note of introduction. It is to be written seriously and professionally.

The letter should be written on your professional letterhead. It should consist of the following components, and may include a brochure outlining your practice.

Paragraph 1: Introduce yourself and tell them the area of practice on which you will focus and specialize. Spell out your specialization in some detail, but yet broad enough to elicit the desired referrals.

Paragraph 2: Give the necessary demographic of your practice, including address. Also, describe the location of your office, especially if it is difficult to find.

Paragraph 3: Give a brief summary of your educational training, internship, and your prior professional practice locations and facilities. Be sure to note your specialized training that supports your intention to focus your practice.

Paragraph 4: Suggest how you can be of help to them as a service provider and improve the services they deliver in the community by working together. Note the unique nature of your professional style in working with your referral sources.

Sign off in a professionally respectful and gracious manner.

THE 14 Ps OF MARKETING A PRACTICE, PROGRAM OR SERVICE

A practice, program or a special service must be regularly and strategically marketed. Your name must be kept out in the public eye and among those that need your services or have a need to refer others to a therapist such as yourself. Essentially, you have a service to render and there are those that need that service. Marketing strategies connect the two needs together at the right time and in the right way. Listed here are the 14 specific Ps of planning and marketing a practice, program or special service.

1. How will the **Practice or Program** be titled or described?
2. What is the **Purpose** that will be fulfilled?
3. What **People** will be served?
4. Where will the services rendered take **Place**?
5. What amenities need to be **Provided** for the services rendered to be successful?
6. What will be the **Period** of time the services will be available?
7. What will be the set up **Procedures** to be followed?
8. What **Personnel** will be needed to make the program happen and go smoothly?
9. What **Payment** will be expected by those that enroll and participate?
10. What **Promotion** strategies will be utilized to get people to come?
11. Who else needs to be involved as **Partners** to the practice, service or program?
12. How will you determine if the service **Packs a Punch** and meet expectations?
13. What is the **Purple Cow,** the unique aspect of the service that will be a draw?
14. What will be the **Plan** to identify the weak spot in the service provided and fix it?

COMMENTS, IDEAS, PLANS OR NEXT STEPS:

MARKETING BY MAIL (1)

Below are several actions you can take to assure that a new practice is recognized in the community and is perceived as a part of the community. A proactive communication pattern is desirable as a practice is being introduced to the community.

Sending an announcement of your new counseling practice opening in their area:

- Doctors
- Lawyers
- Agencies
- Schools
- Churches
- Organizations

Making community service announcements (every 4 months, 1 page in length):

- New workshops
- New training/expertise achieved by staff
- New focus groups available
- New clinical services available
- New group therapy sessions available
- New training seminars available

Sending letters or cards as a "Thank You" for referring clients:

- A letter of appreciation
- A pre-printed card
- A brief report of the consultation results

Speeches/workshops offered on related "hot" topics:

- Send announcements of workshops being offered
- Give handouts at speeches and workshops you give
- Attend, as a guest, the functions that your target clients or referral sources attend

Written communications to put your name in the public eye:

- Write Letters to the Editor of your local newspaper
- Distribute handouts on selected topics at speeches you give in the community
- Give handouts to patients as a "take home"
- Place articles you have written in your Waiting Room
- Place brief articles you have written on selected topics in all mailings from your office
- Periodically, mail out articles you have written to a select mailing list of referral sources

MARKETING BY MAIL (2)

The following action steps are taken to launch a new practice in a community. They can also be used to revitalize a practice going through a downturn in business.

Announcement: "A new counseling practice is opening in your area!"

- Letter to physicians, lawyers, clergymen, and other professionals
- Letter to agencies, organizations, and clubs

Service updates!

Send out one every 4 months, and not more than one page in length:

- New workshops
- New training seminars
- New focus groups and group therapy

Thank you for referring a client!

A formal letter of appreciation

A professional letter of results of consultation

Handouts

Prepare handouts to give to clients and as billing stuffers:

- Give the handouts to patients and ask them to pass them along to others.
- Put the handouts in all billing envelopes and in all mailings from the office.

Speeches, written articles, workshops, and seminars on selected "hot" topics!

- Give handouts at speeches and workshops you give.
- Attend as a guest any function that may generate a referral and where your target clients go.
- Write an article, Letter to the Editor or editorial for the local newspaper.

MARKETING YOUR PRACTICE: A TRIAL EXERCISE

ADVANCE PLANNING

Complete the incomplete sentences below as you think through your practice development over the next year. Remember, it may not be so much *what* you do, but *how* you do it. Image is a major issue in professional practice. Patients are your best PR representatives. Satisfied patients tell a positive story to others.

1. Am I reliable? My patients know that I am reliable when I _____

   _____

2. Do I give needed assurance? My patients know that I express assurance to them when I _____

   _____

3. Am I empathic? My patients know that I am empathic when I _____

   _____

4. Am I responsive? My patients know that I am responsive to their needs when I _____

   _____

5. Am I respectful? My patients know that I am respectful when I _____

   _____

6. Am I one to offer positive tangibles? My patients know I offer positive tangibles when I _____

   _____

GENERAL MARKETING GUIDELINES
- Be pleasant in all your dealings with patients, their family, staff and vendors.
- Be attentive to all requests and promises.
- Be sure your staff know you, your services, practice style, and orientation.
- Be sure all people are treated with respect and are made to feel important.
- Be not indifferent to the needs of your patients and your referral sources.
- Be a person that follows through and goes the extra mile for others.
- Be sure you fulfill the promises you make with patients, staff, vendors, and others.

FREE USE OF THE MEDIA

1. **Call local newspaper** and ask for an interview about your great new counseling practice.

2. **Call local radio stations** and ask if they will do a public service announcement about your new community counseling center. Fax them the details.

3. **Milk a statistic!**
   a. Pick an interesting topic, like the high number of marital separations that happen in January.
   b. Call the newspaper in November with your "hot topic" for them.
   c. Have a phone interview, meet face to face, or offer to submit an article.
   d. Always include your business identification materials so that the world will know more about you and how to contact you (and two business cards!)

4. **Send a fax to radio stations** with an interesting "factoid." Best if it's a local problem and has a possible community solution. Do this every few months. Again, don't forget to clearly identify your business!

5. **Go see someone at the local radio station about doing an on-air segment.** Once a relationship has started with the radio stations this will more likely result in a contract.

6. **Look for opportunities to link people together.**
   a. Offer to call your newspaper contacts about the annual picnic held by the community agency that you are promoting yourself through.
   b. Keep good records of all other local services that your clients might need; build your community by referring clients to other businesses.

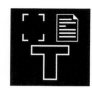

SAMPLE LETTER FOR A PROPOSED COMMUNITY WORKSHOP

DATE

ABC President/Chairman
Church/School/Club
Address
City
State, Zip

Re: **FREE WORKSHOP ON PARENTING**

Dear _____

Would you be interested in a free workshop on a great and helpful program for effective parenting? If so, you may be interested in sponsoring a workshop on Child Management in the Home for young parents in your organization or as a community outreach.

For the past 15 years I have provided classes to parents on a variety of topics, but especially on Child Management in the Home. This topic has always been well attended and over 2400 parents have been participants in these classes over the years.

To help you be sure you will be bringing in a well-qualified presenter and program, I can provide you a list of references you may call. I am sure you will learn that this proposed workshop is one of the best available for young parents.

At this time, I am offering to do this program for you and your families at no charge. If you would like to consider such an opportunity, please call me at your earliest convenience to establish a date. I am also available to answer any questions you may have as you consider this offer.

I look forward to hearing from you.

Respectfully,

NAME
TITLE

GOING GREEN IN THE OFFICE

The following changes in office procedures can make a huge difference in our environment and also save you operational money in your budget. By going green you can be a help to the future and to your bottom line.

GOING GREEN TIPS

- Use energy-efficient fluorescent lights throughout the office.
- Replace incandescent bulbs with compact fluorescent bulbs.
- Use coffee mugs instead of foam or paper cups.
- Use reusable coffee filter baskets when brewing coffee.
- Unplug equipment that is not in use for lengthy periods of time.
- Turn off lights, computers, chargers and other energy-draining equipment at day's end, especially on weekends.
- Keep the AC unit temperature to be comfortable (73–78°F degrees, 23–26°C), but not cool or cold. (Likewise with the heat, 72–68°F, 22–20°C during the winter months.)
- Use the central fan for a portion of the day, before turning on the main unit.
- Make good use of open/closed doors and windows at strategic times during the day and evening office hours.
- If possible, increase the insulation in the walls and ceiling of the office.
- Use e-mail, voicemail, and text messaging to avoid the use of envelopes, letters, and stamps.
- Avoid extra printing by storing documents on the computer rather than downloading and then printing hardcopies not needed.
- Use recycled paper and reuse paper from your fax and printer; use both sides when possible.
- Recycle paper and cans, bottles and other such recyclables from the office and lunchroom.
- Have empty ink cartridges re-filled or traded for printer paper at the local office supply store.
- Utilize electronic billing systems.
- Send reports and letters by e-mail whenever possible.
- Recycle all phone books, catalogues, books, and documents no longer needed.
- Replace appliances and heating/AC units that are more energy-efficient.
- Arrange for employees to car pool to work or use alternative methods of travel.
- Consolidate errands such as trips to the bank and office supply store.
- Other ...

PROGRAM DEVELOPMENT
Process Checklist

When developing a new program or project, the following steps will increase the probability of its success. A systematic process is essential to the early planning stages of development.

ESTABLISH THE PHILOSOPHY OF A NEW PROGRAM:
1. Mission statement
2. Objectives of the program
3. Goals to be achieved
4. Values to be honored

ESTABLISH THE POLICY TO GUIDE IT:
1. The plan or strategy to be followed
2. The point person to guide the process
3. The advisors to be consulted

ESTABLISH THE BUSINESS PLAN TO IMPLEMENT IT:
1. What ads, newsletters, flyers, mailings, and announcements to utilize?
2. What contacts to make by phone or personal letter?
3. How to conduct a follow-up plan?
4. What will the organizational chart look like?
5. What are the costs and the potential income?
6. What accounting and record system needs to be put in place?
7. What professional charts and patient files need to be kept?
8. What is the number of patients needed to be signed up to make the program a "go?" Can the program start with fewer patients?
9. Other …

COMMENTS OR ACTION PLAN:

MODELS AND PROCEDURES FOR PROGRAM PLANNING

When planning future directions for an organization, a program or a professional office, the process can be facilitated and the discussion structured by using one of the following three models of planning and strategic thinking. Use any of them to guide the discussion and keep notes of all ideas suggested. Keep notes on a paper with the letters of the selected model across the top of the page or down the left side of the page.

   When engaging in the planning process, one could follow the Strategic Planning format or the Vision Thinking format, as outlined below. The two are difficult to engage in simultaneously. Choose one or the other. They are not right or wrong, just different ways to engage in planning. The nature and personality of the people involved may decide which process is selected and which model is used for note taking.

MODELS OF PLANNING

D   Direction
O   Organization
C   Cash (Resources)
T   Tracking
O   Overall evaluation
R   Refinement

P   Purpose
O   Objective
G   Goals
A   and
S   Standards

M   Methods utilized
I   Information distribution
D   Development plan for future growth
O   Operation of programs
L   Leadership development

STRATEGIC PLANNING VS. VISION THINKING

	Strategic Plans:	**Vision Thinking:**
1.	Directional step-by-step planning	End-state and ultimate orientation
2.	Linear and chronological planning	Holistic view/a snapshot
3.	Reaction to trends and competition	Desire to create a new perspective
4.	Work forward into the future	Work backwards from the future
5.	Must know how to get there	Unclear how to get there from here
6.	Complete plan with details	Dynamically incomplete on purpose
7.	Plan language (rational, bureaucratic)	Vision language (intuitive, poetic)
8.	Secret and private	Public and open for input from anyone
9.	Calculated and careful discussion	Brainstorming and interactive discussion

A SWOT ANALYSIS OF THE PRACTICE

Every professional must take time to assess the position of the practice in the local market place. The SWOT analysis provides a format to review a practice, and future growth plans can be set forth.

STRENGTHS

1.
2.
3.
4.
5.
6.
7.
8.
9.
10.

WEAKNESSES

1.
2.
3.
4.
5.
6.
7.
8.
9.
10.

OPPORTUNITIES

1.
2.
3.
4.
5.
6.
7.
8.
9.
10.

THREATS

1.
2.
3.
4.
5.
6.
7.
8.
9.
10.

MY ACTION PLAN FOR A STRONGER FUTURE:

Forms Related to Fees

Chapter Contents

A clinical practice is considered a small business. To be successful, care must be taken to reduce costly errors, appropriately bill for services rendered, collect fees for services rendered, and assure expenditures are kept within the levels of income.

Unfortunately, many clients have a knack of nonpayment. There are always insurance company hassles and difficulties in collecting on the claims submitted. These factors must be monitored closely.

Having an array of forms, templates, and procedures in place and ready for use, as included in this chapter, will help make the process of collecting on the fees charged for services rendered more effectively managed and in keeping with standard business practices.

Many therapists are not trained in the financial concepts of running a business, and have to rely on book keepers and accountants to help manage their practice. This chapter includes the necessary forms to assist a therapist in learning how to self-manage the practice and keep it financially sound and viable.

STRUCTURING PAYMENT PLANS FOR PATIENTS WHO CANNOT AFFORD STANDARD FEES

There are patients in active therapy who run into hard times and need a financial break so they can continue their therapy progress. Likewise, there are new referrals that come to you who cannot afford the standard fees but they are referrals you would like to accept for some reason. Here are a few of the options by which you can structure a financial plan that might be workable for these patients. When accepting some modified payment plan or structure, you are urged to consult the Ethics Committee of your professional association.

1. **Time limited therapy.** Propose a brief therapy intervention program of 3–5 sessions. Hit the ground running and stay focused on an agreed purpose for the therapy.

2. **Establish a flexible appointment schedule.** Arrange for appointments during the slow periods of your practice, at a lower cost. Propose to see them once or twice monthly as they are able to come for appointments.

3. **Refer the patient to a group you conduct or a colleague conducts.** Group therapy can be effective for many patients, even from the start of therapy. Group therapy can supplement the progress made in individual therapy.

4. **Contract for two hours of homework and in-vivo therapy for every one hour of individual therapy in the office:** Some patients will be happy to conduct a homework assignment between sessions if you will draft an assignment for them and integrate it with the office based therapy.

5. **Propose a payment plan.** Structure any delayed payment plan as a contract with the payment agreement specified.

6. **Offer a sliding scale of fees.** While this can be a risky policy it may be reasonable to propose in some situations. Lowering fees beyond the minimum payment of Medicare and private insurance companies is a way to jeopardize the fees you submit to any and all insurance companies.

7. **See them pro bono.** This is a practice embraced by the APA Ethics Code. You may limit the number of pro bono sessions, but specify that before therapy begins.

8. **Accept what a patient or family can pay.** A limited number of patients will gladly accept this arrangement and honor its intent. However, be careful when you accept fees even lower than what insurance companies pay.

9. **Refer them out to an appropriate alternative therapist or agency.** The emphasis is on the word "appropriate." Don't just dump them on any therapist. Referral needs to be thoughtful and diligent.

10. **Barter for services rendered.** While this is acceptable under the APA Code of Ethics, it is difficult to establish the relative value of service. The value of services to be exchanged needs to be established ahead of time and be non-exploitative. The value of services exchanged is reportable and taxable at the end of the year in which they were received.

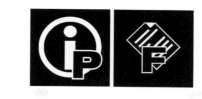

OFFICE FINANCIAL POLICY

I understand that charges are based on a clinical hour defined by insurance carriers as 45–50 minutes with the doctor. I understand that the usual hourly fee is applied for a failed appointment without 24-hour notice of cancellation: This charge is not paid by insurance. Other services including phone calls, review of records, consultation with doctors, attorneys or others at the patient's request, and any other professional services, either requested by the patient or necessary for treatment, but outside of the clinical face-to-face setting are usually the responsibility of the patient. These other services are charged on a quarter-hour basis. Custody cases and court-related referrals and/or charges are the full responsibility of the individual.

I hereby authorize payment of insurance benefits to this office for services rendered to me and/or my dependants. I authorize the release of any medical/psychological information necessary to process claims and/or comply with record keeping requirements.

In cases where prior authorization is required after the initial allotted visits, I will be responsible for additional sessions if my insurance company denies the claims.

I understand that I am financially responsible to this office for all copayments and charges not covered by the assignment of benefits above. It is the office policy to collect at each visit the amount not covered by insurance directly from the patient/responsible party. When the patient is a minor, copayment will be collected from the person scheduling the appointments as it is that person's responsibility to make arrangements with the responsible party for timely payments.

I authorize the release of name, address, telephone number, and outstanding balance in collection matters.

In order to avoid usual time charges at the time of a missed appointment, a 24-hour cancellation notification will be required.

Signature: _____   Date: _____

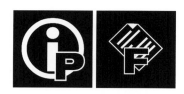

CANCELLATION AND MISSED APPOINTMENTS NOTICE

CONTINUITY OF CARE IS AN IMPORTANT ASPECT OF PROVIDING MENTAL HEALTH THERAPY. Frequent cancellations and/or failing to show for sessions may cause long periods between therapy sessions and impacts the effectiveness of your treatment. For your convenience, I try to accommodate your schedule by working with you to choose session times best suited for you. I strive to provide quality care, but your cooperation in keeping your appointments is of the utmost importance. I would like to take this opportunity to inform my clients regarding my office policy on cancellations (contacting my office prior to your appointment time) and no-shows (failure to notify me prior to your appointment time.)

- If you are unable to keep your appointment and wish to cancel, PLEASE contact my office. I appreciate at least a 24-hour notice, but please call even if it is a couple hours before your scheduled appointment. This allows me enough time to schedule a client that may be waiting for an appointment.
- I attempt to contact clients who have no-showed for an appointment. However, if you no-show and I am unable to contact you, your next scheduled appointment may be given to another client as needed.
- If during the course of treatment you no-show for two appointments in a row, you will receive a letter informing you that your session slot will be made available to other clients but to call if you're interested in making another appointment. I will do my best to accommodate your needs at that time.

Sincerely,

DR NAME

I have read and understand the above scheduling policy.

Client signature: _____   Date: _____

NOTICE OF MISSED APPOINTMENTS

DATE

Dear _____

I regret that you missed your recent scheduled appointment on

_____ at _____.

Please be advised that it is my office policy to make time slots available to other clients once that time allotted for your appointment has not been kept with no advance notice for two consecutive weeks or more. If you wish to schedule an appointment, please call me at _____. If there is a time slot open, I would be happy to accommodate you.

I appreciate your cooperation in this matter. Your advance notification allows me to offer your scheduled time to other clients.

Sincerely,

DR NAME

ACTIONS TO TAKE WHEN PATIENTS MISS APPOINTMENTS

When patients miss appointments, especially if they have missed several appointments without proper notice, it is important to handle such patients in a legal, ethical, and business-like manner. Here are some actions you might consider:

1. Be sure you have a printed policy about missed appointments.

2. Be sure you print the policy on a card, flier or sign so patients are informed of your policy and urged to follow it.

3. Be sure to include this topic when you go over office policies with the patients during their first appointment.

4. After the first missed appointment, inform them that you will bill them for the lost time if they miss again without 24 hours' notice.

5. On the second missed appointment, bill for one half or the full appointment per your policy. Send out the bill immediately.

6. On the second or third missed appointment, tell them that future appointments will not be scheduled but you will see them on a "same day" service plan. In this arrangement, they will be given an appointment if they call in and a time slot is available on the same day. Likewise, you could call them and offer a time slot for the same day.

7. Do not let the bill accumulate very high due to missed appointment charges.

8. Advise them to find another therapist; refer them to another therapist, but with fair notice that finances are an area of difficulty. In such situations, be sure to get the proper release of information. Be helpful in such a transfer of care.

9. Tell them you will resume treatment after the outstanding bill has been paid in full.

10. Allow a reasonable time for payment of the bill to be made in full and services resumed.

11. Be sure not to hold a grudge or ill feelings against them in the event they return or need your services in the future.

PAYMENT AGREEMENT FOR PAST SERVICE RENDERED

_____

The agreement shall be between _____ and _____.

The agreement is in effect as of _____ and shall go forward until _____.

_____ agrees to:

1.

2.

3.

_____ agrees to:

1.

2.

3.

PAYMENT SCHEDULE:

_____ agrees to pay _____ according to the following payment plan:

The agreement shall be a binding agreement and can be amended by mutual consent of both parties or cancelled by 30-day written notice and upon mutual agreement. Failure to comply will result in other courses of collection being undertaken.

Signatures:

_____   Date: _____
Patient

_____   Date: _____
Therapist

PAST DUE LETTER REQUESTING PAYMENT

DATE

NAME

ADDRESS

Re: Past Due Balance of $ _____

Dear _____

The office staff recently brought your outstanding balance to my attention. You have not responded to the billing statements that have been sent during the past months and your account is seriously overdue.

If your balance is not paid in full within **10 working days** of the date of this letter, your account will be forwarded to our collection agency. Since this generally has major significance on your future credit, I would urge your immediate payment of your longstanding, overdue account. Please give me a call if you wish to discuss this billing.

Regrettably, if your account is sent to our collection agency, I will not be able to provide any further services to you. I will be pleased to make your files available to any new therapist you select in the future. However, I must have a bona fide "Release of Information" signed by you with the name and address of your new therapist. There will be the usual charge for photocopying records at that time.

Respectfully,

DR NAME

enc. Billing statement

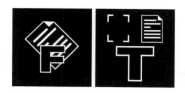

DOCTOR'S LIEN AND AUTHORIZATION OF PAYMENT

To: _____   For:_____
(Attorney)   (Client)

_____   _____

_____   _____

Re: **A Doctor's Lien**

I do hereby authorize Dr _____ to furnish you, my attorney, with a full report of his/her examination, diagnosis, treatment, prognosis, etc., of myself in regard to the injury, mishap or accident in which I was involved.

I hereby authorize and direct you, my attorney, to withhold and pay directly to Dr _____ such sums as may be due and owing him/her for professional service rendered me both by reason of this accident and by reason of any other bills that are due his/her office and to withhold such sums from any settlement, judgment or verdict as may be necessary to adequately protect Dr _____ . And I hereby further give a lien on my case to Dr _____ against any and all proceeds of any settlement, judgment or verdict which may be paid to you, my attorney, or myself as the result of the injuries for which I have been evaluated and/or treated or injuries in connection therewith.

I fully understand that I am directly and fully responsible to Dr _____ for all bills submitted by him/her for the professional service rendered me and that this agreement is made solely for Dr_____'s additional protection and in consideration of his/her awaiting payment. And I further understand that such payment is not contingent on any settlement, judgment or verdict by which I may eventually recover said fee.

Signature:_____   Date: _____
Patient

Signature:_____   Date: _____
Witness

The undersigned, being attorney of record for the above patient, does hereby agree to observe all the terms of the above and agrees to withhold such sums from any settlement, judgment or verdict as may be necessary to adequately protect said doctor above named.

Signature:_____   Date: _____
Attorney

Note to the Attorney: 1. Please sign and return one copy to my office. Keep
                             one copy for your records.
                          2. Periodic billing statements will be sent for your
                             records and to be submitted for payment.
                          3. Periodic progress reports can be provided upon
                             request.

OFFICE DAILY BILLING SHEET

Doctor _____ Date: _____

	To:	❑ Hospital
#1		❑ WC
		❑ Corresp
#2	Pt:	❑ Testing
		❑ Legal
	Re:	**Billable:**
		❑ Yes
		❑ No

	To:	❑ Hospital
#1		❑ WC
		❑ Corresp
#2	Pt:	❑ Testing
		❑ Legal
	Re:	**Billable:**
		❑ Yes
		❑ No

	To:	❑ Hospital
#1		❑ WC
		❑ Corresp
#2	Pt:	❑ Testing
		❑ Legal
	Re:	**Billable:**
		❑ Yes
		❑ No

	To:	❑ Hospital
#1		❑ WC
		❑ Corresp
#2	Pt:	❑ Testing
		❑ Legal
	Re:	**Billable:**
		❑ Yes
		❑ No

	To:	❑ Hospital
#1		❑ WC
		❑ Corresp
#2	Pt:	❑ Testing
		❑ Legal
	Re:	**Billable:**
		❑ Yes
		❑ No

	To:	❑ Hospital
#1:		❑ WC
		❑ Corresp
#2:	Pt:	❑ Testing
		❑ Legal
	Re:	**Billable:**
		❑ Yes
		❑ No

Doctor _____ Date: _____

	To:	❑ Hospital
#1		❑ WC
		❑ Corresp
#2	Pt:	❑ Testing
		❑ Legal
	Re:	**Billable:**
		❑ Yes
		❑ No

	To:	❑ Hospital
#1		❑ WC
		❑ Corresp
#2	Pt:	❑ Testing
		❑ Legal
	Re:	**Billable:**
		❑ Yes
		❑ No

	To:	❑ Hospital
#1		❑ WC
		❑ Corresp
#2	Pt:	❑ Testing
		❑ Legal
	Re:	**Billable:**
		❑ Yes
		❑ No

	To:	❑ Hospital
#1		❑ WC
		❑ Corresp
#2	Pt:	❑ Testing
		❑ Legal
	Re:	**Billable:**
		❑ Yes
		❑ No

	To:	❑ Hospital
#1		❑ WC
		❑ Corresp
#2	Pt.	❑ Testing
		❑ Legal
	Re:	**Billable:**
		❑ Yes
		❑ No

	To:	❑ Hospital
#1		❑ WC
		❑ Corresp
#2	Pt.	❑ Testing
		❑ Legal
	Re:	**Billable:**
		❑ Yes
		❑ No

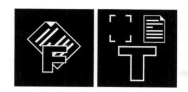

FEE AGREEMENT FOR PSYCHOLOGICAL EXPERT WITNESS SERVICES

This document constitutes a contract between _____ and the undersigned law firm or individual attorney for services performed by Dr _____ in the matter entitled:

_____

I/We agree to prompt payment of Dr_____'s bills for his/her work performed according to the following fee schedule:

I. For work of a non-testimonial nature, including but not limited to psychological evaluations, written or oral reports, consultations with attorneys or their agents, review of records, and any travel pursuant to the above, the fee will be $_____ per hour or portion thereof. Appointments missed without cancellation will be billed at the usual rate.

II. For work of a testimonial nature, including travel to the site at which testimony shall be given and any time spent waiting to give testimony, the fee will be $_____ per hour or portion thereof.

III. For any work requiring travel outside of _____, reasonable travel costs will be reimbursed. A day rate of $_____ will be charged in lieu of the hourly fee for time spent of less than eight hours.

IV. Costs for materials, photocopying, duplication of tapes and other costs incidental to the performance of work that the client requests will be charged separately and are the client's responsibility.

I/We understand that I, an individual attorney, or we, this law firm, constitute Dr _____'s client and hold direct responsiblity for payment of bills to him/her. I/We understand that any arrangements that I/we make with my/our client to obtain funds for my/our payments to Dr _____ are independent of this agreement. I/We will not ask Dr _____ to enter into fee agreements with any other parties, including my/our client, to satisfy my/our indebtedness to Dr _____. I/We understand that Dr _____ cannot bill for his/her work on a contingent fee basis.

I/We understand that any bills in arrears at the end of the calendar month will be charged a late fee of ____ % per month. I/We understand that any bills in arrears for more than three months may be sent to collection at Dr _____'s discretion. If this becomes necessary, I/we understand that I/we will also be responsible for any additional costs incurred by Dr _____ in order to collect fees due. I/We understand that Dr _____ may decline to do further work on any matter where the bill is more than three months past due until payment has been made.

In the event that litigation is necessary to enforce this agreement the prevailing party shall be entitled to reasonable attorney's fees and costs of collection. Venue shall be in _____.

Signature: _____   Date: _____

For (Name of firm): _____

Address: _____

Phone: _____   Fax: _____   E-mail: _____

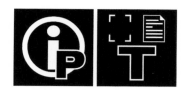

FEE SCHEDULE FOR CLINICAL SERVICES

90801	PDE initial appointment (per hour)	_____
99245	WC Initial Consultation/Evaluation with report	_____
90806	Individual Psychotherapy (50–60 minutes)	_____
90804	Individual Psychotherapy (25–30 minutes)	_____
99040	Missed or Late Appointment (First missed appointment usually pro bono and letter sent to patient)	_____
99049	Late Cancellation (less than 24 hours)	_____
90853	Group Therapy	_____
96100	Psych Testing (see separate listing) (per test)	_____
Ret Check	Returned Check Fee	_____
Materials	Books, Training Tapes, CDs, DVDs, etc. (per item)	_____
Records	Copy Records Fee/Copy Service Office Copy	_____
	less than 20 pages	_____
	20–40 pages	_____
	41 pages or more	_____
	Review of Records	_____
	Case-related Research	_____
99080	Reports (Legal) (per page)	_____
	Reports (Non-legal) (per page)	_____

SKILLED NURSING FACILITIES/HOSPITAL/JAIL

90801 H	Initial Patient Evaluation (80–90 minutes)	_____
	(50–60 minutes)	_____
	(25–30 minutes)	_____
90818	Individual Psychotherapy (50–60 minutes)	_____
90816	Individual Psychotherapy (25–30 minutes)	_____

CONTRACT EVALUATIONS

Law Enforcement Evaluation   _____

    Testing, evaluation, RR, report

    *Second Opinion

Police Officer (Pre-Employment)

Evaluation   _____

Critical Incident Debriefing

    On site (per hour)   _____

    Office (per hour)   _____

Gastric Bypass Surgery Evaluation   _____

    Evaluation, testing, report

Surrogate Parent Evaluation   _____

    Evaluation, testing, report

Fitness for Duty   _____

Child Custody Evaluations   _____

Other   _____

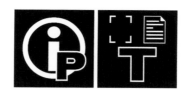

FEE SCHEDULE FOR MEDICAL/LEGAL SERVICES

RETAINERS

Retainer required prior to Neuropsychological Consultation   _____

Retainer required prior to Psychological Consultation   _____

Retainer required prior to Court Testimony   _____

The retainer is not intended to cover the full amount of fees for services rendered, but is considered an initial payment applied as a credit against future billings. Dr _____ reserves the right to charge interest at a rate of 12% per annum on unpaid balances over 30 days old.

HOURLY RATES

Initial phone consultation   _____

Initial diagnostic interview   _____

Neuropsychological/Psychological testing   _____

Review of records, medical/legal report, deposition/court preparation   _____

Meetings/Consultation   _____

Deposition (1 hr minimum)   _____

Court appearances, arbitrations and mediations (2 hr minimum)   _____

Case conferences after normal business hours   _____

Travel time (plus any expenses incurred)   _____

Court stand-by   _____

Other …   _____

ADDITIONAL FEES

Preparation, travel time, and any expenses incurred for depositions will be billed to the retaining attorney per _____ [*appropriate legislation*].

Half day (_____) or full day (_____) charges may be billed to the retaining attorney for depositions conducted out of town.

For less than a 5-day notice on scheduled evaluations, depositions, trials, and related matters, or a patient "no show" on scheduled evaluations, a cancellation charge will be applied based on the time reserved.

Preparation, travel time, and any expenses incurred for depositions will be billed to the retaining attorney per _____ [*appropriate legislation*].

Payment for all services will be the sole responsibility of the retaining attorney or law firm. All invoices are due and payable on receipt. Payment of any unpaid balance is due prior to deposition and trial appearances, including expected fees for preparation and travel.

INSURANCE AUTHORIZATION LOG

Name: _____   Insurance Co.: _____

Copay: _____

Authorization number	From	To	No. of sessions	Session used

NOTES: _____

_____

_____

_____

_____

_____

_____

_____

_____

_____

_____

INSURANCE DIRECT PAYMENT AUTHORIZATION
Direct Payment Request

_____

Name of beneficiary: _____ Plan #: _____

Insurance carrier: _____

Please be informed that I request payment of authorized insurance benefits to be paid on my behalf to Dr _____ directly for any and all professional services he/she rendered to me. I also authorize the holder of any medical and psychological information about me to be released to the relevant insurance carrier to determine those benefits or the benefits payable for related service.

Beneficiary signature: _____ Date: _____

HIPAA/Patient Privacy Forms

Chapter Contents

Privacy and confidentiality are no strangers to the field of psychotherapy. The counseling professional has always performed services while giving full protection to patient's personal information. Historically, patients have appreciated the confidentiality they have been provided when receiving services from a psychotherapist.

Recently, however, a second layer of privacy protection was introduced with the onset of HIPAA (Health Insurance Portability and Accountability Act of 1996) rules and regulations. Even more tightly, the rights and personal information of a patient came under protection. Now a therapist must not only take into account the general ethical guidelines of confidentiality and privacy, but must follow the specific legal guidelines set forth under HIPAA.

This chapter provides information, guidelines, and the essential forms to initiate the implementation of the HIPAA requirements relative to patient care delivery, and when communicating with others on behalf of a patient.

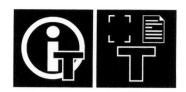

HIPAA OFFICE STAFF GUIDELINES

CONFIDENTIALITY

- All staff shall read and sign the office confidentiality statement.
- All files are to be locked by _____ at the end of the workday.
- We follow the office confidential policy regarding files, communication, etc.
- No files or information shall be released without appropriate release of information forms being signed, filed and permission granted by _____.
- At this time, no clinical records are kept electronically.
- Billing records are electronically maintained and discs appropriately stored in a confidential file cabinet.
- Records may be released only under the signature of _____.

PROFESSIONAL APPEARANCE

- The building, the décor, and the dress of the staff shall be professional at all times.
- The office shall be maintained in an orderly and a clean manner. All staff shall relate to and address each other with respect and professional integrity.

SECURITY

- Whenever the building is unattended, all doors shall be locked and the burglar alarm set.
- The office complex maintains an independent security company that provides guard duties for the complex during off hours.

THIRD PARTIES

- All third party vendors shall be prescreened before business is conducted.
- Business shall not be conducted by door-to-door solicitation vendors.

COLLECTIONS

- All collections shall be under the direction of _____.
- Collection services and agencies shall be used sparingly and only after thorough attempts have been made to collect outstanding accounts from the office. _____ shall give final approval of any accounts being sent for collection to our collection agency.

HIPAA COMPLAINT AND RESOLUTION FORM

_____

(Complete all applicable items)

Name of person bringing the issue to our attention: _____

Address: _____

City/State/Zip: _____

Phone: _____ Fax: _____ E-mail: _____

Date and place of service: _____

Level of service coded (CPT Code): _____

Type of service: _____

Regarding issue: _____

_____

_____

_____

Name of employee completing this form: _____

Date issue first brought to our attention: _____

Was the person referred to another staff?   Y   N

If yes, Name of employee: _____

Cont.

What did the person say: _____

_____

_____

What was the person told: _____

_____

_____

_____

What was done to resolve this issue: _____

_____

_____

AUTHORIZATION FOR RELEASE OR EXCHANGE OF INFORMATION

I, _____ hereby authorize and direct _____

Dr _____ to:

    DISCLOSE the following information: _____

_____

_____

    EXCHANGE the following information: _____

_____

_____

TO/WITH: _____

_____

_____

For the following purpose(s): _____

_____

_____

I understand that my records contain information regarding my mental health. I give specific permission for this information to be released. I understand that my records are protected under State and Federal law and cannot be disclosed without my written consent unless otherwise provided for by law.

This authorization expires on _____ or in 90 days, whichever date is sooner. I understand that I may revoke this authorization in writing at any time.

Signature: _____ Date: _____

PERMISSION TO ALLOW INFORMATION FROM A SESSION TO BE USED FOR RESEARCH, TEACHING, LECTURING, AND/OR PUBLICATION PURPOSES

I, _____ , consent to the use of the personal and psychological information and material from my evaluation and/or therapy by Dr _____ .

I understand that these materials will be kept anonymous so that I am not personally identifiable. Any use will be by Dr _____ only, for professional purposes, following the guidelines of the Ethics Code of the American Psychological Association.

I understand that I may revoke this permission at any time in the future.

ANTICIPATED USE:

Research   ☐

Teaching   ☐

Writing   ☐

Lecturing   ☐

I have read the above conditions and agree thereto:

Patient signature: _____   Date: _____

Doctor signature: _____   Date: _____

PATIENT RECORDS ACCESS FORM

Patient name: _____ Date of birth: _____

I would like to ☐ inspect
            ☐ obtain a copy of
            ☐ both inspect and obtain a copy of
            my protected health information records at this practice.

☐ **Inspection**

I would like to visually inspect the following:
  ☐ My complete record at this practice
  ☐ My record at this practice for time period _____ through _____
  ☐ A specific section of my record (please designate) _____
_____

I would like to inspect my records on the following date and time:
_____

☐ **Requesting a Copy**

I would like to obtain a copy of the following:
  ☐ My complete record from this practice
  ☐ My record at this practice for time period _____ through _____
  ☐ A specific section of my records (please designate):
_____

I request the record in the form of:
  ☐ Readable hard copy
  ☐ A summary in lieu of receiving the complete record
  ☐ Other format agreed to by this practice and myself:
_____

Delivery

  ☐ I would like to pick up the copy of my records on the following date and time:
_____

☐ Please mail the copy of my records to: _____
_____

Your agreement will be requested in advance for any copying or mailing fees that the practice incurs to fulfill your request. This practice has the right to deny access, in whole or in part, to protect health information if the records are psychiatric notes, are a matter of national security or public health policy, are part of legal proceedings, were provided by a non-provider under promise of confidentiality concerning their identity, or could place in danger your life or the lives of others.

Signature: _____ Date: _____
       (Patient/Representative)

If signed by a personal representative of patient, state relationship: _____

REQUEST FOR NO RECORDS TO BE KEPT

I am exercising my right under the Health Care Information Act of 1992, as described to me, to request that no record of the content of our therapy sessions be kept. I understand that I may change this request at any time.

Signed: _____

Date: _____

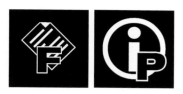

LIMITS ON PATIENT CONFIDENTIALITY

We are required to disclose confidential information if any of the following conditions exist:

1. You are a danger to yourself or others.
2. You seek treatment to avoid detection or apprehension or enable anyone to commit a crime.
3. Your therapist was appointed by the courts to evaluate you.
4. Your contact with your therapist is for the purpose of determining sanity in a criminal proceeding.
5. Your contact is for the purpose of establishing your competence.
6. The contact is one in which your psychotherapist must file a report to a public employer or as to information required to be recorded in a public office, if such report or record is open to public inspection.
7. You are under the age of 16 years and are the victim of a crime.
8. You are a minor and your psychotherapist reasonably suspects you are the victim of child abuse.
9. You are a person over the age of 65 and your psychotherapist believes you are the victim of physical abuse. Your therapist may disclose information if you are the victim of emotional abuse.
10. You die and the communication is important to decide an issue concerning a deed or conveyance, will or other writing executed by you affecting as interest in property.
11. You file suit against your therapist for breach of duty or your therapist files suit against you.
12. You have filed suit against anyone and have claimed mental/emotional damages as part of the suit.
13. You waive your rights to privilege or give consent to limited disclosure by your therapist.
14. Your insurance company paying for services has the right to review all records.

*If you have any questions about these limitations, please discuss them with your therapist.

Signature: _____ Date: _____

I am consenting to my (or my dependant) receiving outpatient treatment.

Signature: _____ Date: _____

RELEASE OF INFORMATION

I authorize _____ to contact my primary care physician (name) _____ regarding an appointment being made for follow-up, as well as information pertaining to psychological and emotional function.

Signature: _____ Date: _____

Therapist's Guide to Clinical Intervention, Second Edition by Sharon L. Johnson (© 2003 Elsevier Inc.)

GUIDELINES FOR THE RELEASE OF PSYCHOLOGICAL TEST DATA

The language in the current standard establishes a presumption that the test data shall be released, pursuant to a client/patient release, unless certain specific exemptions are met. The exemptions are limited to:

- protecting the client/patient or others from substantial harm
- protecting the client/patient or others from misuse or misrepresentation of the data or the test.

The following advice is provided:

- follow the APA Ethics Code informed consent procedures
- if you receive a subpoena for test data from an attorney's office or from a legal copy service, but you do not have a valid written release from the client, do not automatically release the test data.

If you receive a valid subpoena for test data, without a valid written release from the client/patient, the following actions are suggested in this Division I guideline:

- do not send a copy of the test data
- send the attorney a letter explaining why you are not releasing a copy of the test data
- explain that you have concerns about the individual being harmed by non-qualified individuals attempting to interpret the test data
- explain that you have concerns about release of copyrighted test materials to non-qualified individuals
- suggest that your test data be sent to another licensed psychologist who may interpret the data for the attorney
- suggest to the attorney that you will cooperate with a court order for release of the test data
- consult your legal counsel if the attorney threatens to file a motion to compel or to seek monetary sanctions against you.

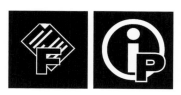

MEDICARE ADVANCE BENEFICIARY NOTICE

Patient Name:

Medicare Number: DOB:

Practitioner:

Dear Patient

Medicare will only pay for services that it determines to be "reasonable and necessary" under Section 1862(a)(1) of the Medicare law. If Medicare determines that a particular service, although it would otherwise be covered, is not "reasonable and necessary" under Medicare program standards, Medicare will deny payment for that service. Even though I believe that the following procedure or service is the best course of treatment for you, I believe, in your case, Medicare is likely to deny payment for the procedure or service for the reason(s) indicated.

Procedure Codes: Charges ($):   Date(s) of Service:

Description:

Expected Denial Reason(s) (from below): (insert corresponding numbers)

Other:

Explanations

According to Medicare guidelines for medically necessary and/or reasonable services and items, Medicare <u>does not usually</u> pay for:

1. Many visits or treatments.
2. Service for certain conditions.
3. Today's office visit unless it was needed because of an emergency.
4. Like services by more than one doctor during the same day or week.
5. Like services by more than one doctor of the same specialty.
6. Many services within period of a week or month.
7. More than one visit per day.
8. Group therapy (if not medically necessary).
9. Legal-related appointments, reports, review of records, etc.
10. Court appearances or stand-bys.
11. Letters, reports, etc.
12. Biofeedback.
13. Consultation with other professionals.
14. Other …

This is a partial list of denial reasons. Other reasons may apply and <u>must</u> be indicated in "Other" above.

Cont.

Patient's Agreement

I have been notified by my psychologist that he/she believes that, in my case, Medicare is likely to deny payment for the services identified above, for the reasons stated. If Medicare denies payment, I agree to be personally and fully responsible for payment. I will also be responsible for copays and unmet deductibles.

Patient signature: _____ Date: _____

Witness signature: _____ Date: _____

Chapter 4

General Informational Handouts for Patients

Chapter Contents

Patients appreciate receiving informational handouts on particular topics relevant to the issues discussed in their therapy sessions. Handouts provide an opportunity to anchor the issues covered in therapy and also give an opportunity to share the insights from therapy with their family or loved one. Handouts help a patient go beyond the issues covered in a given therapy session.

The handouts in this chapter are both for direct use and may serve as samples to the therapist to make up a series of handouts for use with their own unique patient population.

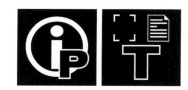

WELCOME BROCHURE

We Welcome you to _____, PhD and Associates

We appreciate the opportunity to provide you with a wide range of behavioral/mental health services.

The information in this brochure is designed to answer many of the questions most often asked. We want you to know our office policies and the manner in which services are rendered. The more you know, the more our services can be of benefit to you.

Everyone in this office operates as a team member to provide quality professional service. If you have questions at any time, please ask. We want to be of help and make your experience here a pleasant one.

Appointments

Everyone is seen on an appointment basis. We ask that you arrange your appointments in advance so we can reserve time for you. Should you not be able to keep your scheduled time, please be courteous and let us know 24 hours in advance.

Appointments that are not cancelled will be charged to your account and not to your insurance.

Business Office Hours

The business office is open for scheduling appointments, financial inquiries, and other matters on Monday–Friday from 9:00 a.m. to 5:00 p.m., except holidays. If you find it necessary to call after office hours, the answering system will take your message. However, if your call is an EMERGENCY, please stay on the line and speak to an attendant.

The answering service will take your message and relay your call at once. **IF YOUR CALL IS LIFE-THREATENING, PLEASE CALL 911 OR GO TO A LOCAL EMERGENCY ROOM** . Please call our office to let us know of your situation. Dr _____ will return your call as soon as possible.

Insurance Coverage

Most mental health benefit plans have been designed only to provide coverage for brief episodes for crisis stabilization. This type of coverage calls for a solution-focused therapeutic intervention aimed at handling problems quickly. However, long-term and intensive psychotherapy is available when problems are chronic and not responsive to short-term therapy. This would be at your expense.

Most insurance plans require a prior authorization and/or referral from your physician before you see a therapist. Please check with your insurance company for their particular requirements.

Finances

The office operates on a fee-for-service basis. We accept cash, check, or payment by insurance. If you are going to utilize your insurance plan there will most likely be a copayment, which is due at the time services are rendered. We will be happy to bill your insurance company or HMO for the balance of your bill.

Please remember that if your insurance contract does not cover the fees for all the services rendered, you are responsible for payment. All insurance payments will be credited to your account.

Many insurance plans require prior authorization for treatment. It is your responsibility to secure authorization before your first appointment. If it is determined that you are not eligible for insurance coverage, you will be responsible for payment, even if that determination is made after services are rendered.

A service charge may be added to accounts carried past 30 days. A collection service may be used when accounts are outstanding beyond 90 days.

The complexities of Managed Care and the many changes taking place in the insurance industry prevent our staff from being knowledgeable of all plans. Yet, we will be happy to do what we can to be of assistance to you in working with your plan.

Treatment Modalities

_____, Phd and Associates offers a variety of treatment modalities for individuals, couples, families, and groups. Examples of the specific modalities include diagnostic evaluations, stress management, anger management, and group therapy, vocational as well as other areas of focus.

Medication and Hospitalization

We will work closely with your referring physician to secure coordination of care and medication management. For those requiring short-term hospitalization, staff privileges are available at a local in-patient health facility.

Please discuss these adjunct treatments with your therapist as needed.

Confidentiality

When patients choose to utilize third party payers, diagnostic information and treatment plans are required to be submitted. Beyond this, information will be released only when you consent to a specific release in writing. There are several legal exceptions to this release, for example, when the therapist has reason to believe you are a danger to yourself or to others or when the therapist has good reason to suspect child abuse or neglect. Periodically your therapist may confidentially consult with another therapist regarding your treatment plan to help you achieve the best outcome for your therapy.

Specialized Services

Dr _____ is available for business consultations, forensic consultations, seminars, lectures, and nursing home consultations.
_____, PhD
Consulting and Clinical Psychologist
_____
_____
Phone: _____
Fax: _____

EMPLOYEE ASSISTANCE PROGRAM
Consultation Areas Needing to be Addressed

An Employee Assistance Program is an excellent tool to assist employers, Human Resource Departments, and employees in coping with issues that they must face every day, and that may well interfere with optimal work performance.

HAVE ONE OR MORE OF THE FOLLOWING PROBLEM AREAS BEEN EXPERIENCED BY YOUR COMPANY IN THE PAST YEAR?

- Death of an employee or employee loved one
- Employee alcoholism or drug use
- Company downsizing
- Violence or threats of violence in the workplace
- Increased customer/client complaints
- Drop in employee productivity
- Increased absenteeism
- Increased company interpersonal conflicts
- Increased employee stress
- Increase in medical or disability claims
- Increase in Workers' Compensation claims
- Accidents on the job
- High employee "counseling" needs from management
- Organizational restructuring
- Other ...

THE WAYS MANAGEMENT MIGHT ADDRESS THESE ISSUES INCLUDE THE FOLLOWING

- Consultation with management
- Employee education seminars
- Use of a flyer or handout on selected topics
- Noon-time bag lunch discussion sessions
- Employee referral for individual consultation
- Other ...

For more information on how we can help your organization at these critical times or with these interfering problems, please call: [PRACTICE DETAILS]

SHALL I SIGN UP WITH AN EAP?

How do EAPs Differ from Mental Health Plans?

OVERVIEW

EAP (Employee Assistance Program) benefits differ from traditional mental health "carve-out" benefits in many ways but can work in tandem to provide the most effective mental health treatment. To begin to understand how the EAP and mental health "carve-out" work together effectively, it is important to first understand the differences:

- EAP is for assistance, **not** therapy. It is a crisis benefit designed to assist an employee in identification of community resources to solve an acute problem or stressor.

- EAP is extremely time-limited, usually resolved in less than 4 visits. EAP's aim is to resolve a crisis within a matter of 4–6 weeks. During that time the intervention is specifically focused on diffusing the crisis by utilizing problem-solving skills, resource referral, practical advice, and limited provision of emotional support.

- EAP utilization is not necessarily expected to resolve the underlying stressor. It is intended to diffuse the crisis situation, and the client is expected to then utilize the resources identified and/or the problem solving skills developed to independently resolve the underlying stressor after completing the EAP sessions. This is where the integrated EAP and "carve-out" can be integrated most effectively, transitioning patients from diffusing the crisis into treatment for issues of an enduring nature.

- Mental Health benefits are intended to provide psychotherapy over a period of either several weeks, months, or years. The goal of treatment is to address problems of a more enduring nature compared to the immediate crisis focus of EAP programs. Typically patients in psychotherapy will be seen for at least 6 visits, but often are seen for longer periods of time.

- Mental Health treatment is appropriate for stresses of an enduring nature, for chronic emotional conditions/mental disorders, and for any evaluation and treatment with psychotropic medications. Additionally, catastrophic traumatic stressors are more appropriately suited to Mental Health treatment (as opposed to EAP intervention) due to the high risk of prolonged psychological effects of trauma.

Example:
The following table gives an example of a common presenting problem and identifies criteria for referral to EAP or Mental Health Treatment. This is only intended to provide guidance in determining the appropriate level of intervention.

Presenting problem/symptoms	Criteria for EAP referral	Criteria for mental health treatment referral
Depressed mood, sadness	1. A single acute loss (such as death of parent or spouse, end of relationship, etc.) which is associated with acute grief (duration less than 6 months since the recent acute loss)	1. Multiple losses, either acutely or sub-acutely, or sub-acute grief (grief has lasted longer than 6 months since the recent acute loss)
	2. Absence of past history of depression needing antidepressant treatment	2. Prior history of significant depressive illness (has required mental health treatment and/or antidepressant medication in the past)
	3. Absence of suicidal ideation/risk	3. Presence of suicidal ideation/risk

DISCLOSURE OF RISKS AND BENEFITS REGARDING THE USE OF PSYCHOTHERAPEUTIC MEDICATIONS

Dear Resident and Family Members,

The following list contains information regarding different classes of psychotherapeutic medications, the brand name by which they are known, the conditions they seek to alleviate, and possible adverse reactions to their use.

It is important to note the following: This information is not intended to supplement any disclosure that the attending physician should make. Informed consent is, and remains, primarily the physician's responsibility. Our staff are not trained to answer any questions that you may have regarding the information contained herein. In this regard, please direct your questions to the attending physician or psychiatrist.

This information is based upon currently available literature regarding the use of psychotherapeutic medications: these may change from time to time. Again, the physician should keep the resident apprised of those changes.

ANTI-PSYCHOTIC DRUGS: Mellaril, Moban, Navane, Prolixin, Thorazine, Haldol, Loxitane, Serentil, Trilafon, Abilify, Geodon, Stelazine, Clozaril, Risperdal, Zyprexa, Seroquel	**BENEFITS:** These drugs alleviate manifestations of psychosis such as hitting, kicking, scratching, grabbing, causing damage to surroundings, injuring self and others, yelling, screaming, insomnia, restlessness, undressing self, hallucinations, delusions, interference with care, throwing objects, and fearful distress	**ADVERSE REACTIONS:** Blurred vision, sedation dry mouth, drowsiness, apathy, constipation, akinesia, muscle rigidity, drooling from the mouth, photosensitivity, weight gain, edema, postural hypotension, akathesia	**OF SPECIAL CONCERN:** Seizure disorder, glaucoma, fever, chronic constipation, skin pigmentation, jaundice, tardive dyskinesia
ANTI-DEPRESSANT DRUGS: Nopramin, Sinequan, Tofranil, Anafranil, Prozac, Serzone, Trazodone, Lexapro, Remeron, Welbutrin, Luvox, Paxil, Zoloft, Cymbalta	**BENEFITS:** These drugs alleviate manifestations of depression such as sleeplessness, sadness, irritability, self pity, weight loss, unhappiness, loss of appetite, poor grooming, being withdrawn, crying, feeling rejected, not socializing, wishing to die, anhedonia	**ADVERSE REACTIONS:** Sedation dry mouth, blurred vision, constipation, postural hypertension, urinary retention, tachycardia, muscle tremors, agitation, headache, skin rash, photosensitivity, excessive weight gain	**OF SPECIAL CONCERN:** Glaucoma, heart disease, chronic constipation, lowering of seizure threshold and edema
ANTI-ANXIETY DRUGS: Xanax, Valium, Tranxene, Ativan, Serax, Atarax, Klonopin, Buspar.	**BENEFITS:** These drugs alleviate manifestations of anxiety such as nervousness, overconcern, restlessness, insomnia, sleeplessness, tension, and tremors	**ADVERSE REACTIONS:** Sedation, morning hangover, ataxia, nausea	**OF SPECIAL CONCERN:** Other sedation, hypnotics, alcohol

RESIDENT-Last Name	First	Room	Med Rec #	Doctor

10 STEPS TO A HEALTHIER BRAIN

The health and functioning of a person's brain is always changing and improving and learning to function more effectively and reliably. When it is working properly, relationships tend to be more healthy and functional. Check out your brain's status and current level of effectiveness. Identify those areas in which you could improve so your brain helps you to be more relational, communicative, analytic, and effective. For example, here are 10 positive steps to make part of your daily life.

- Are you protecting your brain from head injuries and toxic exposure?
- Are you putting good food into your brain every day?
- Are you taking a 100% RDA multiple vitamin everyday?
- Are you being selective about what you watch on TV so that you are constantly learning new things?
- Do you do physical exercise at least 3–4 times a week for at least 20 minutes at a time?
- Are you de-stressing your brain daily?
- Are you correcting your negative thinking patterns that put your brain at risk for anxiety, depression, relationship problems, and job related problems?
- Do you make love regularly and thereby exercise your brain?
- Do you make sure you are getting enough sleep each night?
- Are you treating your brain problems early on and not letting problems eat away at your well-being?

What I need to do to strengthen my brain over the next few weeks:

1.

2.

3.

4.

5.

ALTERNATIVE MEDICINE: GUIDELINES

TYPES OF HERBALS AND SYNTHETIC MEDICINE

St John's Wort – for moderate depression, dysthymia, sleep; 300 mg, tid
Gingko Biloba – for dementia, depression; 60–120 mg bid, has side effects
SAMe – for depression and pain, from 200 to 1600 mg daily; can cause mania
Valerian plant – for insomnia and anxiety; at least 500 mg and up to 12 g
Omega 3 fatty acids – for mood stability, as in bipolar disorder, and brain and heart

WORDS OF CAUTION

- Quality control is not known
- Side effects are not clearly known
- Not sure what brands can be trusted and there is often variability between them
- Generally used for mild and moderate problems
- Not sure of their preventative impact
- Not sure of their interactions with other herbs, foods, and other medications
- Professional consultation is usually at the level of a clerk
- May delay someone from getting more effective treatment for serious problems

POTENTIAL BENEFITS

- Usually less expensive than the alternatives
- Need not reveal their use to an insurance company or other agency
- Usually have fewer side effects
- Compliance is usually higher
- More helpful for mild and moderate problems

USER GUIDELINES

- Use at your own risk
- Evaluate relative benefits periodically
- Ask your physician to assess for any adverse effects if used over a long time
- Tell your physician of your use of herbal or alternative medicines if other medications are being considered
- Read and study the research on the herbs you are taking
- Be aware of their benefits and side effects as you take them over time

ADVICE FOR PATIENTS SEEKING SERVICES ON THE INTERNET

Individuals who claim to be psychologists and who provide psychological services on the Internet must be licensed as a psychologist. This means that if a California resident accesses psychological services via the Internet, the individual providing the psychological services must be licensed as a psychologist in California. Licensing requirements may vary by state or province but, generally speaking, if psychological services are accessed via the Internet, the provider of those services should be licensed to legally practice psychology in the state or province in which the consumer is a resident.

If you communicate with someone, or access a website that purports to provide psychological services, make sure you have and can verify at least the following information:

- The full name, address, and phone number of the individual providing the "service."
- What types of services or advice he/she is qualified to provide.
- Where and as what type of provider he/she is licensed.
- To what extent you can expect your communications with him/her to be confidential and whether his/her website and e-mail use encryption methods to protect confidentiality.
- Payment arrangements.
- How to terminate services.
- Any record of the therapist with the Better Business Bureau? The state licensing board?

PERSONAL BILL OF RIGHTS

1. I have the right to ask for what I want.
2. I have the right to say no to requests or demands that I cannot meet.
3. I have the right to express all of my feelings – positive and negative.
4. I have the right to change my mind.
5. I have the right to make mistakes and do not have to be perfect.
6. I have the right to follow my own values and beliefs.
7. I have the right to say no to anything if I feel that I am not ready, if it is unsafe, or if it conflicts with my values.
8. I have the right to determine my own priorities.
9. I have the right not to be responsible for the actions, feelings, or behavior of others.
10. I have the right to expect honesty from others.
11. I have the right to be angry at someone I love.
12. I have the right to be myself. To be unique.
13. I have the right to express fear.
14. I have the right to say, "I don't know."
15. I have the right not to give excuses or reasons for my behavior.
16. I have the right to make decisions based on my feelings.
17. I have the right to my own personal space and time.
18. I have the right to be playful.
19. I have the right to be healthier than those around me.
20. I have the right to feel safe, and be in a nonabusive environment.
21. I have the right to make friends and be comfortable around people.
22. I have the right to change and grow.
23. I have the right to have my wants and needs respected by others.
24. I have the right to be treated with dignity and respect.
25. I have the right to be happy.

If you are not familiar with your personal rights then take the time to read this daily until you are aware of your rights and begin to assert them. It may be helpful to post a copy of this where you have the opportunity to see it intermittently for reinforcement.

Therapist's Guide to Clinical Intervention, Second Edition by Sharon L. Johnson (© 2003 Elsevier Inc.)

PATIENT BILL OF RIGHTS

As an individual patient receiving services from the offices of _____, your following rights will be upheld to the best of our ability:

1. To participate in the decisions regarding the nature and scope of your treatment/therapy.
2. To access after-hours emergency attention.
3. To be made aware of all fees for services rendered and payment policies.
4. To express concerns and grievances or recommended modifications to your care plan and services being rendered.
5. To have your patient records treated with confidentiality and, except where required by law, the opportunity to approve or refuse their release.
6. To receive truthful and honest care by a licensed therapist.
7. To be provided consultation, evaluations, treatments, and preventative care within a reasonable period of time.
8. To have the freedom to report any illegal, unethical or competency errors to the Board of Consumer Affairs.
9. To receive any and all medically necessary services in a professional manner without regard to age, race, gender, religion, national origin or any other basis that would constitute illegal discrimination.
10. To be treated by all staff with friendliness, courtesy, and respect.

Chapter 5

Forms Related to Referral and Consulting Services

Chapter Contents

Every therapist is a consultant. While most therapy is directed to the individual or family unit, a therapist is often sought out when a larger system fails or comes upon hard times. When a therapist is invited to serve in the role of a consultant, whether it be to a company, office, agency, organization, or corporation, the "therapist-consultant" provides a similar service as is provided to a family.

The identification of a problem, the source of the problem, the identification of the issues to be addressed and the correction of the problem is the expectation placed on any consultant. Suggestions and ideas that would change the landscape of the behavioral patterns contributing to the problem are highly valued.

As a consultant, be it as a coach, career builder, or as an organizational think-tank leader, numerous forms are utilized to help identify problems, understand the scope of the problems and assist in providing an avenue for improved performance and production. This chapter includes the forms, handouts, templates, exercises, and guidelines utilized by consultants to create organizational change and make the necessary improvement in a dysfunctional multi-dimensional system. The goal of the consultant process is to help a good organization become better.

CONTRACT FOR CONSULTING SERVICES: BRIEF FORM

The parties to this agreement are:

Consultant:_____

Client:_____

The consultant will conduct the following procedures and tasks and advise in the following matters:

FEES AND EXPENSES:

The consultant's fee for services rendered as stated above is $_____. This is based on an estimated time duration of:

_____.

A retainer of $_____ is now due and payable. Future payments will be made upon completion of this agreement, or at agreed timely intervals. Expenses will be reimbursed upon receipt of the invoice.

Consultant signature: _____ Date: _____

Client signature: _____ Date: _____

CONSULTING SERVICES AGREEMENT WITH OTHER PROFESSIONALS

This constitutes an agreement between _____ (consultant) and _____ (consultee) for the provision of consultation services by Dr _____ to the consultee. We agree to meet at an interval to be mutually arranged. The fee for a consultation session, based on a minimum of 50 minutes, will be $_____. Fees will be raised $ _____ in even-numbered years. Extra time spent in consultation will be charged at a prorated fee.

We agree to the following rights and responsibilities in this consultation relationship:

1. Notification of risk. If the consultation is on clinical case work, the consultant will be informed during regular consultation session, or by phone or fax in an emergency, of any client currently the subject of consultation who is at imminent risk of harm to self or others, and of any client who is the subject of consultation who reports suspected child or vulnerable adult abuse. The consultant may be available between scheduled consultation session for additional consultation in person or by phone as needed on an emergent basis.

2. Liability. The consultee will maintain her/his own professional liability insurance coverage at all times. The consultee will not be covered by the consultant's liability insurance. The consultant is not the employer or supervisor of the consultee, and is not responsible for any acts or omissions of the consultee. The consultee will maintain licensure or certification in state of practice appropriate to her/his training.

3. Confidentiality. The content of consultation sessions will be held in confidence with the following exceptions: (a) If the consultee releases the consultant in writing to share information for specific purposes; (b) If the consultant receives a court order requiring release of information; (c) If the consultee persists in actions that consultant has advised are ethically or legally potentially actionable. The consultant reserves the right at this time to report the consultee to regulatory or ethical authorities, and to terminate consultation services.

The consultee is free to terminate consultation services at any time.

I understand and agree to the terms of this consultation agreement.

Signature: _____ Date: _____
        Consultee

Signature: _____ Date: _____
        Consultant

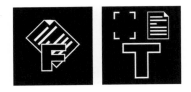

MEMO OF UNDERSTANDING FOR PROFESSIONAL SERVICES
A Sample Contract

DATE

ADMINISTRATOR NAME
SKILLED NURSING FACILITY NAME

_____
_____
_____

Dear _____

In response to your request for a Memo of Understanding, please review the following. If agreeable to you, please sign and return a copy to me.

1. (THERAPIST'S PRACTICE NAME) _____ will provide monthly psychological services to the (NAME OF FACILITY) _____, especially the (SKILLED NURSING FACILITY NAME) _____ on an as-needed basis. Typically, a visit would be at least once monthly.

2. This agreement shall commence on _____, and shall be for an initial period of one year, and will renew itself annually unless either party cancels this agreement by giving thirty (30) days' written notice before any expiration date.

3. The parties agree that the Provider is to provide mental health consultation services, in accordance with any applicable requirements of federal, state or local laws, rules and/or regulation, third party reimbursement sources (public and private), or other reimbursement sources covering the Provider's services. The Provider agrees that services will be rendered with regard to conditions of participation and reimbursement coverage required by governmental and third party reimbursement sources.

   The Facility is responsible for making the necessary arrangements for a patient to be seen for any and all services rendered so that said services qualify for appropriate third party reimbursement, private or public. This shall include, but not be limited to, arrangement for appropriate physician referral, having the patient available at the time of a scheduled visit, and making available the patient's clinical chart.

4. The services provided will be billed to the patient's insurance carrier. In the event that the patient does not have an active insurance plan covering mental health services and on which Dr _____ is not a paneled provider, such as in the case of Medical only, the facility will be billed at the rate of $_____ per hour. The Facility may seek reimbursement from the Responsible Party.

5. Prior to a visit from Dr _____, the Director of Social Services or the Director of Nurses will provide a copy of the patient's fact sheet and a brief notation as to the purpose of the consultation.

6. The Director of Social Services or the Director of Nurses or their staff will obtain the necessary referral for mental health services from the patient's Attending Physician.

7. The Facility will be billed $_____ per visit to the facility to assist in the escalating cost of gas and the _____ reduction in Medicare reimbursement rates.

8. Staff training, corporation consultation, and staff meetings will be provided, as needed, for a fee of $_____ per hour.

9. All services will be provided following the procedures outlined in the attached brochure.

10. A current copy of Dr _____'s professional resume, professional license, and insurance coverage will be provided annually.

11. The Provider shall be an Independent Contractor, who shall retain sole and absolute discretion and judgment in the manner and means of providing services to the Facility. The Provider agrees to comply

with all policies, rules, and regulations of the Facility in relation to the provision of the Provider's services. All services shall be rendered in a competent, efficient, and satisfactory manner, and in strict accordance with the currently approved methods and practices in the Provider's professional specialty.

12. In the desire to provide effective, competent and appropriate services, Dr _____ will work with the staff of each facility to assure that services are provided within context of the professional culture and procedures prevailing in each facility.

13. The Provider agrees to keep and maintain such records on the services rendered by the Provider to patients in the Facility as may be required by fiscal intermediary, federal, state or local governmental agency, facility or other party to whom billings for the Provider's services are rendered.

14. If any action at law is necessary to enforce or interpret the terms of this agreement, the prevailing party shall be entitled to reasonable attorney's fees, costs, and necessary disbursement in addition to any other relief to which he/she may be entitled. Arbitration is to be used as the first means of dispute resolution.

Respectfully Submitted: Read and Approved:

_____   _____
Clinical Psychologist   Administrator

Tax ID: _____

Date: _____   Date: _____

encs: Professional Resume
        Professional License
        Insurance Policy

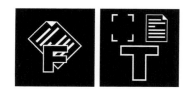

AGREEMENT FOR PSYCHOLOGICAL EXPERT WITNESS SERVICES

This document constitutes a contract between _____ and the undersigned law firm or individual attorney for services performed by Dr _____ in the matter entitled:

_____

I/We agree to prompt payment of Dr _____'s bills for his/her work performed according to the following fee schedule:

> I. For work of a non-testimonial nature, including but not limited to psychological evaluations, written or oral reports, consultations with attorneys or their agents, review of records, and any travel pursuant to the above, the fee will be $_____ per hour or portion thereof. Appointments missed without cancellation will be billed at the usual rate.

> II. For work of a testimonial nature, including travel to the site at which testimony shall be given and any time spent waiting to give testimony, the fee will be $_____ per hour or portion thereof.

> III. For any work requiring travel outside of _____, reasonable travel costs will be reimbursed. A day rate of $_____ will be charged in lieu of the hourly fee for time spent of less than eight hours.

> IV. Costs for materials, photocopying, duplication of tapes and other costs incidental to the performance of work that the client requests will be charged separately and are the client's responsibility.

I/We understand that I, an individual attorney, or we, this law firm, constitute Dr _____'s client and hold direct responsiblity for payment of bills to him/her. I/We understand that any arrangements that I/we make with my/our client to obtain funds for my/our payments to Dr _____ are independent of this agreement. I/We will not ask Dr _____ to enter into fee agreements with any other parties, including my/our client, to satisfy my/our indebtedness to Dr _____. I/We understand that Dr _____ cannot bill for his/her work on a contingent fee basis.

I/We understand that any bills in arrears at the end of the calendar month will be charged a late fee of ____ % per month. I/We understand that any bills in arrears for more than three months may be sent to collection at Dr _____'s discretion. If this becomes necessary, I/we understand that I/we will also be responsible for any additional costs incurred by Dr _____ in order to collect fees due. I/We understand that Dr _____ may decline to do further work on any matter where the bill is more than three months past due until payment has been made.

In the event that litigation is necessary to enforce this agreement the prevailing party shall be entitled to reasonable attorney's fees and costs of collection. Venue shall be in _____.

Signature: _____   Date: _____

For (Name of firm): _____

Address: _____

Phone: _____   Fax: _____   E-mail: _____

_____

CONFIDENTIAL REFERRAL

Dear _____

Re: PATIENT NAME
DOB:

Reason for Referral/Identifying Information: You referred this man/woman for a psychological assessment on _____. He/she has a history of_____ .

You requested my impressions of the mental health factors that underlie these problems along with recommendations for interventions to help.

Assessment Methodology/Sources of Information: After I met with _____ at our professional offices on _____, I interviewed him/her and gave him/her some psychological tests. The latter consisted of:
_____

I consulted with the following professionals about this case:
_____

I also reviewed the following documents:
_____

In explaining the purpose and nature of this assessment to both _____ and his/her parents I clarified that the information obtained by me would not be held confidential. In indicating that he/she understood and agreed to this condition Mr/Mrs/Ms _____ signed a Release of Information authorizing me to send you this report. The youth/child agreed to this condition as well.

Medical and Developmental History:

Family History and Current Functioning:

Physical abuse/sexual molestation history?

Risk of out of home placement:

Risk of family disintegration:

Social/Adaptive Functioning:

Client Substance Abuse (History and Current):

Cont.

Tobacco Use:

Client Legal Issues:

Academic Functioning:

Mental Status/Test Results:

Mental Health Concerns (History and Current):

Diagnosis: AXIS I Clinical Syndrome
AXIS II Personality Disorder
AXIS III Physical Disorder
AXIS IV Psychosocial Stressors
AXIS V Global Assessment Functioning
Current
Past Year

Medical Necessity: The AXIS I disorders noted above cause significant impairments in _____'s functioning at home, in school, and in the community. Interventions are needed to diminish these impairments. His/her condition would not be responsive to physical healthcare based treatment.

Discussion of impressions:

Recommendations:

If you have any questions, feel free to contact me at:

Sincerely,

DR NAME

TITLE

EXPERT WITNESS GUIDELINES

1. **Learn the Rules of Evidence.** These are the rules the govern testimony and evidence in court.

2. **You Begin Preparing for Testimony When You First Take the Case.** Everything you do in the case is subject to challenge.

3. **Be Truthful in Everything You Do – Assessments, Reports, and Testimony.** If you are competent and truthful with the data, conclusions, and your testimony, you are unlikely to get tripped up.

4. **Write Your Report with Cross-Examination in Mind.** You will be cross-examined on your report. Can you defend everything in it?

5. **Insist on Meeting with the Attorney Who Retained You Prior to Testifying.** You and the attorney must be on the same page.

6. **You Can Never Know the Facts Well Enough – But Keep Trying.** A command of the facts is essential for effective testimony.

7. **Remember that as Experts, Our Job Is to Teach.** We are allowed to offer opinions because we have expertise that will be useful to the jury.

8. **Let the Weaknesses in the Case Be Presented on Direct Testimony.** There are no perfect cases.

9. **Cross-Examination Is Supposed to Challenge Your Work and Credibility – It's Not Personal.** If you did excellent and defendable work and testified about it honestly on direct testimony, there should be few surprises on cross-examination.

10. **On Cross-Examination, Be Willing to Admit the Truth, but Only the Truth.** Denying the truth will make you appear biased.

CONTRACTING WITH MANAGED CARE COMPANIES

The terms of any contract with a private managed care company will affect all aspects of your practice, including, but limited to where you may practice, with whom you may provide services, how much you will be paid for services rendered and which services you may provide. The contract will also indicate for how long and/or how many times you may provide such services, and how many minutes you may devote to a patient in a session. Before signing a contract, read it carefully and be sure it is a fit for you and how you practice.

WHAT TO LOOK FOR WHEN REVIEWING A CONTRACT

1. All managed care contracts are not alike.
2. Renewal contracts may be different from the original contract you signed.
3. A contract does not include all restrictions on your practice and all features of the company's expectations. They may be included in the appendices, and various attachments.
4. Be sure to note the allowed locations in which services may be rendered, especially if you have a hospital practice, have more than one clinic location, or consult out of the office in other locations.
5. Note if the contract allows services to be rendered in a private practice setting and a public practice setting.
6. Can you sever your relationship with the company easily and with proper notice?
7. Do they have a reasonable and timely process for appealing disputed claims?
8. Does the contract restrict your service billing procedures and make it difficult to collect on claims submitted?
9. Are the credentialing procedures excessive and intrusive?
10. Study the manual for the policies related to utilization review, pre-authorization, formulary restriction, access to the peer reviewer, and appeal procedures.
11. Know the company's policy regarding on-site review of your practice and files.
12. Look for the procedures to obtain authorization on weekends, holidays, after hours, and in emergencies.
13. Before signing up for another year, be sure your efforts are worthy of the compensation.
14. Asking questions is permissible: a contract's terms are subject to negotiations.
15. Any agreements or modifications are to be obtained in writing.
16. Seek advice from your attorney, if necessary, or from your professional association, from the state's insurance commissioner, or your malpractice carrier.
17. Is retroactive authorization possible when services were provided in good faith and in an unusual situation?
18. Can your patient be seen by another mental health provider at the same time and in the same week or month and all claims are honored?
19. If a patient is seen in a special setting, such as their home, a skilled nursing facility, assisted living facility, office setting or in vivo, will a claim be accepted?
20. Other ...

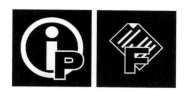

FORENSIC PSYCHOLOGICAL ASSESSMENT CONSENT

This statement is a disclosure of certain information about the process of psychological assessment. It details certain rights and responsibilities that you have in this process and gives you some information about me.

MY TRAINING AND LICENSURE

I have a PhD in Clinical Psychology, earned in [YEAR] from [INSTITUTION]. I am licensed as a psychologist by [STATE] and hold a Diplomate in Clinical Psychology. My expertise is in the assessment of the psychological consequences of trauma, abuse, victimization, harassment, and discrimination.

APPROACH TO ASSESSMENT

The assessment process is designed to help me answer questions about the possible causes of problems or distress that you may be currently experiencing. It is not meant to be psychotherapy, and will be brief and focused on the legal questions raised by the attorney who made this referral. The assessment process usually has two parts that require your participation: a structured interview, which normally takes between three and eight hours, and the administration of psychological testing, which normally takes from three to five hours. The times vary depending on how much information you have to share with me, and the complexity of the issues being assessed. I will also probably be reviewing your medical and psychological records, and other written materials relevant to your case. I may also ask you for permission to speak to other people who have known you well who may help me to understand you.

I am conducting this assessment process because you are, or are planning to become a party in a legal matter. If that is the case, I will be consulting with the attorney who referred you to me regarding my findings. Your consent to this evaluation includes a consent to release information to that attorney and/or their agents (for example, their paralegal). If I am called upon to testify in a deposition or courtroom proceedings, the findings of this evaluation and all supporting materials can be subpoenaed for examination by the opposing attorney, and it is very likely that this will happen. When you raise the issue of your mental status in a legal case, you may have waived your right to confidentiality of these records. In addition, if I am deposed by the opposing attorney, I will be required to respond to questions regarding my evaluation of you and my findings.

I will take all possible steps to protect your privacy at any time when I am not required to render opinions or share information. It is important that you be as candid and open with me as you can possibly be during this assessment. Information that is concealed from me is potentially far more damaging than if it is revealed here so that I can integrate it into the complete findings of my evaluation.

I may be asked to write a report of my findings. If so, you will receive a copy of a draft of that report to check for factual accuracy. If you find that what I say misrepresents you or the facts in some way, you may request that I make changes so as to more accurately reflect your perceptions. However, I retain my right to include those of my professional opinions and observations that I believe to best represent my findings in your case. You are not obligated to use any report that I write.

I will be audio-recording all of our meetings. This is standard practice in a forensic evaluation and preserves an absolutely accurate record of what you say to me. You have the right to request that I turn off the tape recorder at any time. However, I cannot be responsible for the accuracy of my reporting of any information that you give me when the tape recorder is not running. In addition, I cannot base my opinions primarily on anything you say when the tape recorder is not running. If you recall something in between or after our evaluation sessions, please call the office and leave that information in detail on my answering machine, and I will record it onto tape.

If during our evaluation you report information to me that causes me to suspect child abuse or vulnerable adult abuse, I must by law report my findings to the appropriate state agencies. I would inform you if I planned to take this step. If I learned that you were likely to harm another person, I must by law inform that person and the authorities. I would inform you if I took that step.

Cont.

FEES

My fee for any work that I do of a non-testimonial nature (for example, assessment interviews, test scoring, reading records, talking with the attorney, report writing) is $ _____.00/hr. My fee for any kind of testimonial work, including any time I spend traveling or waiting to testify, is $ _____.00/hr. If any of my work requires me to travel outside of _____ [DEFINED AREA] I will charge a daily rate of $ _____.00/day for whatever work I do of less than eight hours in place of the hourly rate, plus reasonable travel expenses. I bill on a monthly basis; fees are payable in full at the end of the month in which services are rendered. Late bills incur a charge of ___% per month on any unpaid balance. I send my bills directly to the attorney who has referred you to me, and who has signed a contract to pay these fees as a cost in your case. I reserve the right to take delinquent accounts to a professional collection agency if your attorney has not paid me after three consecutive unpaid monthly bills. Your insurance will not pay for forensic evaluations, since they do not meet insurance company definitions of medical necessity.

COMPLAINTS

If you have reason to believe that I have acted in an unethical or unprofessional manner, I encourage you to discuss this directly with me. If you do not feel that I have been responsive to your concerns, there are several formal routes by which you can bring a complaint against me. You can write to the Examining Board of Psychology, Department of Health, _____ [STATE] or to the Ethics Committee of the American Psychological Association, 750-1st Street NE, Washington DC 20002-4242.

Client's Consent to Assessment

I have read the above disclosure statement and understand its terms. I have discussed any questions that I have with Dr _____, and he/she has answered them to my satisfaction. I agree to my participation in the assessment process as described above. I understand that my statements in this process will not be kept confidential because I have raised the issue of mental health in a legal case, but I understand that Dr _____ will keep these materials private when he/she is not required by law to share this information. I agree to the release of information to the attorney who has referred me for this assessment. I agree to the fees quoted above. I am over the age of eighteen and competent to enter into this agreement OR I am the parent of a minor signing on behalf of my minor child.

Signature: _____   Date: _____

If signing on behalf of minor state relationship: _____

Minor's name: _____

Address of signatory: _____

City: _____   State: _____   Zip: _____

Phone: _____   DOB of signatory: _____

Witness signature: _____   Date: _____

ETHICAL GUIDELINES IN INTERDISCIPLINARY CARE

Most psychologists leave graduate school with a compartmentalized view of our professional role. To a psychologist fresh out of training, interdisciplinary care typically means a psychodynamic therapist consulting with a behavioralist. But over the past decade, there has been an increased emphasis on treating patients using a more holistic and comprehensive approach to their psychological care. Most psychologists working with patients who experience psychological distress as a result of a primary physical problem find themselves collaborating closely with an array of medical specialists who are not psychologically trained. While the multidisciplinary approach to health care has taken hold, psychologists unfortunately come to this arena with little information about how to navigate our roles and at the same time adhere to our own ethical guidelines.

Following are 10 recommendations to navigate common ethical challenges in interdisciplinary care scenarios:

1. **Clarify your professional role in the medical team and the patient.** Define your function: assessment, case management, surgical readiness, forensic evaluator, ongoing treater, medication monitoring, disability rating, medication detox, etc.

2. **Set and maintain clear boundaries regarding medications input.** Monitor medication responses, give feedback to the physician, be informed of potential side effects and alert the patient where appropriate, and consider recommending certain medication options but ensure that instructions about medication dosing occur between patient and doctor.

3. **Use testing appropriately.** Ensure that testing data are incorporated with your clinical impressions, but watch out that other medical professionals do not use your test findings as a shorthand for medical treatment or disability impressions.

4. **Define the edges of your competence.** Recognize the need for medical input. Broaden your expertise to include a working knowledge of common medical procedures so you can help patients prepare for medical treatment.

5. **Maintain clear communication.** Be precise about the words you use. Explain testing results. Provide differential diagnostic considerations. Avoid jargon.

6. **Address individual differences.** Be alert to cross-cultural issues. Help both patient and physician understand the impact of personal differences on expectations for each other.

7. **Maintain adequate records.** Assure you will have to testify in open court about every case. Be prepared to recreate patient's care and the communication involved in that care. Use written consent forms.

8. **Understand the power differentials between patients and clinicians.** Realize that many patients harbor feelings of mistrust about medical care and this may be transferred to your relationship as well. Maintain a therapeutic alliance with the patient and act as an advocate.

9. **Be a responsible psychologist.** Redefine the usefulness of psychologists in medical treatment. Broaden the concept of patient management to include behavioral management.

10. **Uphold the ethics code.** Keep a copy of the ethics code handy and consult it often. If you have a question about how to apply the code to your clinical predicament, call the state Ethics Committee for a live consultation.

GUIDELINES FOR MEDICATION REFERRALS

1. Only physicians (preferably a psychiatrist) prescribe a course of treatment that includes psychopharmacology. Not nurses, dentists, psychologists, chiropractors, herbalists, curanderos or other folk healers, or other health professional. However, psychologists play a significant role in the management of medications and are able to prescribe in some States and in some health care jurisdictions.

2. Be ready to discuss the notion in general of how psychotropic medication essentially works.

3. Be able to discuss in general the length of time needed for the medication to begin to work.

4. Be able to discuss in general terms the side effects most often associated with the medication.

5. Be able to link the positive side effects that the client may need to be aware of so that they can monitor improvement with you. For example, sleep, energy, concentration, appetite, anxiety, mood etc.

6. Have a brief descriptor text outlining psychotropic medication use, dosage, and side effects handy to use with your client on monitoring their progress and addressing questions that you are able to answer.

7. Sometimes, the fear of seeking out a psychiatrist and being placed on medication is so great the client may drop out of treatment altogether. It is important at times to stress the immediacy in the need for improvement to the client. Often times sharing with the client the likelihood that the medication will help with sleep, anxiety, stress, and rest is a viable enough incentive to seek out and continue with treatment.

8. Be prepared to give your client a "what to expect" scenario when he/she goes to see the psychiatrist. Psychiatrists like most professionals come in all shapes, sizes, and sensitivity levels. Many times, your client may be limited by their HMOs as to who can offer them treatment. If this is the case, give them the gist of what to expect. Remind them that many times psychiatrists are busy, and are often times trying to get to the etiology of their problem from a biological and behavioral standpoint. Often times their approach is from a medical model and not always empathic from a therapeutic standpoint. Encourage the client to ask questions, be assertive, and disclose as much information as possible regarding their case to equip the physician in their diagnostic and treatment recommendations.

9. If you do not like your interaction or results from your meeting with the psychiatrist, get a second opinion. Psychiatrists have been wrong in the past. Just because they say it, label it, and prescribe for it, does necessarily make it true or part of the best treatment plan for your client. Share with your client that you would be willing to discuss the diagnosis and treatment plan with them if they desired.

10. When you and your patient have decided that a visit to a psychiatrist is part of the patient's treatment plan, have the patient make the appointment. You can have them call from your office. That way you know when their scheduled appointment is, with whom, and you can follow up with the client on their meeting. At times, when it is appropriate and with the client's permission, you can contact the client's HMO directly, identify your relationship with the client, and make your way through the HMO maze of calls until you get to the psychiatric division of the HMO. Once there you may be able to share permitted background information and try to schedule an appointment for your client. You can do the scheduling yourself or hand the phone over to the client, at the HMO's request, for them to schedule.

NETWORKING TO TAP THE HIDDEN JOB MARKET

Given the competitive nature of today's market place, job seekers must utilize strategies that will help them tap into the hidden job market. The key to discovering this pool of employment opportunities is personal networking; this refers to contacting friends and acquaintances that can help you access information concerning job leads and potential job openings. You can start by making a preliminary list of contacts that include:

- relatives, friends, and neighbors
- current and former instructors
- people you met during summer jobs
- people you meet at on-campus events
- members of your alumni (Career Information Network)
- business/professional groups related to your career goals.

Once you have prepared your list, begin by informing your contacts that you are conducting a job search campaign. Your goal is not to secure a job but rather to create visibility for yourself. Ask your contacts to suggest some good companies whom you can contact. They can also give you feedback on the companies you have already targeted as well as helpful advice on strategies you might incorporate into your job search. Most importantly, remember to follow up every job lead promptly. Based on the studies of the Career Placement Council, the following list provides helpful hints for developing an effective networking strategy in seeking out "the hidden jobs."

10 NETWORKING TIPS

1. KNOW EXACTLY what it is you want from others. Prepare questions in advance of a meeting or telephone conversation. Be succinct, courteous, and appreciative.
2. HAVE A POSITIVE ATTITUDE when you network.
3. TALK TO STRANGERS and mingle with people you don't already know at meetings and events. Introduce yourself!
4. SHARE INFORMATION, ideas, resources, and contacts with others. Networking is a two-way process.
5. DON'T ASK for too much at one time. Limit the amount of assistance or information you seek from one person.
6. DON'T NEGLECT to follow up on leads you have been given. You don't want to embarrass those who have made connections for you.
7. DON'T BETRAY other people's confidentiality. Trust is a vital part of networking.
8. DON'T MONOPOLIZE other people's time when networking. Keep your conversations brief and make arrangements to call or meet at another time if you discover areas of mutual interest.
9. CONTINUE NETWORKING even after you've found a job. There will be ways an active network can help. Everyone needs a person and professional support system. Keep yours in place throughout your career.
10. INCORPORATE NETWORKING into your everyday life. It is a powerful tool for marketing yourself, but also a powerful tool for enriching your life and the lives of those in your network.

Chapter 6

Fitness for Duty and Workers' Compensation Forms

Chapter Contents

In servicing the needs of patients, a therapist must know and appreciate the patient's work world and the specific issues related to fitness for duty and workers' compensation for the injured or impaired worker. While these types of evaluations are conducted in a similar manner to most comprehensive evaluations, the final product, a report, must be provided in a specific format. Payment for services rendered must be requested on the proper forms and submitted in the required time frame.

The chapter provides the forms and notice formats for communicating with employers, insurance companies, and the Workers' Compensation Appeals Board. Helping a patient through the process of recovering from an injury and returning to work after an illness or injury is a significant service to patients.

NOTICE OF UNFITNESS FOR DUTY

Date: _____

Re: _____

DOB: _____

Employer: _____

DOI: _____

To whom it may concern:

The above named employee has been under my care since _____. My professional services have focused on his/her work stress related concerns.

At this time, my assessment indicates that he/she is UNABLE to return to work and assume normal duties. It is anticipated that he/she will be able to return to work on or about _____. Work restrictions and/or special accommodations are/are not anticipated.

My additional comments for your consideration:

_____

_____

_____

Respectfully submitted,

DR NAME
TITLE

NOTICE OF RETURN TO DUTY

Date: _____

Re: _____

DOB: _____

Employer: _____

DOI: _____

To whom it may concern:

The above named employee has been under my care since _____. My professional services have focused on his/her work stress related concerns.

At this time, my assessment indicates that he/she is ABLE to return to work and assume normal duties. It is anticipated that he/she will be able to return to work on or about _____. Work restrictions and/or special accommodations are/are not requested.

My assessment indicates that the following restrictions or special accommodations will facilitate a successful return to full and productive employment:

_____

_____

_____

Respectfully submitted,

DR NAME
TITLE

WORKERS' COMPENSATION INFORMATION INTAKE FORM

Full Name	SS #
Address	Case #
City, State, Zip	DOB

Telephone
Home _____ Work: _____ Other: _____

Date of Loss/Injury

Total Disability from: to:	Partial Disability from: to:

Return to Work Indicator ❑ Limited ❑ Normal ❑ Conditional

Percent Disability

Attorney	Telephone
Address	

Employer	Telephone
Address	

Employer's Attorney	Telephone
Address	

Insurance Carrier	Telephone
Address	

Adjusting Agency, if agency administered	Telephone
Address	

ADDITIONAL INFORMATION:

WORKERS' COMPENSATION LIEN COVER LETTER

DATE:

WORKERS' COMPENSATION APPEALS BOARD
Attn: Assistance Officer
ADDRESS

RE: CLIENT NAME
     WCAB Number:

     Claim Number:

     Date of Injury:

Gentlemen

Enclosed herein for filing, please find a **Notice and Request for Allowance of Lien** for reasonable expenses regarding the above-referenced matter. Please properly stamp the copy attached and return to our office at your earliest convenience in the envelope provided.

A copy of the lien has been served on the interested parties listed on the attached proof of service.

Thank you for your attention to this matter.

Respectfully submitted,

DR NAME

TITLE

encs

Chapter 7

Forms Related to Patient Services

Chapter Contents

One of the important roles of the therapist is to manage the treatment plan and assure that the patient is cared for and treated in a meaningful, helpful, and satisfying manner. Every appointment should count and contribute towards achieving the objectives and goals agreed upon at the beginning of therapy. Every patient should feel satisfied and valued in the manner therapeutic care was delivered. By managing the agreed treatment plan on a case-to-case basis, the therapist remains in charge of the sessions and is allowed to make adaptations as necessary, helpful, and cost-effective.

The forms, templates, homework assignments, and guidelines set forth in this chapter allow the therapist to clearly and easily manage the treatment plan for the ultimate improvement and good of the patient and those important to them.

"WELCOME TO THE OFFICE" PATIENT SIGN IN

We Value Your Trust

Please sign in and know you are welcome and appreciated.

Full Name	Time In	Time Out	Copayment?	Payment on Account

Comments:

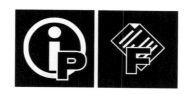

PSYCHOTHERAPY INFORMATION DISCLOSURE STATEMENT AND CONSENT TO TREATMENT

Therapy is a relationship that works in part because of clearly defined rights and responsibilities held by each person. This frame helps to create the safety to take risks and the support to become empowered to change. As a client in psychotherapy, you have certain rights that are important for you to know about because this is your therapy, whose goal is your well-being. There are also certain limitations to those rights that you should be aware of. As a therapist, I have corresponding responsibilities to you.

MY RESPONSIBILITIES TO YOU AS YOUR THERAPIST

I. Confidentiality

With certain specific exceptions described below, you have the absolute right to the confidentiality of your therapy. I cannot and will not tell anyone else what you have told me, or even that you are in therapy with me without your prior written permission. Under the provisions of the Health Care Information Act of 1992, I may legally speak to another health care provider or a member of your family about you without your prior consent, but I will not do so unless the situation is an emergency. I will always act so as to protect your privacy even if you do release me in writing to share information about you. You may direct me to share information with whomever you chose, and you can change your mind and revoke that permission at any time. You may request anyone you wish to attend a therapy session with you.

You are also protected under the provisions of the Federal Health Insurance Portability and Accountability Act (HIPAA). This law insures the confidentiality of all electronic transmission of information about you. Whenever I transmit information about you electronically (for example, sending bills or faxing information), it will be done with special safeguards to insure confidentiality.

If you elect to communicate with me by email at some point in our work together, please be aware that email is not completely confidential. All emails are retained in the logs of your or my internet service provider. While under normal circumstances no one looks at these logs, they are, in theory, available to be read by the system administrator(s) of the internet service provider. Any email I receive from you, and any responses that I send to you, will be printed out and kept in your treatment record.

The following are legal exceptions to your right to confidentiality. I would inform you of any time when I think I will have to put these into effect:

1. If I have good reason to believe that you will harm another person, I must attempt to inform that person and warn them of your intentions. I must also contact the police and ask them to protect your intended victim.

2. If I have good reason to believe that you are abusing or neglecting a child or vulnerable adult, or if you give me information about someone else who is doing this, I must inform Child Protective Services within 48 hours and Adult Protective Services immediately.

3. If I believe that you are in imminent danger of harming yourself, I may legally break confidentiality and call the police or the county crisis team. I am not obligated to do this, and would explore all other options with you before I took this step. If at that point you were unwilling to take steps to guarantee your safety, I would call the crisis team.

4. If you tell me of the behavior of another named health or mental health care provider that informs me that this person has either (a) engaged in sexual contact with a patient, including yourself or (b) is impaired from practice in some manner by cognitive, emotional, behavioral, or health problems, then the law requires me to report this to their licensing board at the _____. I would inform you before taking this step. *If you are my client and a health care provider, however, your confidentiality remains protected under the law from this kind of reporting.*

The next is not a legal exception to your confidentiality. However, it is a policy you should be aware of if you are in *couples therapy* with me.

If you and your partner decide to have some individual sessions as part of the couples therapy, what you say in those individual sessions will be considered to be a part of the couples therapy, and can and probably will be discussed in our joint sessions. *Do not tell me anything you wish kept secret from your partner.* I will remind you of this policy before beginning such individual sessions.

Cont.

II. Record Keeping

I keep very brief records, noting only that you have been here, what interventions happened in session, and the topics we discussed. If you prefer that I keep no records, you must give me a written request to this effect for your file and I will only note that you attended therapy in the record. Under the provisions of the Health Care Information Act of 1992, you have the right to a copy of your file at any time. You have the right to request that I correct any errors in your file. You have the right to request that I make a copy of your file available to any other health care provider at your written request. I maintain your records in a secure location that cannot be accessed by anyone else.

III. Diagnosis

If a third party such as an insurance company is paying for part of your bill, I am normally required to give a diagnosis to that third party in order to be paid. Diagnoses are technical terms that describe the nature of your problems and something about whether they are short-term or long-term problems. If I do use a diagnosis, I will discuss it with you. All of the diagnoses come from a book titled the **DSM-IV**; I have a copy in my office and will be glad to let you borrow it and learn more about what it says about your diagnosis.

IV. Other Rights

You have the right to ask questions about anything that happens in therapy. I'm always willing to discuss how and why I've decided to do what I'm doing, and to look at alternatives that might work better. You can feel free to ask me to try something that you think will be helpful. You can ask me about my training for working with your concerns, and can request that I refer you to someone else if you decide I'm not the right therapist for you. You are free to leave therapy at any time.

V. Managed Mental Health Care

If your therapy is being paid for in full or in part by a managed care firm, there are usually further limitations to your rights as a client imposed by the contract of the managed care firm. These may include their decision to limit the number of sessions available to you, to decide the time period within which you must complete your therapy with me, or to require you to use medication if their reviewing professional deems it appropriate. They may also decide that you must see another therapist in their network rather than me, if I am not on their list. Such firms also usually require some sort of detailed reports of your progress in therapy, and on occasion, copies of your case file, on a regular basis. I do not have control over any aspect of their rules. However, I will do all that I can to maximize the benefits you receive by filing necessary forms and gaining required authorizations for treatment, and assist you in advocating with the MC company as needed.

MY TRAINING AND APPROACH TO THERAPY

I have a PhD in Clinical Psychology earned in _____ at _____. I am a licensed psychologist (No. _____) in _____[STATE]. My areas of special training and expertise include women's and gender issues in general, and specifically working with survivors of trauma, abuse, and victimization, and people in recovery from alcohol and drugs.

My approach to therapy is called _____ Therapy. This is a philosophy of psychotherapy which looks at the _____. If you would like to learn more about this approach, I have books about it that I will lend to you. I use a variety of techniques in therapy, trying to find what will work best for you. These techniques are likely to include dialogue, interpretation, cognitive reframing, awareness exercises, self-monitoring experiments, visualization, journal keeping, drawing, and reading books. If I propose a specific technique that may have special risks attached, I will inform you of that, and discuss with you the risks and benefits of what I am suggesting. I may suggest that you consult with a physical health care provider regarding somatic treatments that could help your problems; I refer both to traditional and non-traditional practitioners, and will be glad to discuss with you the pros and cons of various alternatives. I may suggest that you get involved in a therapy or support group as part of your work with me. If another health care person is working with you, I will need a release of information from you so that I can communicate freely with that person about your care. You have the right to refuse anything that I suggest. I do not have social or sexual relationships with clients or former clients because that would not only be unethical and illegal, it would be an abuse of the power I have as a therapist.

Therapy also has potential emotional risks. Approaching feelings or thoughts that you have tried not to think about for a long time may be painful. Making changes in your beliefs or behaviors can be scary, and sometimes disruptive to the relationships you already have. You may find your relationship with me to be a source of strong feelings, some of them painful at times. It is important that you consider carefully whether these risks are worth the benefits to you of changing. Most people who take these risks find that therapy is helpful.

You normally will be the one who decides therapy will end, with three exceptions. If we have contracted for a specific short-term piece of work, we will finish therapy at the end of that contract. If I am not in my judgment able to help you, because of the kind of problem you have or because my training and skills are in my judgment not appropriate, I will inform you of this fact and refer you to another therapist who may meet your needs. If you do violence to, threaten, verbally or physically, or harass myself, the office, or my family, I reserve the right to terminate you unilaterally and immediately from treatment. If I terminate you from therapy, I will offer you referrals to other sources of care, but cannot guarantee that they will accept you for therapy.

I am away from the office several times in the year for extended vacations or to attend professional meetings. If I am not taking and responding to phone messages during those times I will have someone cover my practice. I will tell you well in advance of any anticipated lengthy absences, and give you the name and phone number of the therapist who will be covering my practice during my absence. I am available for brief between-session phone calls during normal business hours. If you are experiencing an emergency when I am out of town, or outside of my regular office hours (after 5 pm weekdays or over the weekend), please call _____. If you believe that you cannot keep yourself safe, please call 911, or go to the nearest hospital Emergency Room for assistance.

YOUR RESPONSIBILITIES AS A THERAPY CLIENT

You are responsible for coming to your session on time and at the time we have scheduled. Sessions last for ___ minutes. If you are late, we will end on time and not run over into the next person's session. If you miss a session without canceling, or cancel with less than 24 hours notice, you must pay for that session at our next regularly scheduled meeting. The answering machine has a time and date stamp which will keep track of the time that you called me to cancel. I cannot bill these sessions to your insurance. The only exception to this rule is if you would endanger yourself by attempting to come (for instance, driving on icy roads without proper tires), or if you or someone whose caregiver you are has fallen ill suddenly.

You are responsible for paying for your session weekly unless we have made other firm arrangements in advance. My fee for a session as of _____ is $ _____. If we decide to meet for a longer session, I will bill you prorated on the hourly fee. Emergency phone calls of less than 10 minutes are normally free. However, if we spend more than 10 minutes in a week on the phone, if you leave more than 10 minutes' worth of phone messages in a week, or if I spend more than 10 minutes reading and responding to emails from you during a given week I will bill you on a prorated basis for that time. My fees go up $ _____every two years. If a fee raise is approaching I will remind you of this well in advance.

If you have insurance, you are responsible for providing me with the information I need to send in your bill. You must pay me your deductible at the beginning of each calendar year if it applies and any copayment at each session. You must arrange for any pre-authorizations necessary. I will bill directly to your insurance company via electronic means for you once a month. You must provide me with your complete insurance identification information, and the complete address of the insurance company. If a check is mailed to you to cover your balance due, you are responsible for paying me that amount at the time of our next appointment. If the insurance over-pays me, I will credit it to your account or refund it to you if you would prefer that. I am a preferred provider with _____
_____.

I am not willing to have clients run a bill with me. I cannot accept barter for therapy, I do not take credit cards or Paypal, nor can I take DSHS medical coupons. I am a Medicare participating provider and accept assignment from them. Any overdue bills will be charged ___% per month interest. If you eventually refuse to pay your debt, I reserve the right to give your name and the amount due to a collection agency.

COMPLAINTS

If you are unhappy with what is happening in therapy, I hope you will talk about it with me so that I can respond to your concerns. I will take such criticism seriously, and with care and respect. If you believe that I have been unwilling to listen and respond, or that I have behaved unethically, you can complain about my behavior to the Examining Board of Psychology, Department of Health, _____ [STATE].You are also free to discuss your complaints about me with anyone you wish, and do not have any responsibility to maintain confidentiality about what I do that you don't like, since you are the person who has the right to decide what you want kept confidential.

Client Consent to Psychotherapy

I have read this statement, had sufficient time to be sure that I considered it carefully, asked any questions that I needed to, and understand it. I understand the limits to confidentiality required by law. I consent to the use of a diagnosis in billing, and to release of that information and other information necessary to complete the billing process. I agree to pay the fee of $ _____ per session. I understand my rights and responsibilities as a client, and my therapist's responsibilities to me. I agree to undertake therapy with Dr _____. I know I can end therapy at any time I wish and that I can refuse any requests or suggestions made by Dr _____. I am over the age of eighteen.

Signed: _____ Date: _____

Witness: _____ Date: _____

PATIENT CONFIDENTIAL INFORMATION FORM

Name: _____ DOB: _____ Sex: _____ Marital Status: _____

SS #: _____ Employed: _____ Student: _____ CDL#: _____

Address: _____ City: _____ State: _____ Zip: _____

Phone: (Home) _____ (Work) _____ (Other) _____

Employer: _____ Referred By: _____

Spouse or Parent Name: _____ DOB: _____ SS #: _____

Address: _____ City: _____ State: ____ Zip: _____ Phone: _____

Person Responsible for Payment: _____ Relationship to Client: _____ CD #: _____

Address: _____ City: _____ State: _____ Zip: _____ Phone: _____

* *

Primary Insurance: _____ Phone: _____ Auth #: _____

Billing Address: _____ City: _____ State: _____ Zip: _____

ID #: _____ Group #: _____ Copay: _____

Employer: _____ Phone: _____

If insured is other than client:

Subscriber: _____ Relationship to client: _____

SS #: _____ DOB: _____ Sex: _____

Address: _____ City: _____ State: _____ Zip: _____ Phone: _____

* *

Secondary Insurance: _____ Phone: _____ Auth #: _____

Billing Address: _____ City: _____ State: _____ Zip: _____

ID #: _____ Group #: _____ Copay: _____

Employer: _____ Phone: _____

If insured is other than client:
Subscriber: _____ Relationship to client: _____

SS #: _____ DOB: _____ Sex: _____

Address: _____ City: _____ State: _____ Zip: _____ Phone: _____

* *

OFFICE USE ONLY

Provider Code: _____ 1st Visit: _____ Procedure Code: _____ Releases signed: _____ Ins Contact: _____

Diagnosis: Axis I _____ Axis II: _____ Axis III: _____ Axis IV: _____ Axis V: _____

CONFIDENTIAL ALTERNATE COMMUNICATIONS REQUEST

Patient name: _____ DOB: _____

I would like to receive communications of my protected health information from this practice by alternate means or at an alternate location.

The information I would like communicated by alternate means or to an alternate location is:

☐ All information

☐ Other (specify) _____

☐ **I request my information be delivered in the following manner:**

☐ US Postal Service other than First Class Mail (please specify)

_____

☐ Express / overnight delivery (specify preferred carrier)

_____

☐ Email address _____

☐ Other (specify) _____

☐ **I request my information be delivered to the following valid mailing address location:**

_____

_____

_____

I understand that I may be required to pay this practice for any non-customary expenses incurred to satisfy my request, and that the address provided is correct and capable of accepting my information. I will be notified and must agree in advance to pay the cost of the alternate communication. The practice reserves the right to deny requests that impose an unreasonable cost or burden.

Signature: _____

Date: _____

Relationship to patient (If signed by a personal representative of patient): _____

_____

DOCUMENTING ALL SERVICES RENDERED

DOCUMENTATION OF SERVICES

Patient Name: _____ Therapist: _____

Current GAF: _____ Highest GAF this year: _____

Interventions this session: _____

Homework: _____ Current meds: _____

Risk issues assessed: _____ Tx Plan: _____

_____

Date of service: _____ Length of session: _____ CPT: _____

Diagnosis: _____

Symptoms this session: _____

Axis IV Psychosocial and Environmental problems addressed:

✂--cut--✂

DOCUMENTATION OF SERVICES

Patient Name: _____ Therapist: _____

Current GAF: _____ Highest GAF this year: _____

Interventions this session: _____

Homework: _____ Current meds: _____

Risk issues assessed: _____ Tx Plan: _____

_____

Date of service: _____ Length of session: _____ CPT: _____

Diagnosis: _____

Symptoms this session: _____

BEHAVIORAL THERAPY PLAN

Patient name: _____ Date: _____

Presenting problem:

Behavioral analysis:

Behaviors to be increased: _____

Treatment methods:

1.

2.

3.

4.

5.

Behaviors to be decreased: _____

Treatment methods:

1.

2.

3.

4.

5.

Comments:

NEEDS APPRAISAL AND SERVICES PLAN

Client name:	DOB:	Age:	Sex: ___ Male ___ Female	Date:

Background Information: Brief description of the client's medical history/emotional, behavioral and physical problems; functional limitations; physical and mental; functional capabilities; ability to handle personal cash resources and perform simple housekeeping tasks; client's/resident's likes and dislikes

NEEDS	OBJECTIVE/PLAN	TIME FRAME	PERSON(S) RESPONSIBLE FOR IMPLEMENTATION	METHOD OF EVALUATING PROGRESS
SOCIALIZATION – Difficulty in adjusting socially and unable to maintain reasonable personal relationships.				
EMOTIONAL – Difficulty in adjusting emotionally.				
MENTAL – Difficulty with intellectual functioning including inability to make decisions regarding daily living.				
PHYSICAL/HEALTH – Difficulties with physical development and poor health habits regarding body functions.				
FUNCTIONING SKILLS – Difficulty in developing and/or using independent functioning skills.				

REVIEW OF BEHAVIORAL MEDICATION BY PHYSICIAN

Patient name: _____   Date: _____

ACTIONS
__ I have reviewed this patient's medication plan.

__ I have consulted the necessary resources to help me assess the relative benefit of the current medication plan.

__ I have met with the patient (or family/responsible party) and considered his/her opinion on its continued use and relative benefits.

__ I am aware of the State Codes and guidelines calling for a periodic medication review.

__ I am aware that State Mandates do not require a medication change, reduction or discontinuance if it is not in the best interest of the patient.

PROFESSIONAL OPINION
__ I am of the opinion that medication dosage reduction or discontinuance is warranted at this time. I am taking action accordingly. See new orders. The patient (or family/responsible party) has been contacted and is aware of my decision.

__ I am of the opinion that medication change at this time is not warranted. No action will be taken. I have so informed the patient and/or the family/RP of my decision.

Signature: _____, MD   Date: _____

MONITORING OF ANTECEDENT EVENTS TO
SELF-DEFEATING BEHAVIOR

There are times when self-defeating behavior is engaged in and needs to be addressed. Examples might be: panic attacks, delusional thinking, cutting, hallucinations, seizures and mood changes, to name a few. Keep track as best as possible so that any pattern can be identified and addressed. Do this exercise for a few weeks to get a clear perspective.

Date	Time	Where was patient at the time?	What seemed to cause the behavior?	Describe specific behavior	Action taken

1.

2.

3.

4.

5.

6.

7.

8.

9.

10.

COMMENTS

COMPONENTS OF A PATIENT'S CHART: A CHECKLIST

Therapist's name _____   Patient's name _____

	Yes	No	N/A
1. Do all pages contain patient name and identification number?			
2. a. Each record includes the patient's address?			
b. Employer or school?			
c. Home and work telephone numbers including emergency contact?			
d. Marital/legal status?			
e. Appropriate consent forms?			
f. Guardianship or Power of Attorney information, if relevant?			
3. Is the provider identified on each entry (i.e., are the case notes signed)?			
4. Is date of initial and routine contact by patient noted in file?			
5. Are all entries dated?			
6. Is the record legible?			
7. Is the Primary Care Physician identified?			
8. Are allergies and adverse reactions to medication prominently displayed?			
9. Are relevant medical conditions listed, prominently identified and revised?			
10. Are presenting problems and relevant psychological and social conditions affecting patient's medical and psychiatric status documented?			
a. Are therapeutic interventions and responses documented?			
b. Are sources of clinical data documented?			
c. Are results of laboratory tests, and consultation reports documented?			
d. Are psychological testing results summarized?			
e. Is the previous medical history, including dates, documented?			
f. Is the previous psychiatric history, including dates, documented?			
g. Is relevant family information documented?			
h. What medications have been prescribed and the dosages of each?			
11. Special status situations, such as imminent risk of harm, suicidal ideation, or elopement potential, are prominently noted, documented, and revised in compliance with written protocols?			
12. If patient over age 12, history of past and present substance use (illicit, prescribed, and over the counter)?			
13. Are past and present smoking habits documented?			
14. Is the history of alcohol and drug use past and present documented?			
15. a. Mental status evaluation documented and includes: b. Affect			
c. Speech			
d. Mood			
e. Thought content			
f. Judgment			

EVALUATION OF THERAPIST

Now that you have had several sessions with me as your therapist, please evaluate the manner in which I conduct myself and provide a meaningful therapy experience. Your name will not appear on this form and it will be confidentially reviewed and evaluated by a third party. The following scale should be utilized:

+ 2 Excellent
+ 1 Very Good
   0 So, So, Nondescript
− 1 Fairly Weak
− 2 Very Weak

TRAITS/CHARACTERISTICS

____ Graciousness, Warmth, Connecting, Interested

____ Engaging, Responsiveness, Approachable

____ Energy, Animation, Alert

____ Orderliness, Flow of sessions, Systematic thinking

____ Depth of experience, Understanding, Knowledgable

____ Voice, Posture, Appearance, Eye contact

____ Compassion, Caring, Empathy

____ Open, Shares common experiences, Tells personal stories

____ Other

COMMENTS

Thank you very much. Others will benefit from your feedback. I am indebted to you.

PATIENT SATISFACTION QUESTIONNAIRE

To ensure that you are receiving the best possible care, please take a moment to complete our anonymous questionnaire and return it in the envelope provided or place it in the box provided in the office. We are committed to improving the quality of the services provided and appreciate your comments, questions and suggestions. This is anonymous; no name please.
Thank you.

Name of Treating Clinician: _____   Date: _____

PLEASE FILL OUT BY PLACING AN 'X' ON YOUR BEST ANSWER:

1. Were you satisfied with our telephone access and ease of scheduling an appointment?
   Very Satisfied   Satisfied   Neutral   Dissatisfied   Quite Dissatisfied

2. Were you satisfied with our ability to meet your language and cultural needs?
   Very Satisfied   Satisfied   Neutral   Dissatisfied   Quite Dissatisfied

3. Were you satisfied with our office location?
   Very Satisfied   Satisfied   Neutral   Dissatisfied   Quite Dissatisfied

4. In general, how satisfied were you with the comfort and attractiveness of our facility?
   Very Satisfied   Satisfied   Neutral   Dissatisfied   Quite Dissatisfied

5. Considering your particular needs, how helpful were the services you received?
   Very Satisfied   Satisfied   Neutral   Dissatisfied   Quite Dissatisfied

6. Do you feel your therapist was supportive and really tried to understand you and your problem?
   Very Satisfied   Satisfied   Neutral   Dissatisfied   Quite Dissatisfied

7. Would you recommend your therapist to a friend?
   Very Satisfied   Satisfied   Neutral   Dissatisfied   Quite Dissatisfied

8. Were your complaints or questions, if any, handled sufficiently?
   Very Satisfied   Satisfied   Neutral   Dissatisfied   Quite Dissatisfied

9. Did you feel respected as an individual?
   Very Satisfied   Satisfied   Neutral   Dissatisfied   Quite Dissatisfied

10. Would you recommend our office to a friend?
   Very Satisfied   Satisfied   Neutral   Dissatisfied   Quite Dissatisfied

COMMENTS, QUESTIONS OR SUGGESTIONS:

_____

_____

_____

PATIENT SATISFACTION: THERAPY'S GREATEST
PUBLIC RELATIONS APPROACH

Patients come to therapy with certain expectations. As in all of life, when our expectations are met, we are satisfied. We say we've had a good experience. If our expectations are exceeded, a level of satisfaction increases experientially.

Satisfied customers spread the word. Satisfied customers come back. Satisfied customers help build any business.

The problem with most therapists is that they never assess a patient's level of satisfaction, let alone their expectations as they come to therapy. Therefore, most therapists are "assessment blind" and are not able to capitalize on this critical aspect of patient satisfaction for public relations purposes.

It is important for a therapist to be trained and to think in terms of patient satisfaction. It is important for a therapist to understand the importance, value, and the impact of a patient's level of satisfaction or, for that matter, dissatisfaction. It is also important for a therapist to know how to assess a patient's level of satisfaction relative to their expectation at different stages throughout therapy.

The patient may be well-satisfied initially but then come to be dissatisfied later on. Conversely, sometimes patients increase in their level of satisfaction as therapy proceeds and as they benefit.

The assessment of the patient's satisfaction is an ongoing dynamic process that should be part of the therapeutic interaction with every patient. If not with every patient, with a sampling of patients, to be sure.

Forms, questionnaires, and surveys are well utilized to provide information on the expectations of therapy and the level of satisfaction of a patient after he/she has engaged in the therapeutic process.

It would be important not to only assess the style and the nature of therapy, but to assess the therapist as a person and as an agent of change. To assess the therapeutic environment relative to cleanliness, safety, comfort level, etc. Further, it is important to assess the manner in which the patient is treated by the office staff, by others in the office, and by the therapist themselves. Lastly, patients have their own expectations and nuances of what they expect when they come. They may not tell you – yet, they know. Opportunity to have a general discussion on this topic or opportunity to provide written feedback in a general way certainly is an appropriate option to be provided the patient.

WAITING ROOM ASSIGNMENT

How has it gone since the last session?

While waiting for your appointment to start, please complete this Homework Review. I hope this will be a constructive and meaningful assignment for you.

1. List the things you were asked to work on after your last session:

2. List the progress and changes you have made since your last session:

3. List the issues and events you would like to discuss in today's session:

4. Other comments or items to clarify:

Name: _____ Date: _____

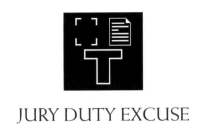

JURY DUTY EXCUSE

DATE

Jury Commissioner

_____ County Superior Court

ADDRESS _____

_____

_____

Re: _____

Dear Commissioner

Please be informed that NAME is undergoing active therapy at this time. Due to his/her current state of emotionality, he/she is unable to serve on a jury effectively. I would anticipate that this will continue to be the case for _____ months.

Respectfully,

DR NAME

TITLE

Chapter 8

Forms Related to Therapist's Professional Activities

Chapter Contents

It behooves all professionals to maintain an active and intentional continuing education program, required or not. Selecting relevant courses and keeping track of courses completed are essential to one's professional effectiveness and reputation. Similarly, keeping track of professional expenses and the supervision of interns is also vital to the accurate and proper operations of an office. Accepted professional business practices are necessary to any office as a clinical practice is more than therapy. It is a small business in a competitive world.

The forms and worksheets in this chapter are designed to help a therapist keep up with the legal and professional accounting demands placed upon the therapist.

CONTINUING EDUCATION LOG

Year_____

Date	Title of Course	Course No.	Credit HR	Provider

WEEKLY TRAVEL EXPENSE SHEET

Weekly Travel Expense Sheet (Mileage and Related Expenses)   Dates _____

Monday	Tuesday	Wednesday	Thursday	Friday	Weekend

EXPENSE ACCOUNT

_____

CONVENTION / MEETING: _____

DATE / PLACE: _____

SUBMIT EXPENSE ACCOUNT TO: _____

TRAVEL: RECEIPT ATTACHED

Parking: _____   _____

Plane: _____   _____

Car rental: _____   _____

Gas: _____   _____

Mileage: _____   _____

 Subtotal: _____

LODGING:

Place / Date: _____   _____

Cost: _____   _____

 Subtotal: _____

MEALS (DATE / COST):

_____   _____

_____   _____

_____   _____

_____   _____

_____   _____

 Subtotal: _____

TELEPHONE, INTERNET, FAXES, SECRETARIAL:

_____   _____

_____   _____

_____   _____

 Subtotal: _____

Signature: _____   Date: _____

SUPERVISION DOCUMENTATION FORM

Supervisee Name:

Date:

Total Time:

Topics:

Date:

Total Time:

Topics:

Managing an Office Staff

Chapter Contents

Therapists impact a huge number of individuals and groups of people. The impact of a therapist begins in the office and may reach around the globe. Therapists along with their office staff are shapers of change in today's world: their influence may be bestowed upon those known for their positive character, expressions of confidence, clarity of communication, forthright courage, and office procedures. Caring for the office staff and operating an office on a sound business model are key factors to a profitable and successful counseling practice.

The forms, templates, handouts, and checklists in this chapter have been designed to help professional therapists establish a well-running office and build a strong and viable practice of psychotherapy. In so doing, the practice will become known for its caring and helpful service to those that work in the office and those that walk the pathway to the therapist's door week after week.

PROGRAM STAFF MEETING MINUTES

Date: _____ Time: _____

Persons present:

Persons absent:

Issues discussed:

Decisions:

Assignments:

Items/Issues for our next or future meetings:

THERAPIST'S EVALUATION OF THE OFFICE STAFF

For Use in a Multi-Staff Clinic

INSTRUCTIONS: For each question, please rate your satisfaction with the office staff by circling the appropriate response.

5 = Very Satisfied 4 = Somewhat Satisfied 3 = Neither 2 = Somewhat Dissatisfied 1 = Very Dissatisfied 0 = Unknown/ Not applicable

BILLING MANAGEMENT

1.	Billing process overall	5	4	3	2	1	0
2.	Professionalism of office staff in collections	5	4	3	2	1	0

WORKING WITH US

1.	Ease of reaching appropriate clerical staff	5	4	3	2	1	0
2.	Ability of clerical staff to make immediate decisions	5	4	3	2	1	0
3.	Appropriate and timely follow-up	5	4	3	2	1	0
4.	Ability to resolve questions or concerns without requiring you to make additional calls or notes	5	4	3	2	1	0

PROBLEM HANDLING

1. If you had a problem with the clerical office in the past 1–3 months, please indicate the specifics of the situation:

_____

_____

2.	Satisfaction with how the problem was handled	5	4	3	2	1	0
3.	Satisfaction with the outcome	5	4	3	2	1	0

PRACTICE INFORMATION

1.	Approximately what percentage of your patients comment on the office staff and office procedures?	76–100	51–75	26–50	1–25	1–10
2.	What percentage of the comments are positive?	76–100	51–75	26–50	1–25	1–10

COMMENTS

In the spaces below, please provide any comments or suggestions.

_____

_____

_____

Thank you for your feedback.

ANNUAL SURVEY OF OFFICE STAFF

Please complete the form below as a way to give your feedback of our office staff and how well they serve you. Do not sign it. Do it anonymously. Thank you.

	How important is this to you?	How satisfied are you?
Easy to work with For example: Office staff helpful, easy to reach by telephone, responsive	__ Very important __ Important __ Not important	__ Very satisfied __ Satisfied __ Neutral or no opinion __ Dissatisfied __ Very dissatisfied
Timelines For example: Time it took to receive a call back or get help from the office	__ Very important __ Important __ Not important	__ Very satisfied __ Satisfied __ Neutral or no opinion __ Dissatisfied __ Very dissatisfied
Billing procedures For example: Easy to understand the documents, billings and letters	__ Very important __ Important __ Not important	__ Very satisfied __ Satisfied __ Neutral or no opinion __ Dissatisfied __ Very dissatisfied
Communication patterns For example: Clear explanations, knowledgeable staff, speak in friendly manner	__ Very important __ Important __ Not important	__ Very satisfied __ Satisfied __ Neutral or no opinion __ Dissatisfied __ Very dissatisfied
Courtesy, politeness For example: Treated with respect and concern; considerate	__ Very important __ Important __ Not important	__ Very satisfied __ Satisfied __ Neutral or no opinion __ Dissatisfied __ Very dissatisfied
Quality of service For example: Everything was correct the first time we did what you expected of us. No mix-ups.	__ Very important __ Important __ Not important	__ Very satisfied __ Satisfied __ Neutral or no opinion __ Dissatisfied __ Very dissatisfied
Overall satisfaction with office staff Give us your general impression and experience	__ Very important __ Important __ Not important	__ Very satisfied __ Satisfied __ Neutral or no opinion __ Dissatisfied __ Very dissatisfied

If you answered "dissatisfied" or "very dissatisfied" in any category, please state the reason:

PEER EVALUATION OF EMPLOYEE

Name of employee: _____

Date form completed: _____

As part of the annual review of the above named employee, you have been selected by the above named employee to provide any comments and observations that you feel might be helpful to the employee's future performance and for the good of the office. Please be specific and constructive. Thank you.

1. Any comments or observations you would like to share about this employee's patterns of communication, both verbal and non-verbal?

2. Any comments or observations you would like to share about this employee's style of confronting and solving problems?

3. Any comments or observations you would like to make about this employee's teamwork and interpersonal relationships?

4. Any comments or observations you would like to make about this employee's professionalism?

5. Any comments or observations you would like to make about this employee's work skills and competency?

6. Any other comments or observations?

Signature: _____ Date: _____

EMPLOYEE SELF-EVALUATION FORM

Department: _____ **Name of employee:** _____

Date of evaluation: _____

1. Areas of excellence:

2. Progress made from time of last evaluation:

3. Areas in which progress is planned for this year:

4. New suggested specific goals to be achieved:

5. My supervisor could help me perform better in the following ways:

6. What I would like to do to help myself and the company/agency this next year:

7. What I would like the company/agency to do differently to make my job and the workplaces a better work environment this next year:

8. Is there anything in the workplace that is unsafe or that places you or anyone else at risk?

9. What did you do this year to advance yourself through personal reading, volunteer work, continuing education, and in-service training, and benefited therefrom?

10. Other comments you would like to have on the record and for consideration:

11. What 2–3 people would you like us to ask to submit a brief evaluation of you and your work performance as they observe you in the work environment?

EMPLOYER FEEDBACK TO EMPLOYEE FROM ANNUAL REVIEW

The following review is for your professional development based on the results of your annual review. We hope this additional information and feedback will be helpful to you this next year in the services you render to our customers/patients.

1. Date annual review was completed: _____

2. Comments from the evaluators:

   _____
   _____
   _____
   _____

3. Recommended classes, seminars, books or in-service training sessions to attend:

   _____
   _____
   _____
   _____

4. Recommended goals to achieve and behaviors to improve this next year:

   _____
   _____
   _____
   _____

5. Other comments that may be of value:

   _____
   _____
   _____
   _____

Employee's signature: _____ Date: _____

Supervisor's signature: _____ Date: _____

EMPLOYEE PROGRESSIVE DISCIPLINE

A Notification System

Employee name: _____   **Position/Department:** _____

VERBAL COUNSELING VERIFICATION:
Summary:

Signature of supervisor: _____   Date: _____

Signature of employee: _____   Date: _____

WRITTEN WARNING NOTIFICATION:
Summary:

Signature of supervisor: _____   Date: _____

Signature of employee: _____   Date: _____

WORK SUSPENSION AND SECOND WARNING:
Summary:

Suspension dates: from: _____ thru _____.

Signature of supervisor: _____   Date: _____

Signature of employee: _____   Date: _____

EMPLOYEE TERMINATION NOTIFICATION:
Summary:

Date of termination: _____

Terms of termination: _____

Signature of supervisor: _____   Date: _____

Signature of employee: _____   Date: _____

ANNUAL EMPLOYEE SATISFACTION SURVEY

As part of our annual employee satisfaction survey, we ask you to complete the following questions. If you would like to discuss any of them in person, please feel free to so indicate this on the form. Your feedback is important to us and to the process of making our company/agency a good place to work. Please complete the survey in the next few days and turn it in to _____.

Employee name: _____ **Date:** _____

1. Please note any cost savings ideas you have had this year. Were you able to try it out and what was your experience?

2. Please note any ideas you have had this year to generate higher levels of income and improved quality of services which would result in an income stream.

3. What was your most important professional accomplishment this year and why?

4. How did you volunteer your time on committees and other ways to improve the operations of the company/agency?

5. How did you go about to improve customer (consumer) satisfaction this year?

6. What are 3–4 areas of professional advancement on which you would like to focus this next year? How can management be of help to you?

   a.

   b.

   c.

   d.

7. If you could change anything about the job or the work environment, what would it be?

8. Is there anything you would like to do differently to make your work environment a better place in which to make a living?

9. Are you aware of any situation in the workplace that is inconsistent with our Code of Conduct, corporate compliance, or ethics?

10. I would like to meet with someone regarding my responses _____ .

My current job satisfaction rating level is _____ (1 = Very Satisfied; 5 = Not At All Satisfied).

UNUSUAL INCIDENT REPORT FORM

Please report any unusual event or incident taking place in the parking lot, waiting room, bathrooms, or any other location in the building or clinic. Be as specific as possible.

Person(s) involved: _____

Exact location: _____

Witnesses: _____

What happened as per your observations: _____

_____

_____

_____

_____

_____

_____

Did anyone intercede: _____

_____

_____

Who was notified of this incident: _____

_____

_____

Suggested action to prevent it from happening again: _____

_____

_____

Other comments: _____

_____

Signature of observer:_____ Date: _____

REQUEST FOR TIME OFF

_____

I _____ would like to request to be off from _____

thru _____

Number of days off requested: _____

Total work hours requested: _____

Reason for the request:
  Personal   ☐
  Paid vacation   ☐
  Holiday pay   ☐
  Bereavement   ☐
  Time without pay ☐
  Paid sick time   ☐
  Comp. time   ☐
  Other   ☐

Signature of employee: _____ Date: _____

Approval signature of supervisor: _____ Date: _____

REQUEST FOR EARLY DISMISSAL OR OVERTIME AUTHORIZATION

Employee name: _____ Date: _____

Requested date/time of early dismissal: _____

Requested date/time for overtime work: _____

Reason for the request: _____

_____

Signature of employee: _____ Date: _____

Approval signature of supervisor: _____ Date: _____

EMPLOYEE EXIT INTERVIEW

Employee's name: _____

Title: _____

Department: _____

Date of interview: _____

What were some of the best things you liked about your current position?

_____

_____

_____

What were some of the things you liked least about your current position?

_____

_____

_____

What were some of the things you liked best about the office/agency?

_____

_____

_____

What were some of the things you liked least about the office/agency?

_____

_____

_____

What are your feelings toward your supervisor or about the supervision you received?

_____

_____

_____

Cont.

Employee Exit Interview (Continued)

Why are you leaving the office/agency at this time? What is the attraction of the office/agency or company and position to which you are now going?

_____

_____

_____

What are your comments about our office/agency's salary, benefits, and working conditions?

_____

_____

Was there any particular incident or event that happened during your employment that made the difference in your decision to stay or leave the office/agency?

_____

_____

_____

What suggestions do you have for improving our work environment, and any other aspects within the office/agency?

_____

_____

_____

Interviewed by: _____ Date: _____

Interviewer's remarks:

_____

_____

_____

_____

_____

_____

AUTHORIZATION TO RELEASE EMPLOYMENT INFORMATION

Dear _____

I have recently applied for a position with _____ .

As part of the process in evaluating my qualifications, I have been requested to provide background information and a list of possible references. I have listed you as one of my references. Therefore, I authorize you to release any information you wish to share about me and my work-related background. They want to know if I will be a fit for the position and the agency/office.

This authorization is valid for 90 days from the date of my signature below. Please keep this copy of my release authorization for your files. Thank you for your willingness to help and cooperate in this new venture with me. Your timely response is requested.

Signature: _____ Date: _____

AUTHORIZATION FOR LETTER OF REFERENCE

Dear _____

Recently, I applied for a position with _____ .

As part of the process in evaluating my qualifications, I have been requested to provide background information and a list of references. I have listed you as one of my references. Therefore, I ask you and authorize you to release any information you wish to share about me, my work performance, and my work-related background. Essentially, they want to know if I will be a fit for the position and their agency/office.

Please keep this copy of my release authorization for your files. Thank you for your willingness to help and cooperate in this possible new venture with me. Would you be so kind as to respond to this request in a timely manner.

Signature: _____ Date: _____

RECOGNIZING EARLY WARNING SIGNALS OF A DANGEROUS EMPLOYEE

The dangerous worker in the work environment is not easy to proactively identify so that preventative actions can be undertaken in a timely manner. Any action plans to disrupt and cause harm in the work environment, once identified, must be swiftly diffused and turned over to those in higher levels of authority within the company or organization and local law enforcement. Each office needs a preventative and safety plan when risk is present.

SIGNS TO NOTICE AND TAKE SERIOUSLY

1. Direct or veiled verbal threats of harm.
2. Intimidation of others (this can be physical or verbal intimidation: harassing phone calls and stalking are obvious examples).
3. Carrying a concealed weapon or flashing a weapon to test reactions.
4. Paranoid behavior. Perceiving that the whole world is against them.
5. Moral righteousness and believing the organization is not following its rules and procedures.
6. Unable to take criticism of job performance. Holds a grudge, especially against a supervisor. Often verbalizes hope for something to happen to the person against whom the employee has the grudge.
7. Expression of extreme desperation over recent family, financial or personal problems.
8. History of violent behavior.
9. Extreme interest in semi-automatic or automatic weapons and their destructive power to people.
10. Fascination with incidents of workplace violence and approval of the use of violence under similar circumstances.
11. Disregard for the safety of co-employees.
12. Obsessive involvement with the job, often with uneven job performance and no apparent outside interests.
13. Being a loner who has a romantic obsession with a co-worker who does not share this interest (this interest will often be so intense that the co-employee will feel threatened and may report the unwanted attention under a sexual harassment policy).

PROFESSIONAL STAFF MEETING AGENDA

Date of Meeting: _____

AGENDA

Call to Order

Roll Call/Appointment of Secretary

Announcements

Approval of the Minutes

Approval of the Financial Report

Unfinished Business

1.

2.

3.

4.

New Business

1. Consent Agenda Items — voted upon without discussion

2. Consideration and Action Items — voted upon after discussion

3. Contemplation Items for Ongoing Discussion and Later Action — with full presentation and exploration of issues; vote delayed, if possible to a time certain.

Adjournment

EMERGENCY ACTION NEEDED: "INA"

There may be a time in any office or agency when a staff member, such as a secretary, is placed at risk and is in need of immediate assistance.

At such times the staff member may be alone and out of sight from others.

As hospitals have Code Blue to summon help at the time of a crisis, so an office or agency needs a "code" to call out when someone is at risk and in need of immediate help.

"INA" means "I need assistance." When "INA" is called out by anyone, all that hear it are to come running and ready to help, as needed.

The emergency could be an unwanted visitor to the office, a waiting room ruckus, an angry patient or some type of threat or high risk situation. If help is needed, "INA" is called out, but only if absolutely needed. There are to be no false alarms or teasing using the code.

WHEN DEPRESSION COMES TO THE OFFICE

CONSIDER THE FACTS

- Depression has been recognized as a major disorder since Hippocrates called it melancholia.
- It is now referred to as the "disease of the decade."
- At least 10% of the population experiences depression; average age is 24–44.
- 3% of short-term disability days are due to depression.
- Untreated depression accounts for $45 billion dollars annually in lost productivity due to absenteeism.
- The cost to business is $600.00 annually per depressed worker.
- Over 200 million work days are lost due to depression.
- Depressed persons spend more days in bed than those with diabetes, arthritis, low back pain, and GI disorders, to name a few.
- 80% of those that seek therapy benefit for the experience; treatment is usually a few months' duration and usually includes psychotherapy and medication use.

WHAT MANAGERS NEED TO KNOW

- Follow the guidelines of the American Disabilities Act and make accommodation appropriate to the situation.
- Help the depressed employee draw upon local resources, such as the EAP Program of the company, a local therapist, and relevant reading materials.
- Lend support to the employee by a call to the spouse or family, offer needed assistance, prepare meals or a person home visit, if desired.
- Develop a return to work plan with a set of guidelines agreed upon, such as light duty, part-time work, etc.
- Annually review the corporate medical, mental health benefits and the EAP program. Make changes as indicated and look into developing stress management programs and policies, as needed.

WHAT DEPRESSED EMPLOYEES NEED TO KNOW

- Correct irrational thinking.
- Learn to be self-complimentary.
- Seek time with healthy and non-depressed colleagues at work and after work.
- Know that you have the right to be assertive and speak up on issues that affect you and others.
- Engage in a problem-solving task on some issue, one step at a time.

LEADERSHIP IN TODAY'S WORLD

Leadership in today's world requires the tapping of all the strengths, skills, and experience one can draw upon to address the high demand of those seeking assistance and direction in their personal and business life. The call is for a fast-paced and focused response on the part of the consultant. Here are a few guidelines to make leadership effective in today's volatile market place.

- A democratic rather than autocratic approach is preferred.
- Foster an active and ongoing learning process both for leading and following.
- Learning of new skills and strategies is best through experience.
- Your own personal style of relationship building is the best beginning point when exercising leadership.
- Your goal is to be good enough as a leader for the situation.
- Embrace challenge and do the best you can; learn from any mistakes made.
- Work on your style of leadership and learn ways to behave so others will follow.
- Take time to learn from others but focus on a few specific points and learn to do them well.
- Come to know your own strengths and weaknesses as a leader and as a follower. Focus on your strengths and learn to do those things even better.
- No person learns on an island. We learn any skill better as we share with others what we have recently learned to do differently.

Based on an article by Tori DeAngelis.

LEADERSHIP IN THE WORKPLACE

DOMINEERING SELFISH LEADERSHIP

- A leader's objective is to be served.
- Interested primarily in the leader's image and advancement. Self-preservation and personal image is at the forefront of most decisions.
- Co-workers are seen and treated as inferiors.
- Creates an atmosphere of dependence.
- Condemns others for mistakes.
- Rejects constructive criticism and takes the credit for accomplishments.
- Does not train others to function effectively.
- Authority is based on external controls in the form of rules, restrictions, and regulations enforced by force.

SERVANTHOOD LEADERSHIP

- A leader's objective is to serve others.
- Seeks to enable subordinates to advance to their fullest potential by downplaying self and exalting others. The team or enterprise and all its members are considered and promoted before self.
- Co-workers are treated with respect as part of a team who work together to accomplish a task.
- Creates an atmosphere in which others see their potential being encouraged and developed.
- Values individual workers and offers praise.
- Encourages input and feedback and shares credit for the results.
- Equips and invests in others with a view to their advancement.
- Authority is based on influence from within through encouragement, inspiration, motivation, and persuasion.

LEADERSHIP IN LARGE CORPORATE AND PROFESSIONAL ORGANIZATIONS

A Check List and Plan for Improvement

THE HEALTHY MENTAL HEALTH AGENCY:

1. Has a high staff retention rate.
2. Has a demonstrated level of positive customer satisfaction.
3. Has a staff leadership that is flexible and adaptable to circumstances.
4. Has a productive and cost-effective growth pattern.
5. Has a pattern of expansion into the community with a positive financial profile.
6. Has a strong influence in a community and on regulatory and government bodies.

THE HEALTHY LEADERSHIP STRUCTURE:

1. Centralize the decision making leadership.
2. Decentralize and diversify the service delivery system.
3. Plan out into the future in stages as far as is reasonable.
4. Plan for advanced staffing patterns both in numbers and type of staff.
5. Ensure budgeting is service oriented.
6. Develop an assimilation plan for new staff.
7. Develop staff and leadership attitudes that are growth and outreach based.
8. Promote attitudes that are positive, analytic, and critical.
9. Build an image that emphasizes friendliness, caring, compassionate, and responsive.

THE HEALTHY LEADER:

1. Finds strength by realizing that he/she has weaknesses.
2. Finds vision by seeing the needs of others and the community.
3. Finds credibility by being an example of integrity.
4. Finds greatness by being a servant leader.
5. Finds loyalty by expressing compassion and being a caring person.
6. Finds direction by laying down plans while inviting others to offer their input.
7. Finds authority by being under authority.

FACING A KEY CRISIS IN A BUSINESS

TYPES OF CRISES IN THE WORK WORLD

Many types of crises can impact a business. Wise executives keep alert for the signs of a forthcoming crisis. They are ready to confront the crisis and deal with it effectively. Here are a few types of crises that can come upon a business concern, with some rather high-profile examples. Management must be alert to what could be before them. Consultants play a key role at such times in the life of a business.

- PUBLIC HEALTH AND SAFETY: The Union Carbide Bhopal disaster, Love Canal, the Kansas City Hyatt accident.
- LEGAL AND POLITICAL TROUBLES: ITT in Chile, the Bank of Boston and money laundering.
- PUBLIC PERCEPTION: The nuclear plant accident at Three Mile Island.
- LABOR: Union problems faced by Eastern Airlines or International Harvester.
- PRODUCT FAILURE: Rely tampons and the problems of toxic shock syndrome.
- MANAGEMENT CONTINUITY: The hotel fire in upstate New York that resulted in death of most top managers of Arrow Electronics.
- TAKEOVER BATTLE: The fight for control of Phillips Petroleum.
- CHANGED ENVIRONMENT: The deregulation of the airline and banking industries, the move towards "for profit" in the health care field.
- MONEY PROBLEMS: Chrysler, Lockheed and their loan guarantees.
- INTERNATIONAL EVENTS: The oil companies and the Arab oil embargo.

REACTING TO A CRISIS

The Cardinal Rule for any communications during a crisis or emergency is:

- Tell it all
- Tell it fast
- Tell it straight

When information gets out quickly rumors are stopped ... nerves are calmed ... and an ongoing, continuous flow of information indicates people are working on the problem.

RULES IN CRISIS COMMUNICATION

1. *It's the boss's show.* The boss gets a lot of money and a crisis is that period of time when he or she earns it. Everybody – the media, the public, employees, the government – will want to hear what's happening directly from the top person.
2. *Control rumors.* Don't let rumors build or fester. Deal with them immediately. Confirm them or deny them.
3. *Centralize all information.* Make sure all sources speak from the same platform about a situation at a specific time.
4. *Don't hold anything back.* Cover all the bases and all the important subjects as long as security and confidentiality are not breached. Make everything possible public.
5. *Update frequently.* It is better to give people too much information than not enough. People are really into details.
6. *Be pre-emptive if necessary.* If you can anticipate something, like a damaging government report or a public attack by a competitor or public organization, the best strategy might be to take the initiative and announce the damaging information before your opponent has a chance to.

PLANNING FOR A CRISIS

In planning for a crisis, it is vital that all information be centralized and all parties are cooperative. It is best to develop a plan to which all can contribute and buy into. It needs to be "our" plan.

A **Crisis Communications Plan** should have the following elements:

- A precise chain-of-command spelling out who is in charge of communications.
- Rules on release of information pending notification of kin.
- A plan for notification of employees, government agencies, stockholders, and suppliers.
- Caveats to employees on offering speculation to the media when speaking as company employees.
- Trained switchboard operators who know what to do in an emergency – who to refer calls to, the importance of speed, and where to track down people.
- Background information on your PROCESSES (how you do things) and PEOPLE (biographical information).

SPECIAL TOOLS FOR CRISIS COMMUNICATIONS

1. Be able to explain anything in five simple charts or less.
2. Empathy is absolutely crucial in crisis communications. *Don't hide your feelings.*
3. Don't be afraid to *follow your human instincts.*
4. Make sure top managers and spokespeople have been rigorously trained in dealing with tough media encounters.
5. Don't use colorful idiomatic language in talking about the crisis. *Maintain professionalism.*
6. Keep everything *on the record.*
7. Have good background material available – fact sheets etc.

DEALING WITH "CONFRONTATIONAL CRISIS"

1. Confrontation is a means to an end; keep the end in focus.
2. Not all groups want discussion; keep it to an essential minimum.
3. Management must be trained in dealing with confrontation and debate; be ready.
4. Rhetoric must be ignored; turn it into functional and operational terms.
5. Perceptions of the same problem differ; known what they are and deal with them.
6. Remember, reasonable people can and do differ; agreeing to disagree can end it.

Chapter 10

Termination of Treatment/Practice Forms

Chapter Contents

In the course of professional practice a therapist must make many decisions regarding patient care and professional service delivery. Two tough decisions relate to the termination of a patient from treatment, and when to terminate a professional practice. Both of these decisions do not come easily. Often they come with much thought, prayer, consultation, and thinking through the "What if …" issues and considerations. Lives are affected, emotions are aroused, lifestyle is changed, career plans are altered, and income is curtailed, to name a few considerations.

This chapter contains forms, templates, and documents that assist the therapist in carrying out these two major decisions at the time when "enough is enough."

RELEASE FROM RESPONSIBILITY FOR DISCHARGE

This is to certify that I, _____, understand the fact that I am terminating treatment and leaving the office/facility of _____ against the advice of Dr _____ and his/her staff. I acknowledge that I have been informed of the risks and possible consequences of my decision. I hereby release Dr _____, his/her staff, office, and facility from all responsibility for any ill effects which may result from the action I am taking.

Signature: _____   Date: _____

Signature of parent/RP if patient is a minor: _____   Date: _____

Witness: _____   Date: _____

LETTER TO TERMINATE SERVICES TO A PATIENT

DATE

ADDRESS

Dear _____

I am writing to inform you that regretfully I will not be able to provide ongoing care and treatment to you any longer after _____.

I do believe you deserve the best possible care and services today and in the future. May I suggest that you proceed to contact another therapist to arrange for your ongoing care and treatment. Should you need a few names to consider let me know or ask your primary doctor.

Please contact my office soon to arrange for the transfer of your records. A small fee will be charged for this transfer of records.

Best wishes to you as you continue to move forward in your life.

Respectfully,

DR NAME

PROFESSIONAL PRACTICE FOR SALE AND PROFILE

PROFESSIONAL PRACTICE IN CLINICAL PSYCHOLOGY
NEW TOWN, STATE

This professional practice in _____, _____ commenced in 1974. Over the years it has become one of the foremost practices in the community and in the Central Valley of _____. Multiple referral sources have been established, numerous insurance and EAP panels have been joined. A broad based local network of support services has also been developed.

The practice has consistently grossed in the six figures for the past 25 years. The practice has had a full five day a week appointment schedule for the past 30 years. The practice includes individual, family, marital, and group therapy, assessments and evaluations, consulting and speaking opportunities.

The practice is known throughout _____ and has been a source of referral for many different professionals seeking psychological services for their clients, especially in the areas of forensics, skilled nursing facilities, churches/clergy, medical facilities/physicians, corporations, non-profit organizations and community service agencies. The practice has growth potential for the motivated and intentional professional.

The practice is available for purchase due to the pending retirement in 20__ of the owner/ clinician. A brief time of transition is potentially workable, if desired. An ongoing consultation relationship is also available, if desired. The assets listed below are available with the purchase of the practice, all subject to negotiation.

Interested parties may initiate a serious confidential communication with the owner/clinician by contacting: _____.

THE PRACTICE PROFILE

VALUED ASSETS:

- Over 1500 active files and over 2000 inactive files on hand
- File of over 200 psychological tests, survey forms, and questionnaires
- Computerized testing capability; license for internet testing can be arranged
- Office equipment, furnishings, and office machines
- Professional office furnishings
- Library of books and professional materials
- Accounts Receivable after a grace period
- Office forms, practice documents, and HIPPA compliance documents
- Billing software has been used for over 10 years. Will help with transfer.

VALUED PROFESSIONAL SETTING:

- Central prime location and easy access to freeways and public transportation
- Desirable professional condo office complex and building
- Office is located near other mental health practitioners and business professionals
- Ample free parking

VALUED CLIENTS/PATIENTS:

- Individuals of all ages
- Skilled Nursing Facilities
- Clients of local attorneys

- Members of selected insurance companies
- POST evaluations, Second Opinions
- EAP members
- Former patients, their family members and friends

VALUED PERSONNEL:

- Professional office staff available, but negotiable
- Professional colleagues have offices and share common area in the office building

VALUED VENDORS:

- Professional typist
- Payroll services
- CPA
- Lawyer
- Insurance plans and panels
- Professional computer consultant
- Professional billing software consultant

VALUED INFORMATION:

- References available upon request
- Office specs are available upon request
- Financial documents are available to serious potential buyers

OTHER:

PSYCHOTHERAPY PRACTICE FOR SALE

Psychologist retiring. Steady history of six-figure income. A full range practice. Great opportunity for a young enterprising professional. Much growth potential. Many consulting contracts and insurance panels are transferable. Friendly and supportive professional community. Several psychiatric units in local hospitals and a host of community resources to serve the needs of your patients.

Practice is located in a growing community in _____. The market area population is about 1 million. The home of a major university and many colleges and trade schools. Many nearby recreational lakes, mountains, and trails. The city is known for its performing arts, restaurants, shopping, and several athletic teams. Quality of life is good.

Practice profile available upon request. Confidential and serious inquiries should be directed to: _____.

You will be contacted within three days of your confidential inquiry.

Forms for Session Notes

Chapter Contents

It is generally understood that, "If it is not recorded in the patient's record or chart, it did not happen." Session notes are essential. All types of therapy require record keeping. There are many ways to keep notes and store them for future reference. There are strong ethical, legal, and professional reasons to maintain a systematic record of each session. Every therapist is well advised to select a format and use it throughout the years of practice. A consistent trail can thereby be laid down. Referring back to the notes of earlier sessions is thereby easier.

Several samples of note taking are provided in this chapter for the therapist.

SESSION NOTES: VERSION 1

Name of patient: _____ Sesssion #: _____ Date: _____

AGENDA FOR TODAY   **TODAY'S SESSION NOTES**
1. Homework in Review

2. Review of Last Session

3. Ongoing Issues Discussed

4. New Issues Arising

HOMEWORK FOR NEXT WEEK/MONTH
1.

2.

3.

4.

5.

Signature of therapist: _____ Date: _____

SESSION NOTES: VERSION 2

_____

Name of patient: _____

Today's date: _____ Session #: _____

Goal for this session:

Outcome from previous session and/or homework:

Description of patient's involvement:

Assessment of patient's status today:

Today's intervention and apparent effectiveness:

Homework:

Future plans and interventions:

Other:

Signature of therapist: _____

SESSION NOTES: VERSION 3

Patient name: _____ Session date: _____

Symptoms Noted or Mentioned:

Observations of Significance:

Assessment of Behavior Needing Change:

Plan of Care Utilized Today to Bring About Change:

Other Considerations or Issues to Be Addressed:

Signature of therapist: _____ Date: _____

SESSION NOTES: VERSION 4

Patient name: _____ Session #: _____

Date: _____ Time: _____ Therapist: _____

Client's report of homework exercise since last session. Stressors since last session. How client processed stress since last session? What methods were used to manage the stress effectively?

Content of this therapy session, such as topics covered, insights gleaned, and new learning:

Assessment of client's participation, insight, and new learning session:

Homework assignment for next week:

Other notes:

RELAXATION TRAINING AND BIOFEEDBACK THERAPY
SESSION NOTES

Name of patient: _____ Session #: _____

Time: _____ Modality: _____ Date: _____

Patient's report of homework, stress levels over last week, nature of stress experienced, response to the stressors, how the stress was managed, use of the relaxation response, and any other events that were successfully managed through the relaxation and/or biofeedback techniques:

Content of the relaxation and/or biofeedback session, including methods utilized and response levels attained. Was deep relaxation achieved?

Assessment of the patient's learning today:

Homework assignment for the next week or two:

Therapist's signature: _____

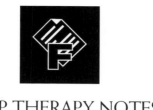

GROUP THERAPY NOTES

Patient: _____

Date of group session: _____

Time of group session: _____

Session #: _____

How many in group today? _____

Today's topic and main points covered:

Patient's participation today:

Patient's status and progress as of today:

Any special observations or happenings today:

Therapist signature: _____

Clinical Errors, Bad Habits, Ethical Complaints, and Law Suits

Chapter Contents

No therapist is perfect. Therapists make mistakes by over-reacting, taking risky actions, failing to think ahead, and engaging in unacceptable behavior. Consequences can be severe. Becoming embroiled in formal adversarial proceedings is not uncommon. Giving grace and allowing for forgiveness is not readily offered and made available to therapists in such situations. While counseling may seem innocuous, there are times when a miss-step can be harmful to a patient. These times represent the most lonely and distressing times in the life of a professional therapist.

A proactive or preventative view is essential for practicing therapists in today's litigious society. Periodic reminders of "good" behavior are important.

The forms, exercises, guidelines, and information sheets in this chapter were selected to help the therapist deal with these unfortunate events in a proactive and positive manner.

12 STEPS FOR REDUCING YOUR RISKS
IN A MALPRACTICE SUIT

1. Keep records current at all times.

2. If more than one therapist is treating a patient, document the dates and content of communications between team members.

3. Use consultants with difficult patients, and clearly identify them as such in your notes. Document the dates and content of the consultations.

4. Hold on to all patients' records for as long as time remains on the liability clock. Remember that in many states the clock only starts ticking when the plaintiff has knowledge of an incident.

5. Support diagnoses with history. If a diagnosis differs from prior records, substantiate your judgment. Cite it in your records if you suspect the patient is an unreliable historian. Clarify that you're making a partial evaluation based on incomplete data – not a lack of investigation. And if you perceive the patient to be unreliable, cite objective supporting data such as resistive attitude, mental status exam, etc.

6. Provide resources for the patient when any member of the treatment team is away – document it.

7. Document your recommendations and patient's noncompliance: refusal to take psychotropic medications; referral to a consultant; cancellations and no-shows; refusal to sign release of information.

8. Before discussing a patient's treatment with their family members, your colleagues, or anyone else, check to see that you have a signed release-of-information form in the chart.

9. Following evaluation sessions, outline the treatment plan in the chart, and note every subsequent change.

10. Document the presence or absence of suicidal ideation or intent, or homicidal ideation/intent at intake. Relate them to past and/or present occurrence. Whenever suicidal intent and/or homicidal intent are noted, indicate the action you've taken, as dictated by legal statute. Document periodic updates of mental status.

11. Include in the treatment contract a clause stating that if patients are considering taking harmful action, they will contact a designated party. The contract should include at least three parties to notify the primary treating therapist, another member of the treatment team, the ER, etc.

12. Document termination reasons and recommendations. If you suspect any misunderstanding regarding termination recommendations, send a letter to the patient via certified mail with return receipt requested.

Adapted from *Psychotherapy Finances*, Vol. 24, No. 7, Issue 291, 1998.

FOUR ISSUES TO BE ADDRESSED IN DETERMINING NEGLIGENCE IN A CIVIL LAW SUIT

1. PROFESSIONAL RELATIONSHIP
- Was a therapeutic atmosphere established?
- What was the therapist's intent?
- Was there a discussion of patient's situation and concerns?
- How clear was therapist about taking or not taking on a patient's case?

2. STANDARD OF CARE
- Degree of care, skill, and devotion that **reasonably** prudent professionals practice under similar circumstances.
- Determined by members of the profession.
- Type of therapy or training of practitioner, patient's condition, codes of ethics, and professional guidelines are all considered by court to determine standard of care.
- Shift has occurred from local standard to national standard.

3. HARM OR DAMAGE
- Patient must have received some injury or harm.
- May be physical, economic or subjective mental injury.

4. PROXIMATE CAUSE
- Therapist's actions or inactions were **legal** proximate cause of injury.
- Proximate means different things in different states.
- General rule is to use the "but for" test. Example: "But for" what the therapist did (did not do), this injury would not have occurred.

Adapted from the American Psychiatric Association, *Practice Guidelines for the Treatment of Psychiatric Disorders*, APA, Arlington, VA, 2006.

WAYS TO RESPOND TO A COMPLAINT

- Start by identifying an attorney that you would utilize. One way to do this is to begin calling one or more of them as consultants when possible problems arise in your practice or when you have questions as to the best way to proceed with a difficult case. Preferably this will be an attorney who specializes in the area of mental health. Check with your insurance carrier as well.
- Be aware of Red Flags:
  - If the Department of Consumer Affairs requests a file for one of your clients.
  OR
  - You are notified by the Department of Consumer Affairs that you are to meet with an investigator.
- Strongly consider consulting an attorney who specializes in Administrative Law and also in mental health, as stated above.
- Keep in mind the following questions about the Licensing Board in your state?
  - What would it look like at the end of the year if the Licensing Board had no (or few) penalties issued?
  - Would the Licensing Board members still have a job the next year?
- Be quick to consult with a wise and trusted professional in the same field of expertise as the area of the threatened action.

MANAGING CLINICAL ERRORS, MISTAKES, AND MISHAPS

Unintended errors do occur. Almost always they happen under unusual circumstances. Therapists do not come to the office on a given day planning to hurt someone or cause them personal pain or distress. Yet, unfortunately, inadvertent mistakes and mishaps do take place.

What to do? Drawing from the experiences of several hospitals that have developed a plan to handle mistakes and minimize the impact of the resulting problem, here are a few guidelines to consider.

GUIDELINES FOR MANAGING UNINTENDED ERRORS AND MISTAKES

1. Acknowledge the error.
2. Analyze the chain of events that led to the problem.
3. Put in place new measures that are aimed at preventing such errors in the future.
4. Communicate with the injured party directly or through a third party.
5. Apologize, and do so quickly and fully.
6. Seek forgiveness; forgive yourself.
7. Offer reasonable compensation for any costs incurred.
8. Engage the injured party or family member(s) to educate you, your staff, and other therapists on error prevention in the future.
9. Consider ways in which something good can come out of the unfortunate situation.
10. Follow through on any promises or plans developed from the event.
11. Seek help and consult other professionals as needed and as appropriate.
12. Other …

BAD HABITS TO AVOID AS A THERAPIST

According to the studies of Dr John Grohol, therapists can develop a series of bad habits that annoy patients and interfere with good business and with therapy effectiveness. Here are a few key bad habits of therapists.

1. Taking notes excessively during a session. It creates the impression of a bad memory and is distracting.
2. Displaying your wealth inappropriately to patients. It implies greed and financial purpose as your motivation.
3. Watching the clock constantly during the session. It can be distracting and implies disinterest in the patient and the issue being discussed.
4. Engaging in physical contact, such as hugging and patting on the back. It can send a mixed signal and mislead a patient.
5. Coming late for appointments when the patient is on time. It teaches poor time management and a casual attitude towards patients.
6. Eating food and drinking coffee or water in front of a patient without offering the same to the patient. It can be seen as selfish and uncaring.
7. Being too personal and offering too many personal disclosures of one's own problems. It takes time away from the patient; it's their hour, not yours.
8. Bringing your pet or baby to the therapy office. They are distracting and may compete for the attention and time of the therapist.
9. Being impossible to reach by phone or email and not returning messages left on an answering machine or with an answering service. This implies, "Out of sight is out of mind."
10. Yawning, dozing, or falling asleep during a session. This implies that the patient is not interesting, important or that you care about their concerns.
11. Allowing a phone, email, pet or noise in the building to distract the focus of therapy. As we want the patient's attention, so do they want our attention.
12. Taking time to discuss personal preferences in music, movies, racial or religious ideas. This can introduce controversy and debate on an irrelevant topic.
13. Taking the patient's time to comment on your own personal problems. The patient needs to feel the focus of their session is on them, not you.

MEDICATION CONSULTATION BY PSYCHOLOGIST

In most states and jurisdictions psychologists cannot legally prescribe medication. There are a few states where limited prescription is legally allowed.

Often consumers seeking mental health services are taking medications or suffering from conditions that could be treated very successfully by medications prescribed by a physician. Psychologists are often the first mental-health-care providers assessing and treating such consumers. Indeed, many psychologists have extensive training and experience in the applications of medications.

Psychologists may discuss medications with a patient. A psychologist may suggest to a physician a particular medication to be prescribed by a physician. However, the ultimate decision as to whether a patient should receive medication lies solely with the physician.

A psychologist may engage in a collegial discussion with a patient's physician regarding the appropriateness of a medication for a condition being treated. A psychologist has primary responsibility to monitor the patient's progress in psychotherapy, which includes assisting in monitoring the changes that may be attributable to the medication in the patient. Psychologists should maintain a close consultative relationship with physician caregivers in order to assure appropriate overall treatment of the patient.

There are many psychological conditions that manifest themselves in physical symptoms. There are physical problems that have psychological symptoms as well. The best interests of the patient demand that psychologists work closely with primary care physicians and psychiatrists who are prescribing medications to the patient of the psychologist. While a psychologist's responsibility can include involvement in limited aspects of a patient's medications, the patient's physician is the only person who may lawfully prescribe the medication for the patient, unless State Codes allow otherwise.

Adapted from the Board of Psychology, California.

Expanding Your Practice

Chapter Contents

Opportunities abound today to expand any clinical practice. The use of technology and the Internet opens the door to many new ways to deliver services and reach a population in need of services. Therapists may take advantage of opportunities to expand their practice and build a small to medium-size business, but need to be creative and entrepreneurial in thinking and drive. The opportunities are endless.

In this chapter the therapist will find forms, guidelines, and informational documents to help a therapist decide if the challenge to expand the practice will be undertaken.

INFORMED CONSENT PROCEDURES FOR TELEMEDICINE

"Telemedicine" means the practice of health care delivery, diagnosis, consultation, treatment, transfer of medical data, and education using interactive audio, video, or data communications. Neither a telephone conversation nor an electronic mail message between a health care practitioner and patient constitutes "telemedicine" for the purposes of this section (section 2290.5*).

For the purposes of this section, "health care practitioner" has the same meaning as "licentiate" as defined in paragraph (2) of subdivision (a) of Section 805*.

1. Prior to the delivery of health care via telemedicine, the health care practitioner who has ultimate authority over the care or primary diagnosis for the patient shall obtain verbal AND written informed consent from the patient or the patient's legal representative. The informed consent procedure shall ensure that at least all of the following information is given to the patient or the patient's legal representative verbally AND in writing.

2. The patient or the patient's legal representative retains the option to withhold or withdraw consent at any time without affecting the right to future care or treatment, nor risking the loss or withdrawal of any program benefits to which the patient or the patient's legal representative would otherwise be entitled.

3. A description of the potential risks, consequences, and benefits of telemedicine.

4. All existing laws regarding patient access to medical information and copies of medical records apply. All existing confidentiality protections apply.

5. Dissemination of any patient identifiable images or information from the telemedicine interaction to researchers or other entities shall not occur without the consent of the patient.

6. A patient or the patient's legal representative shall sign a written statement prior to the delivery of health care via telemedicine, indicating that the patient or the patient's legal representative understands the written information provided pursuant to subdivision (a), and that this information has been discussed with the health care practitioner, or his or her designee.

7. The written consent statement signed by the patient or the patient's legal representative shall become part of the patient's medical record.

8. All existing laws regarding surrogate decision making shall apply. For purposes of this section "surrogate decision making" means any decision made in the practice of medicine by a parent or legal representative for a minor or an incapacitated or incompetent individual.

---

*Business and Professional Code, State of California.

THERAPIST'S GUIDELINES FOR CONFLICT RESOLUTION

Mental health professionals are often asked to mediate conflicts between parents and children, adult children and their parents, fellow workers, friend to friend, and neighbor to neighbor, to name a few. Instead of Court, it is often preferred to undergo a lower level of mediation or negotiation. It is an area in which a therapist could specialize. Training in conflict resolution is necessary. Below are a few guidelines for the therapist to help resolve a conflict should there be opportunity to intercede in such situations.

RESOLVING CONFLICT

1. Guide the parties in asking for opportunity to appeal an unfavorable decision; help them do so respectfully.
2. Ask the parties to be prepared to go their half way to bring about a peaceful resolution.
3. Help the parties to respond to each other in a manner that will not cause more conflict, such as blaming others.
4. Ask the parties to think ahead as to why they want to discuss this decision and how they will express it.
5. Assure that the parties appeal in an honorable way, such as not raising the voice, talking over the other, walking off.
6. Help the parties be prepared to accept the final decision humbly with understanding of the reason.
7. Help the parties overlook the minor offenses.

MAKING A CONFESSION

1. Prepare the parties to state where they were wrong in what they said or did.
2. Help the parties apologize for how their actions, statements or decisions affected the other person.
3. Prepare the parties to accept the consequences of their actions with understanding and humility.
4. Help them ask the other party for their forgiveness.
5. Help them commit to changing their way of handling these types of situations in the future.
6. Ask if there is any action that could be taken to help the healing process progress.

NEGOTIATING SUCCESSFULLY

1. Help all parties be rational and stay focused on the issue.
2. Be well prepared before entering into the negotiations, especially if the parties are hostile.
3. Guide the parties in thinking through all their alternatives and options; the more the better.
4. Spend more time listening and asking probing questions; times of silence can be helpful.
5. Determine which side makes the first offer to set the upper limit.
6. Be prepared to change your perspective or mindset about the problem as you guide them in changing their perspective.
7. Remind all parties that resolution is reached by compromise, accommodation, mutual agreement or by agreeing to disagree, yet keeping the peace between them.

INTERNET-BASED THERAPY: IS IT FOR ME?

Increasingly, patients are asking for the option to use Internet therapy when they are out of town, traveling or have a job that makes it difficult to come to your office weekly. There may be some patients, some problems, and some therapist components that render Internet therapy an option. While no research is known to address this issue, here are some general guidelines:

THERAPIST VARIABLES

1. Are you savvy in the use of computers?
2. Are you able to take time and deal with a patient in writing out answers in good detail and answer all of the patient's questions?

COMPUTER VARIABLES

1. Are your computer and the computer of the patient of the same technological level so that e-mail and attachments can be used to their fullest extent?
2. Can confidentiality be maintained in the computer files devoted to the patient?

PROBLEM VARIABLES

1. Is there any research data or anecdotal evidence for Internet therapy use with the given problem of the patient?
2. Is the problem clean cut and can it be addressed simply and forthrightly by e-mail messages?

PATIENT VARIABLES

1. Is the patient computer savvy?
2. Is the patient a good communicator and can he/she express himself/herself emotionally and factually in writing?
3. Has a doctor–patient relationship been established before Internet therapy began?

PROFESSIONAL VARIABLES

1. Does your state have any prohibition against the use of Internet therapy if the patient is living or visiting in a different state from the state of the therapist?
2. Is Internet therapy allowed in your state if you are a licensed therapist?
3. Is this approach to be used in rural America or a foreign country to reach an unreachable population?

What is my general conclusion? _____

_____

What steps are to be taken now? _____

_____

TELEPHONIC COUNSELING: IS IT FOR ME?

The following issues and questions will help you decide if telephonic counseling is for you. Enter this arena slowly and be sure it is legal, ethical, and practical for you. Be sure it fits with your 5-year plan for the development of your practice also.

AREAS OF CONSIDERATION

- Do you have a need for it in your practice?
- Do you have time for it as part of your practice schedule?
- Do you have a good phone voice?
- Do you demonstrate a feeling of concern and empathy on the phone?
- Do you have the ability and experience to think quickly as a problem is presented?
- Do you have the time and interest to learn the legality and ethics of this approach?
- Do you have the interest to continue this approach to therapy for the long haul?
- Do you have the staff and technical support system to make this program work?
- Do you have sufficient interest to attend ongoing workshops on this approach?
- Do you know someone who will train and supervise you during the start-up time?
- Do you have the billing and administrative back-up to make it profitable?
- Do you know of a virtual office with lease space available for an Internet service?

MY PLAN TO GO FORWARD

Steps I need to undertake to develop a business plan for a telephonic counseling service:

Steps I need to take to launch a telephonic counseling service:

Steps I need to take to market a telephonic counseling service:

Steps I need to take to build the necessary support system to make it profitable:

Other:

COACHING MANAGERS AND EXECUTIVES

One-on-one instruction and strategic skill development on-site in the client's office is a good way to make the greatest impact. Meeting someone on their own turf is more likely to yield a buy-in and support for the eventual plan agreed upon.

Why Coaching?

- More capabilities and flexibility are required of managers and executives than ever before.
- With rapid promotion there is a matching demand for rapid skill development.
- Today, if you are not developing you are falling behind!

One-to-one Coaching is Preferred Over "Training" Classes:

- Individualized curriculum to fit your current work challenges.
- Immediate application and practice of skills.
- Personalized attention, flexible scheduling, and private meetings on your site.

Coaching is the Executive Development Tool of Choice Because it is:

- Individually focused, intensive, and results-oriented.
- Tailored to the participant's learning style and personality.
- Solves immediate work problems first.
- Strategic development designed for career progression and success.

Coaching Includes Your Choices of:

- Strategic planning meetings with your coach to fast-forward your career development.
- Data based, 360° feedback for errorless identification of key areas for development.
- Role play and feedback for rehearsal of new skills.

EXECUTIVE COACHING TO ACCELERATE LEARNING

The five necessary conditions that define the *"active ingredients"* of personal development are:

1. *Insight.* The extent to which the person understands what areas need to be developed in order to be more effective.
2. *Motivation.* The degree to which the person is willing to invest the time and energy it takes to develop oneself.
3. *Capabilities.* The extent to which the person has the skills and knowledge that are needed.
4. *Real-world practice.* The extent to which the person applies those capabilities where it matters.
5. *Accountability.* The extent to which there are internal and external mechanisms for monitoring progress and providing meaningful consequences.

Coaches can use a variety of tools and techniques to address each of the conditions. A sampling of some of the most useful approaches is presented here.

1. To facilitate greater *insight*, coaches can:
   - Help people clarify what matters most to them – their personal goals, values, and motivators.
   - Help people understand what others expect of them and what it takes to be successful in their environment.
   - Teach people to get feedback from others.
   - Identify where skill enhancement or development of new capabilities will have the greatest payoff.
2. To enhance *motivation* to develop, coaches can:
   - Identify both personal and organizational reasons for change.
   - Identify personal and organizational environmental barriers that will make change difficult.
   - Seriously examine the trade-offs and make a realistic decision to proceed.
   - Discuss specific steps for addressing barriers and challenges.
3. To help the person *build* their capabilities, coaches can:
   - Share new ideas and best practices.
   - Help people find appropriate resources and opportunities for learning.
   - Explore alternative ways to handle difficult situations.
   - Provide opportunities for the person to practice new skills and behaviors in realistic situations.
4. To improve *real-world practice*, coaches can:
   - Identify specific situations where change is most relevant.
   - Help people determine how they will put small changes into practice every day.
   - Work with people to create personal strategies for assessing what is working well and what they need to do differently the next time they are in a similar situation.
5. To increase *accountability*, coaches can:
   - Encourage people to make specific commitments for action.
   - Follow up on learning assignments and personal commitments for action.
   - Encourage people to enlist others to give them feedback and discuss progress.

ESTATE AND HEALTH CARE PLANNING WITH PATIENTS

The following suggestions are proposed to help a patient engage in advanced estate planning so that his best interests are protected and he is better able to come to terms with his own mortality and wishes. Essentially, the patient should be referred to his own attorney or estate planner or to one that specializes in this area of the law and could be of help to him.

THE GENERAL STEPS TO BE FOLLOWED

1. Help the patient obtain an advanced directive document from their physician or from the Health Department. You may choose to have a few copies available if you serve a number of aging patients. A copy may be obtained online also.

2. Help the patient think through what they want in the document and what they do not want done when facing the end times. This includes life support and the donation of organs, for example.

3. Help the patient update their advance directive if it is out of date or they wish to make any changes. Ask them the status of their advanced directive in an open and forthright discussion. It should be kept up to date at all times.

4. Help facilitate awareness on the part of the extended family so that any issues can be discussed and resolved in a timely and constructive manner.

5. Help the patient name the person they trust and want to be the health care proxy so their wishes are carried out. The proxy should be someone they trust and is easily available for decision making when needed.

6. Help the patient fill out the form if needed. An attorney is not necessary to fill it out, but a copy should be filed with their attorney of record.

7. Help the patient understand that the advanced directive is only one document needed to be completed and on file before mental decline sets in or circumstances make it beyond consideration at that time. The sooner the better.

8. Help the patient contact their physician and file a copy with his/her office so it is readily available to be followed. Help the patient be sure the physician is agreeable to the terms of the document and will follow them. Have the patient ask the physician to explain any procedures that might be confusing or offensive.

9. Help the patient think through the charities to which the patient has given in the past and may wish to leave a charitable donation at the time of death in the form of a Charitable Gift Annuity or some such instrument.

PART II

Intake Forms and Initial Assessment Tools for Evaluating Patients

The field of assessment has generally been the historical domain of psychometrics. Its historical use revolved around the practice of measurement and testing, generally conducted by master's level psychologists, identified as a psychometrist.

Psychometrics relates to the field of informal assessment and evaluation, as well as more formal psychological testing. The value and importance of the results are based on the premise that an accurate diagnosis can be reached and a targeted treatment plan can then be formulated. The initial assessment is the foundation stone for subsequent effective and cost-efficient treatment, whatever "problem in living" is presented to the therapist at the time of the referral.

The forms in Part II are informal assessment tools guidelines, exercises, checklists, and questionnaires that can be utilized, along with formal and standard psychological tests, to determine the nature of the primary problem to be the focus of treatment. The forms also provide ways to economically and efficiently obtain a breadth of information through the sample of informal procedures and instruments as contained in this section.

Armed with information gathered from the various informal and formal assessment procedures, the therapist is now in a strong position to analyze and conceptualize the patient's presenting problem and design a structured treatment plan to meet the needs of the patient. In so doing, the patient's social, personal, and psychological history are also taken into account. Likewise, the therapist considers the relative strength of the patient's personal resources, support system and learning potential to acquire a new and healthier lifestyle and behavioral patterns.

Chapter 14

Organizing Your Charts and Evaluations

Chapter Contents

The therapist is responsible for producing, gathering, and strategically organizing an array of personal and clinical information on every patient. This information must be organized in a manner that is helpful to the therapist in providing therapeutic services in a timely and effective manner. It is not sufficient to conduct a comprehensive evaluation on a patient. The data obtained must be readily available, usable, and helpful to the therapist to assist patients in achieving their goals in therapy.

The forms, templates, charts, and guidelines in this chapter have been selected to assist the therapist in their assessment and therapeutic efforts to help patients attain their desired goals and lifestyle changes.

OUTLINE FOR A COMPREHENSIVE CLINICAL EVALUATION

Identifying information:

Client name: _____   Client #: _____ DOB: _____

Reason for referral:

Medical/Developmental Hx (Mark Y if present: Elaborate as needed)
Medical condition (Describe if present):
Current medications:
Pregnancy, birth, or neonatal complications:
Motor delays:
Problems with toilet training:
Delays in language development:
Head trauma or other neurological risks (toxins, losses of consciousness, seizures, high fevers, etc.):
Problems with sleep:
Sleep disturbance:
Current health, complaints:

Individual Hx (Mark Y if present: Elaborate as needed)
ADHD:
Anxiety or panic:
Posttraumatic stress disorder:
Grief:
Bipolar:
Depression:
Psychosis:
Suicide gestures or attempts:
Anger problems:
Teen parent:
Hx psych meds:
On psych meds:

Family Hx (Mark Y if present: Elaborate as needed)
Both parents in home:
Single parent:
Step family:
Multiple move:
Parent–child conflict:

Deaths/Grief:
Verbal abuse:
Neglect:
Sexual abuse:
Physical abuse:
Domestic violence:
Out of home placements:
Child Welfare Services involvement:
Parental health problems:
Parental mental illness:
Parental substance abuse:
Parentified child:
Parental criminality:

Educational Hx (Mark Y if present: Elaborate as needed)
Spec. Education (active IEP):
Spec. Education in past:
Learning disorder:
Gifted:
Truancy:
Grade retention/School failure:
School avoidance:
Other:

Social and Adaptive Functioning (Mark Y if present: Elaborate as needed)
Formal job:
Informal work outside home:
Vocational or pleasurable interests:
Self-reported aptitudes:
Antisocial peers:
Impaired social judgment ("Street-smart" Naïve Heedless Victimized

   Victimizing Poor social cue decoding, anticipation, or reasoning
   Unaware or heedless of social norms Vengeful)

Poor response to authority figures:
Misattributions of hostility:
Difficulty predicting consequences:
Views violence as acceptable or desirable:
Fails to take responsibility:
Arousal-seeking:

Drug/ETOH Hx (Mark Y if present: Elaborate as needed)
ETOH:
MJ:
Meth:
Cig:
Other:

Cont.

Criminality Hx (Mark Y if present: Elaborate as needed)
> *Property:*
> *Violent crimes:*
> *Weapons:*
> *Sexual offenses:*
> *Gang:*
> *Drug sales:*
> *Fire setting:*
> *Animal cruelty:*
> *Shows empathy or remorse for harm:*
> *Family Hx:*

Strengths (Individual + Family), e.g.:
> Prosocial values, Religious faith, Effective discipline style, Motivation for change, Participation in (programs, sports, etc.), Positive role models, Has "street smarts"/survival skills, Can make friends, Has some skills to cope with severe stressors, Resilient, Likes to talk, Interested in family dynamics, Has family loyalty, Shows insight, Sense of humor, Physically healthy, Athletic, Creativity, Desire for change, Independent, Open to outside assistance, Extended family, Pride in culture

Mental Status/Cognitive Functioning

Appearance and self-care:

Relating: Eye contact, facial expression, attitude

Affect and mood:

Attention: Normal   Unaware   Inattentive   Distractible   Confused
Persistent   Vigilant

Concentration: Normal   Scattered   Variable   Preoccupied
Anxiety interferes   Focuses on irrelevancies

Orientation: Time   Person/Place   Situation/Purpose   Familiar objects   Familiar persons

Recall/memory: Normal/Defective in: Immediate/short-term   Recent   Remote

Fund of knowledge: Average Impoverished by (specify):

Intelligence: Below average to Average   Above average   Needs investigation

Thought process: Impoverished   Hesitant   Normal   Rapid flight of ideas
Incoherent   Loose   Idiosyncratic   Clear   Dissociative

Ideation: Not grossly disordered Delusions (reference, persecution, grandeur, control)
Thought broadcasting etc.

Thought content (note topics):   Personalized   Idiosyncratic   Odd   Trivial
Obscene   Overly detailed   Preoccupations   Overvalued ideas
Selective   Self-doubting   Phobic Suicidal   Depressive
Suicidal   ideation   Homicidal ideation etc.

Abstraction: Similarities, Opposites, Differences, Proverbs

Proverbs to use: Spilled Milk, Glass Houses, Rolling Stone, Bird in Hand …

Similarities: (e.g., Apple/Orange, Cow/Giraffe, Car/Plane, etc.)

Normal   Concrete   Functional   Popular   Abstract   Overly abstract

Cont.

Comprehensive Clinical Evaluation (*Continued*)

Judgment: (e.g., Smoke in crowded theater, Find stamped/addressed envelope)

Normal   Common-sensical   Fair   Poor   Dangerous

Able to make routine decisions/Able to make stressful decisions/Impulsive

Reality testing: Realistic   Adequate   Distorted   Variable   Unaware

Insight: (causes and effects, evaluation of risks, ability to make hypotheses about own and others' behavior)

Uses connections Gaps Flashes of   Unaware   Nil   Denial

Decision making: Normal   Only simple   Impulsive   Vacillates   Confused   Paralyzed

Speech and word usage: Normal   Pressured   Retarded   Mute   Logical
Coherent   Rambling   Circumstantial   Looseness of associations
Neologisms   Flight of ideas   Perseverations   Tangential

Executive Functioning: Inhibition of behavior/impulses   Shifting attention/responses as situation changes
Emotional control   Initiating ideas or activities   Working memory   Planning/Organizing (goals,
strategies, key ideas)   Organizing materials (workspace, material resources)   Monitoring performance
(can assess effectiveness)

Diagnosis
Axis I
Axis II
Axis III
Axis IV
Axis V Current:
          Past Year:

Additionally, a determination has been made regarding the following medical necessity criteria. That the identified mental health condition results in:

(Mark Y)

_____ A significant impairment in an important area of life functioning.

_____ A probability of deterioration in an important area of life functioning.

_____ A probability of not progressing developmentally as appropriate.

The initial care plan noted below will target interventions with an expectation that they will:

(Mark Y)

_____ Significantly diminish the impairment.

_____ Prevent significant deterioration in an important area of life functioning.

_____ Promote developmental progress as individually appropriate.

OR

(Mark Y)

_____ It has been determined that the identified condition WOULD NOT be responsive to physical healthcare-based treatment.

COMPONENTS OF A CLINICAL CHART

FILE ORGANIZATION

- Is the file available and in a secure area?
- Are the patient name and authorization to treat in the file?
- Is the file in order and secured?

CLINICAL ASSESSMENT

- Is Initial Clinical Summary complete and in file?
- Is presenting problem identified?
- Is medical history and current medication documented?
- Is pertinent primary care physician information documented?
- Is substance abuse history documented?
- Is diagnostic impression noted?

TREATMENT PLAN

- Is there a descriptive problem statement?
- Are goals and interventions stated?
- Are timeframe and frequency of visits stated?
- Are community resource/adjunctive referrals noted?
- Has the treatment plan been signed by patient and therapist?

PROGRESS NOTES

- Does each page contain patient identification and session information?
- Is the problem stated with impairment noted?
- Is there a specific intervention stated?
- Is outcome of intervention documented?
- Is the intervention tied to treatment plan goals?
- Are medication and other evaluations documented?
- Are ancillary referrals noted?
- Is homework information documented?
- Has the practitioner fully signed each page?

DISCHARGE

- Is the discharge summary complete and in the file?
- Is a detailed aftercare plan documented?

DISCLOSURE FORMS

- Is there detailed financial and copayment information?
- Are there necessary signed releases of information?
- Is there a written and signed cancellation policy?
- Are limits of confidentiality explained?
- Is there a statement of brief treatment philosophy?
- Is there signed consent for treatment for medication and/or minors?
- Is there a description of how to utilize appeals/grievance procedures?
- Is there a detailed emergency access procedure?
- Are there signatures on forms from both patient and provider?

OUTLINE FOR A STANDARD CLINICAL EVALUATION AND SUMMARY REPORT

Statement of the reason for the referral:

Brief statement of the presenting problem:

Family history:

Educational history:

Marital and family history:

Medical history:

Social history:

Occupational history:

Mental health history:

Drugs and alcohol history:

Any other addictions:

Any unusual events or experiences in the past:

Mental status exam:

Third party interviews:

Assessments, past and current:

Diagnostic impressions (Axis I–V):

Potential to achieve:

Recommendations:

Other:

Chapter 15

General Assessments: Intake, Brief, Comprehensive, and More

Chapter Contents

Undertaking a comprehensive assessment of a new patient is one of the most important skills of a therapist. A comprehensive assessment brings understanding to the patient's presenting problem and exposes its personal and historic roots. Only then is a therapist ready to begin the process of therapy and creating behavior change. While the time devoted to assessment may seem less than justifiable, especially in a managed care system of limited services, it is actually the means by which a therapist can expedite therapy and bring about needed and desired change in a cost-effective manner.

This chapter provides the therapist forms, templates, guidelines, questionnaires, and checklists to conduct intake assessments and gain critical information on which to build an effective treatment plan. As the specific care plan is designed to target areas of impairment and dysfunction, producing desired behavior change to correct the identified problems is the ultimate objective of the therapist. Effective outcome is more likely to result when there is a well-designed assessment from the start of therapy.

GETTING TO KNOW YOU

My name is …

I was born in …

My family is made up of …

The best thing I did during the past year was …

Some of my nicknames are …

I feel happy when …

What I do for fun is …

The greatest person I have ever met was …

I am anxious or afraid of …

What I dislike is …

Something I regret is …

I feel sad when …

My major disappointment last year was …

If we have time, I would like to tell you the following about myself …

THE INTAKE PROCESS – ISSUES TO ASSESS

1. Greeting and clarifying confidentiality.

2. Getting background information:
   a. Client name
   b. Client age
   c. Client nationality
   d. Client spiritual orientation
   e. Working? Where?
   f. Major in school
   g. Plans after school

3. Sharing the problem(s)
   a. What's the area of difficulty today?
      OR
   b. Where do you feel overwhelmed today?

4. Getting a history of the problem(s)
   a. What are some of the symptoms?
   b. How severe has it been?
   c. How often has this been going on?
   d. How long has this been going on?

5. Suicidal/homicidal ideation: Rule out.

6. Theme: What's the theme (if there is one), i.e., relationship, work, school, family etc.?

7. Sharing the theme: Relay the theme back to the client and see if the theme makes sense.

8. Session summary: Offer to the client a sense of what can be worked on in the future, i.e., a plan:

   We talked about a number of issues today, [a. b. c.], there also appears to be a theme [if there is one] and I think you and I can work on these together if you feel comfortable about this process. Would you like to come back next time and work on these issues?

9. Offer the client the opportunity to ask questions, provide feedback about the session.

10. Plan next session's topics or issues and assign homework.

LEGAL INTAKE FORM

DATE: _____

Name: _____   DOB: _____

Address: _____

Telephone: Home _____ Work _____

Whom do we bill? _____

Address: _____

Are fees needed upfront? Yes _____   No _____   Partial Fee? _____

Total agreement amount $ _____   Fees _____

What it covers: _____

Type of case: [Psych Evaluation, Criminal, WC evaluation for Attorney, IME, QME, MV Accident, Personal Injury, Employment, Other] _____

If criminal case, is client in custody and where? _____

If need to be seen out of town, where? _____

Date of injury, incident or onset: _____

Date last worked: _____ Date returned to work: _____

Who is plaintiff/defendant/injured party? _____

What Court? [Federal, Municipal, WC, Superior, Other] _____

Do they need Vitae or our fee schedule? _____

Are we seeing plaintiff or defendant? _____

When do they need evaluation and/or report? _____

To whom do we send report? _____

Address: _____

E-mail: _____ Fax: _____

Do they have settlement conference date? _____

Report due date? _____

Court/trial date? _____

Will there be records to review? _____ If Yes, please arrange for them to be sent as soon as possible.

Who is Deposing Attorney for deposition? _____

Address: _____

Telephone: _____ Fax: _____ E-mail: _____

Comments: _____

_____

_____

_____

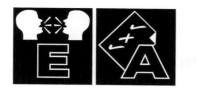

INTAKE ASSESSMENT AND PROPOSED TREATMENT PLAN

Name: _____ DOB: _____

Address: _____

_____

Telephone: Home _____ Work _____ Cell _____

Fax: _____ E-mail: _____

PRIMARY PRESENTING PROBLEMS:

PROBABLE CAUSE OR THE BASIS OF THE PROBLEMS:

EXPECTATIONS, GOALS, PLANS, AND DESIRED OUTCOME:

DIAGNOSTIC IMPRESSION:

Interviewer: _____ Referred to: _____

Community resources recommended: _____

Follow-up plans or agreement: _____

_____

PATIENT NAME: _____

PATIENT NUMBER: _____

AREAS FOR EXPLORATION FOR A COMPREHENSIVE MENTAL HEALTH ASSESSMENT

BRIEF CLINICAL ASSESSMENT

DIAGNOSTIC SUMMARY OF CURRENT CLINICAL STATUS

1. **Reason for Referral/Identifying Information:**

2. **Methodology Utilized:**

Medical/Developmental Hx (Describe if present)
Medical condition:

Current medications:

Pregnancy, birth, or neonatal complications:

Prenatal drug or alcohol exposure:

Motor delays:

Problems with toilet training:

Delays in language development:

Neurological risks:

Sleep disturbance:

Obesity, overweight, or underweight:

Appetite or eating disturbance:

Physical disability:

Hx or current enuresis:

Hx or current encopresis:

Allergies/medication reactions:

Additional:

Family Hx (Mark Y if present: Elaborate as needed)
Both parents in home:

Single parent:

Stepfamily:

No. of siblings and client's position in birth order:

Multiple moves:

Parent–child conflict:

Deaths/Grief:

Verbal abuse:

Neglect:

Sexual abuse:

Physical abuse:

Domestic violence:

Out of home placements:

Child Welfare Services involvement:

Parental health problems:

Parental mental illness:

Parental substance abuse:

Parentified child:

Parental criminality:

Low income:

High income:

Monolingual (self or parents):

Housing problems:

Other noteworthy:

Family Strengths (Mark Y if present)

Caring parents:

Caring siblings:

Prosocial family values:

Effective approach to discipline:

Good communication skills:

Effective at resolving conflicts or problems:

Parent(s) employed:

Insightful family:

Extended family support:

Family motivated and willing to participate:

Family resourceful:

Family bilingual/bicultural:

Other:

Educational Hx (Mark Y if present: Elaborate as needed)

Spec. Education (active IEP):

Spec. Education in past:

Grades/Academic performance:

Learning disorder:

Gifted:

Cont.

Truancy:

Grade retention/School failure:

School anxiety-avoidance:

Discipline issues:

Other:

Social and Adaptive Functioning (Mark Y if present: Elaborate as needed)

Formal job:

Informal work outside home:

Vocational or pleasurable interests:

Self-reported aptitudes:

Boyfriend/girlfriend, dating behavior:

Antisocial peers:

Impaired social judgment:

Poor response to authority figures:

Misattributions of hostility:

Difficulty predicting consequences:

Views violence as acceptable or desirable:

Fails to take responsibility:

Arousal-seeking:

Social skills and ability to resolve conflict:

Drug/ETOH Hx (Mark Y if present: Elaborate as needed)

Caffeine:

ETOH:

Cannabis:

Methamphetamine:

Tobacco:

Inhalants:

Prescription or OTC meds:

Other:

Criminality Hx (Mark Y if present: Elaborate as needed)

Property crimes:

Violent crimes:

Weapons:

Sexual offenses:

Gang involvement:

Drug sales:

Fire setting:

Animal cruelty:

Shows empathy or remorse for harm:

Family Hx:

Other:

Comprehensive Mental Health Assessment (*Continued*)

Individual Hx (Mark Y if present: Elaborate as needed)
  ADHD:

  Anxiety or panic:

  Posttraumatic stress disorder:

  Grief or losses:

  Depression:

  Mania/bipolar:

  Psychosis:

  Suicide gestures or attempts:

  Anger or aggression:

  Mood regulation:

  Teen parent:

  Hx psych meds:

  Currently on psych meds:

  Prior treatments and their effectiveness:

  Hx of running away:

  Hx of psychiatric hospitalizations:

  Ethnic identity or acculturation problems:

Strengths (Individual)

Mental Status/Cognitive Functioning
  Appearance and self-care:

  Attitude: Eye contact:

  Sensorium:

  Orientation:

  Attention:

  Concentration:

  Recall/memory:

  Fund of knowledge:

  Intelligence:

  Abstraction:

  Judgment:

  Reality testing:

  Insight:

  Decision making:

  Speech and word usage:

  Executive functioning:

  Mood:

  Affect:

  Perception:

  Thought form/process:

  Thought content:

Cont.

Specific Impairments

Living arrangements:

Educational:

Vocational:

Social/community relationships:

Daily activities:

Developmental:

Physical health:

Other:

3. **Summary of Symptoms Resulting in Diagnostic Formulation:**

4. **Recommendations for Interventions:**

5. Service Plan Goals and Recommendations:

6. **Diagnostic Impressions:**

CLIENT'S STATED GOALS (including those for treatment):

"_____"

GAF (Current):
SOFA (Current):

PATIENT NAME: _____

PATIENT NUMBER: _____

BRIEF ASSESSMENT AND DIAGNOSTIC SUMMARY

Name: _____ DOB: _____ Date of exam: _____

BASIC INFORMATION AND STATUS:

He/She is: Mentally ill ___ ; Chemically dependent ___ ; Mentally retarded ___ ; Personality disorder ___; Psychopathic ___ ; Sex Offender ___ ; Other _____

Safety assessment: Risk of self harm ___ ; Risk of harm to others ___ ; Suicide intent ___ ; Impulse control problems ___ ; Irrational thought disorder ___ ; Other _____

Substance abuse/Dependence: Alcohol ___ ; Illegal drugs ___ ; Prescriptive drugs ___ ; OTC drugs ___ ; Poly-substance abuse ___ ; Other _____

Mental status exam: (Areas of impairment) Speech ___ ; Mood ___ ; Affect ___ ; Thought content ___ ; Delusional thinking ___ ; Judgment ___ ; Insight ___ ; Attention ___ ; Impulse control ___ ; Memory ___ ; Concentration ___ ; Bodily tension ___ ; Other _____

Treatment potential: Very good ___ ; Fair ___; Poor ___ ; Rejects proposed treatment ___ ; Will be cooperative/compliant ___ ; Will need to be imposed ___ ; Other _____

Level of support: Positive support ___ ; Inconsistent support ___ ; Little to none ___ ; Mostly unhealthy support ___ ; Available support is rejected ___ ; Other _____

DIAGNOSTIC IMPRESSIONS:

Axis I _____

_____

_____

Axis II _____

_____

_____

Axis III (Medical factors) _____

_____

_____

Axis IV (Social factors) _____

_____

_____

Axis V GAF (Current) ___ ; GAF (Past six months) ___ ; GAF (Past year) ___

GAF (Highest during past 5 years) ___; GAF (Potential level) ___

Observational Comments:

Recommendations:

Respectfully submitted,

NAME OF EXAMINER

DATE OF SUBMISSION

PATIENT NAME: _____

PATIENT NUMBER: _____

BRIEF DIAGNOSTIC STRUCTURED CLINICAL INTERVIEW

Client name: _____   Date: _____

Therapist: _____   Session #: _____

Identifying Information and Mental Status (II): _____

_____

Presenting Issue or Referral Issue (PI): _____

_____

Symptom Profile (Sx) : _____

_____

Psychiatric or Psychological History (PSY): _____

_____

History of Presenting Issue (HPI): _____

_____

     Family History (FHx): _____

     Social History (SOHx): _____

     Work – Occupational History (WHx): _____

     Relationship – Marital History (RMhx): _____

Substance and or Alcohol Use/Abuse (SubETOH): _____

Suicidality or Homocidality Issues (SHI): _____

Medical Issues (MI): _____

Legal Issues (LI): _____

Assessment (A): _____

Initial Diagnosis (DX):

     Axis I: Diagnostic label and corresponding DSM IV-TR code

     Axis II: Diagnostic label and corresponding DSM IV-TR code

     Axis III: Client report or medical report on related conditions

     Axis IV: Psychosocial stressors and severity rating (1–5)

     Axis V: GAF Current: _____ and GAF Highest/Past year: _____

Treatment recommendations (Tx): _____

Signature of therapist: _____

Name of therapist: _____

SENTENCE COMPLETION-WORK

Name: _____ Date: _____

DIRECTIONS

This form contains a series of incomplete sentences. Your task is to finish each sentence in any way you wish. Complete each sentence as quickly as you can.

1. The work I enjoy doing most is _____

2. Good work is hard to do when _____

3. I become unhappy in my work when _____

4. When talking before other _____

5. I could work better if _____

6. My future career goals are _____

7. In my opinion those that I have worked with in the past _____
_____

8. When I was younger I thought I would like _____

9. To lead other _____

10. A major obstacle in my career goals is _____

11. My bosses have been _____

12. What motivates me _____

13. At work I feel upset when _____

14. People in authority _____

15. When my work plans are upset _____

16. At work I could lose my temper if _____

17. If I could be anything I wished _____

18. My major weakness _____

19. Taking orders _____

20. I criticize others when _____

Cont.

21. Paperwork _____

22. My main problem at work _____

23. If given the opportunity, I would prefer to be _____

_____because _____

PATIENT NAME: _____

PATIENT NUMBER: _____

For the therapist:
OBSERVATIONS, ATTITUDES, AND PATTERNS OF NOTE:

PSYCHOPATHY CHECKLIST

Please complete the form as you know the person and how he/she generally behaves.

Key:
0 = Does not apply	1 = Slightly applies	2 = Mostly applies; true
3 = Very much applies	4 = Definitely applies	5 = Totally applies; has become a lifestyle

FACTOR 1: Selfish, Callous, and Remorseful Use of Others

1. Glibness, superficial charm   _____
2. Egocentricity/grandiose sense of self-worth   _____
3. Pathological lying and deception   _____
4. Conning/Lack of sincerity   _____
5. Lack of remorse or guilt   _____
6. Lack of effect and emotional depth   _____
7. Callous/Lack of empathy   _____
8. Failure to accept responsibility for own actions   _____
9. Drug or alcohol abuse not direct cause of anti-social behavior   _____

            Subtotal   _____

FACTOR 2: Chronically Unstable and Anti-Social Lifestyle

10. Proneness to boredom/low frustration tolerance   _____
11. Parasitic lifestyle   _____
12. Short tempered/poor behavior controls   _____
13. Early behavior problems   _____
14. Lack of realistic long-term plans   _____
15. Impulsivity   _____
16. Irresponsible behavior as a parent   _____
17. Frequent marital relationships   _____
18. Juvenile delinquency   _____
19. Poor probation or parole risk   _____
20. Many types of offense   _____

            Subtotal   _____

            TOTAL   _____

NOTE: The higher the score the more likely the person has a psychopathic behavioral pattern and lifestyle. Extensive treatment is required.

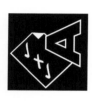

CRITICAL EVENTS TIME LINE

Name of patient: _____

Fill in the critical events in the patient's history and analyze the relative impact and influence on the person.

(yr___)	(yr___)	(yr___)	(yr___)	(yr___)	(yr___)	(yr___)	(yr___)

Chapter 16

Assessments Related to Specific Tests and Scales

Chapter Contents

Therapists are asked to summarize a patient's status at the beginning of treatment and at the end of the time services were rendered. Hopefully, progress can be documented. Further, therapists also need to help their patients understand the results of various tests and questionnaires administered and how the relevant results can be interpreted so they are helpful to the patient and aid in the achievement of their personal goals.

The forms, scales, templates, and guidelines provided in this chapter will assist the therapist draft a profile of their patients and be able to demonstrate the changes that have occurred in therapy. The education of patients regarding their testing results and their personal history will be easier if therapists utilize the forms in this chapter and other tools similar to them.

PRACTICAL MODEL FOR INTERPRETING MCMI-III TEST RESULTS

INTRODUCTION

Sharing test results is an ethical principle in the American Psychological Association's code of conduct. However, studies indicated that 69% of psychologists are unlikely to share results of assessments with clients. One reason given for this exclusion is that psychologists have not found adequate methods to share delicate, theoretical, and complex information with a client whose ability to process the information may be impaired and the consequential distortion could create greater emotional trauma.

The following model, called the Iceberg Model (IM), for visually interpreting results of the Millon Clinical Multiaxial Inventory-III (MCMI-III) should not only be easy to understand for clients but also supply a structured protocol for psychologists. As seen in Figure 16.1, the IM is designed to add understanding and clarity to idiosyncratic information available on the MCMI-III and provides a link to Millon's theoretical underpinnings of the MCMI-III.

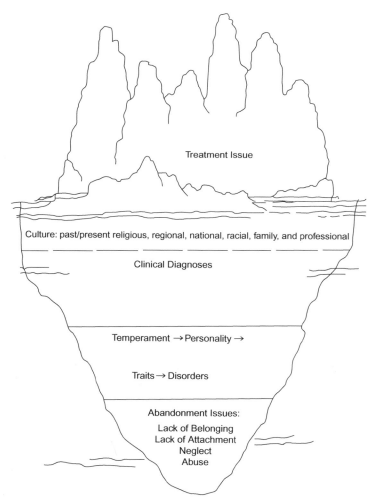

Figure 16.1 Iceberg Model for Interpreting Results of MCMI-III

PROCEDURE TO EXPLAIN THE ICEBERG MODEL OF TEST INTERPRETATION

After the testing is completed and the MCMI-III results are available, the clinician starts the process of explaining the IM. In Figure 16.1, the jagged parts above the waterline represent the presenting problems, stressors, or symptoms (such as a relational problem, problems with a child, or a grief reaction) that are impacted by a vast, deeper core of issues submerged "under the waterline." Just as only 10–15% of an iceberg is visible, in much the same way a client's treatment issues are often the "seen and known part" of larger underlying psychological and pathological elements. The hidden or unconscious parts of a person's life gravely impact symptoms but often become less injurious when they are exposed to therapy and treatment.

VISIBLE LAYER

The clinician then allows the client to name the presenting problems, writing each on the iceberg's above-water part, called Treatment Issues. At this time, clinicians will often discover data that were not obvious or clear during the initial interview or on the intake form. Although not as vast as the underlying part, a ship captain never minimizes the iceberg's upper parts nor should the symptoms and concomitant pain be minimized.

ABANDONMENT LAYER

Due to its critical place as a foundation of much dysfunction, IM's lowest layer, labeled Abandonment Issues, is discussed with the client, including any sexual, spiritual, physical, verbal, emotional, financial, and mental abuse experienced. Abandonment can be subtle or understated, such as not belonging among peers, neglect, or lack of attachment to parents who are deceased, divorced, or work out of town. For the child, all of these involve abandonment. These abuses can also exist in adult relationships, school or work settings, and marriages, and can be teased out at this time (e.g., neglect of a partner or lack of belonging).

PERSONALITY LAYER

Just as the client's experiences of abandonment influence symptomatology, so does the genetic template of temperament, i.e., the "raw biological material from which personality occurs." Just after conception, the fetus begins to experience and interact with the environment, first with mother and then with outside influences such as social roles, culture, socioeconomic status, and family environment. All these interactions cause changes to the basic temperament of the child, and a personality develops. Children play an active role in this, creating their own environmental conditions, which, in turn, serve as a basis for reinforcing their biological tendencies, a recursive phenomenon theory. Furthermore, personality traits can appear and form clusters of symptoms to become personality disorders. By definition, disorders eventually impair work, school, social, and home life. Since personality labels can be deleterious, the psychologist writes on the IM handout general terms and explanations for personality traits (scores 85 or under) or disorders (over 85) such as "avoids social situations" rather than "Avoidant."

CLINICAL SYNDROME LAYER

Subsequently, personality dynamics form the substrate of the next IM level, i.e., Axis I Clinical Diagnoses. Personality disorders can be vulnerabilities that predispose a person to developing an Axis I clinical syndrome, such as dysthymia.

CULTURAL LAYER

The clinician now focuses on the next level, an individual's culture, which is a filter of all the other underlying layers of the IM, including both past and present religious, regional, national, racial, family, and professional culture.

PERMEABLE BOUNDARIES

Noteworthy, the IM has permeable boundaries between each section symbolized by the dotted lines. As Millon stated, "psychopathology develops as a result of an intimate *interplay* [italics added] of intraorganismic and environmental forces. Such interactions start at the time of conception and continue through life."

GLOBAL ASSESSMENT OF RELATIONAL FUNCTIONING (GARF) SCALE

By using the rating scale below, rate the patient's relational unit and level of functioning at this time in his/her life. Rate the patient's relational unit on Problem Solving Skills, Organizational Skills, and Emotional Climate.

81–100 Relational unit functioning satisfactorily. Optimistic, good communication, sharing of values, minimal conflict, low stress, good decision making, and are employed.

61–80 Relational unit somewhat unsatisfactory, with some conflict unresolved, some tension, fairly or usually competent in handling life circumstances. Relational unit functioning fairly well.

41–60 Relational unit functioning satisfactorily occasionally. Clearly dysfunctional and have unsatisfying relationships. Prevailing problems. Much unresolved conflict.

21–40 Relational unit fairly dysfunctional. Much hurt prevails. High stress, poor communication patterns, unfair treatment of each other, poor decision making and planning.

1–20 Relational unit extremely dysfunctional. Very loose associations, disconnected, boundary violations, detachments, lack of concern for the best interest of each other.

	Problem solving	Organization	Emotional climate
81–100			
61–80			
41–60			
21–40			
1–20			
0			
Inadequate information to rate			

Total Score _____ _____ _____

Average Score _____

GAF EVALUATION

The GAF score is derived for a patient based on the patient's social, psychological, and occupational functioning on a daily bases in all areas of his/her life. The rating is based on a 100-point scale. When rating a patient, do not take into account any physical or environmental limitations the patient may have. The scale should reflect the patient's mental health status.

Evaluation:	Minimal	Fair	Adequate	Good	Best Possible	Score
1. Working	20	40	60	80	100	_____
2. Leisure	20	40	60	80	100	_____
3. Eating	20	40	60	80	100	_____
4. Sleeping	20	40	60	80	100	_____
5. Social contact	20	40	60	80	100	_____
6. Earning	20	40	60	80	100	_____
7. Parenting	20	40	60	80	100	_____
8. Loving	20	40	60	80	100	_____
9. Environment	20	40	60	80	100	_____
10. Self-acceptance	20	40	60	80	100	_____

Average Score _____

	Date	Index
First evaluation		
Last evaluation		
Current evaluation		

COMMENTS AND CLARIFICATION:

SOCIAL AND OCCUPATIONAL FUNCTIONING ASSESSMENT (SOFA) SCALE

The SOFA scale is used to estimate a person's level of functioning with respect to his/her mental and physical problems. The scale is completed as to how the patient is able to actually function in occupational (school) settings and in social settings. The time period on which the rating is based should be this past month, or some other designated time frame.

THE RATING SCALE:

100   Doing super well
90   Doing well, good
80   Slightly improved
70   Some difficulty noted
60   Moderate impairment
50   Serious problems
40   Major problems and impairment in functioning
30   Markedly impaired; unable to function independently
20   Unable to function in most situations
10   Cannot function without much external support; at risk

MY RATINGS:

Occupational/School functioning: _____

Social and interpersonal functioning: _____

Average level of functioning: _____

Time period considered in making the ratings: _____

Name of rater: _____ Date: _____

Title: _____

Chapter 17

Assessments Related to Risk, Competency, Health, and Neuropsychology

Chapter Contents

Therapists must assess patients with a variety of presenting problems and areas of difficulty in their daily lives. It is the clinical task of a therapist to come to know the behavioral patterns and personal background information of their patients so that certain therapeutic actions and decisions can be carried out, as well as relevant psycho-educational concepts being implemented.

The forms, guidelines, questionnaires, and templates included in this chapter are provided to assist the therapist in assessing their patients accurately for appropriate care planning and the initiation of treatment.

COMPETENCY TO STAND TRIAL STATUS EXAM

Name: _____   Date: _____   Site of interview: _____

DEGREE OF INCAPACITY:

1 = Total   *2 = Severe*   *3 = Moderate*   *4 = Mild*   *5 = None*

1. Appraisal of available legal defenses   _____

2. Unmanageable behavior   _____

3. Quality of relating to attorney   _____

4. Planning of legal strategy, including guilty plea to lesser charges where pertinent   _____

5. Appraisal of role of:
   a. Defense counsel   _____
   b. Prosecuting attorney   _____
   c. Judge   _____
   d. Jury   _____
   e. Defendant   _____
   f. Witnesses   _____

6. Understanding of court procedure   _____

7. Appreciation of charges   _____

8. Appreciation of range and nature of possible penalties   _____

9. Appraisal of likely outcome   _____

10. Capacity to disclose to attorney available pertinent facts surrounding the offense including the defendant's movements, timing, mental state, actions at the time of the offense   _____

11. Capacity to realistically challenge prosecution witnesses   _____

12. Capacity to testify relevantly   _____

13. Self-defeating vs. self-serving motivation (legal sense)   _____

Signature of examiner: _____   Date: _____

ASSESSING LIFESTYLE AND HEALTH

A. CURRENT RISK FACTORS

Check all that apply:

__ hypertension   __ elevated triglycerides   __ elevated cholesterol

__ overeating   __ excess salt, sugar, fat   __ lack of exercise

__ chronic stress   __ smoking   __ overweight

__ alcohol abuse   __ sleep disturbance   __ prescription medication abuse

B. NUTRITION

When you review your diet and compare it to one year ago and five years ago, is it the same, less healthy, or more healthy?

1. The positive changes made are

2. Changes that need to be made are

C. STRESS MANAGEMENT

1. Current level of stress is _____ low   _____ moderate   _____ high

To the following, respond never (N), sometimes (S), often (O), or always (A):

2. In an effort to deal with stress:
   a. Exercise is used to decrease tension _____
   b. Relaxation techniques are helpful for releasing tension _____

3. Characteristics I have in common with those who manage stress well:
   a. Daily moments of peace and solitude _____
   b. Playfulness and humor to improve mood _____
   c. Positive relationships with family and friends _____
   d. Distracting activities _____
   e. Good level of frustration tolerance _____
   f. Good ability to manage criticism _____
   g. An ability to avoid overloaded scheduling _____
   h. A good balance of work and pleasure _____

Cont.

Therapist's Guide to Clinical Intervention, Second Edition by Sharon L. Johnson (© 2003 Elsevier Inc.)

D. NEGATIVE LIFESTYLE HABITS

Answer each of the following questions regarding your negative lifestyle habits:

1. How is it a problem?

2. How did it begin and develop?

3. What could be some appropriate substitutes?

4. What do you want to change?

E. PLAN OF CHANGE

Name: _____ Date: _____

INFORMAL DIAGNOSTIC EXERCISES OF APHASIA

Aphasia is a language disorder that can affect the expression of language or the reception of language. Aphasia has a major effect on the lifestyle of the person and requires major multi-dimensional therapeutic intervention.

THE SQUARE:
Copy a square
Say "square"
Spell "square"

THE KEY:
Draw a key
Say "key"
Demonstrate the use of a key

WORD RECALL:
Repeat "triangle"
Repeat "Massachusetts"
Repeat "Methodist Episcopal"
Repeat "seven"
Repeat "he shouted the warning"

SOUND RECOGNITION:
Make 5–6 different sounds to be named.

BASIC SKILLS:
Ask the patient to carry out 5–6 basic skills or actions, i.e., fold a piece of paper three times

OBJECT IDENTIFICATION:
Select 5 random objects in the room to be identified and their use specified

THE CROSS:
Copy a cross
Say "cross"
Spell "cross"

THE TRIANGLE:
Copy a triangle
Say "triangle"
Spell "triangle"

LATERALITY:
Read "Place left hand to the right ear"
Place left hand to right ear
Place left hand to right elbow

COMPREHENSION:
Read a paragraph and ask 4–5 questions about the details of the paragraph

ROTE SPEECH:
Name the days of the week, months of the year, alphabet, count to 20, and name 5 colors

HISTORY:
Conduct an interview of the person's history of language development, pathology, intelligence, handedness, head trauma, medical profile, and educational experience

NEUROPSYCHOLOGICAL ASSESSMENT: PATIENT INFORMATION

WHAT IS CLINICAL NEUROPSYCHOLOGY AND PEDIATRIC NEUROPSYCHOLOGY?

Clinical neuropsychology is a specialty profession that focuses on brain functioning. In clinical neuropsychology, brain function is evaluated by objectively testing motor, sensory, memory, and thinking skills. A very detailed assessment of abilities is done and the pattern of strengths and weaknesses is used to assist with diagnosis and treatment planning. Pediatric neuropsychology also addresses how learning and behavior are associated with the development of brain structures and systems.

WHY ARE CHILDREN AND ADULTS REFERRED FOR NEUROPSYCHOLOGICAL ASSESSMENT?

Children are typically referred because of difficulty in learning, attention, behavior, socialization, or emotional control. They also may be referred for neuropsychological assessment because of a disease or developmental problem that affects the brain in some way. Both adults and children may be referred when there is a brain injury from an accident, illness, or other trauma, or there is some unexplained change in the person's concentration, organization, reasoning, memory, language, perception, coordination, or personality.

WHAT IS ASSESSED?

A typical neuropsychological evaluation will involve assessment of the following:

- General intellect
- Executive skills such as organization, planning, reasoning, and problem-solving
- Attention and concentration
- Learning and memory
- Language
- Visual–spatial skills (e.g., perception)
- Motor and sensory skills
- Behavioral and emotional functioning
- Achievement skills such as reading and math

Some abilities may be measured in more detail than others, depending on the individual's needs. Emerging skills can be assessed in very young children. However, the evaluation of infants and preschool children is usually shorter in duration, because the child has not yet developed many skills.

WHAT WILL THE RESULTS TELL ME?

Test results can be used to understand the patient's situation in a number of ways.

For adults:

- Testing can identify weaknesses in specific areas. It is very sensitive to mild memory and thinking problems that might not be obvious in other ways. When problems are very mild, testing may be the only way to detect them. For example, testing can help determine whether memory changes are normal age-related changes or if they reflect neurological disorder. Testing might also be used to identify problems related to medical conditions that can affect memory and thinking, such as diabetes, metabolic or infectious diseases, or alcoholism.

- Test results can also be used to help differentiate among illnesses, which is important because appropriate treatment depends on accurate diagnosis. Different illnesses result in different patterns of strengths and weaknesses on testing. Therefore, the results can be helpful in determining which areas of the brain might be involved and what illness might be operating. For instance, testing can help to differentiate among Alzheimer's disease, stroke, and depression. Your physician will use this information along with the results of other tests, such as brain imaging and blood tests, to come to the most informed diagnosis possible.

- Sometimes testing is used to establish a "baseline," for documenting a person's skills before there is any problem. In this way, later changes can be measured very objectively.

- Test results can be used to plan treatments that use strengths to compensate for weaknesses. The results help to identify what cognitive problems to work on and which strategies to use. For example, the results can help to plan and monitor cognitive rehabilitation therapies following a stroke or traumatic brain injury.

- Studies have shown how scores on specific tests relate to everyday functional skills, such as managing money, driving, or readiness to return to work. Your results will help your doctors understand what problems you may have in everyday life. This will help guide planning for assistance and treatment.

For children:

- Testing can explain why your child is having school problems. For example, the child may have difficulty reading because of an attention problem, a language disorder, an auditory processing problem, or a reading disability. Testing also guides the pediatric neuropsychologist to design interventions that draw upon your child's strengths. The results identify what skills to work on as well as which strategies to use to help your child.

- Testing can help detect the effects of developmental, neurological, and medical problems, such as epilepsy, autism, attention deficit hyperactivity disorder (ADHD), dyslexia, or a genetic disorder. Testing may be done to obtain a baseline against which to measure the outcome of treatment or the child's development over time.

- Different childhood disorders result in specific patterns of strengths and weaknesses. The profiles of abilities can help identify the child's disorder and the brain areas that are involved. For example, testing can help differentiate between an attention deficit and depression, or determine whether a language delay is due to a problem in producing speech, understanding or processing language, social shyness, autism, or cognitive delay.

- Most importantly, testing provides a better understanding of the child's behavior in learning and school, at home, and in the community. The evaluation can guide teachers, therapists, and you to better help your child achieve his or her potential.

WHAT SHOULD I EXPECT?

A neuropsychological evaluation usually includes an interview and testing. A detailed intake history form and symptom checklist is filled out by adult patients or parents of children prior to the initial visit. During the interview, information that is important for the neuropsychologist to consider will be reviewed. The testing involves taking paper-and-pencil or computerized tests and answering questions. The time required to complete the testing depends on the problems being assessed. In general, several hours are needed to assess the many skills involved in processing information. Some tests will be easy while others will be more complex. It is important that the person being tested gets a good night's sleep before the testing. Also, it is important that glasses or hearing aids be used during the evaluation. Any medications that are being taken at the time of testing should be reported to the examiner.

KEY BENEFITS

- More sensitive than CT, MRI or EEG in detecting brain impairment/dysfunction.
- Provides objective information regarding functional limitations.
- This information can be used to develop helpful treatment interventions.

Forms, Exercises, and Information for Treating Specific Disorders

Understanding how to bring about the behavioral changes needed to produce emotional healing and a higher quality of life is the hallmark of a mental health therapist. Therapists assist individuals, groups, and organizations to change a wide variety of dysfunctional behavior patterns and emotional states, such as anxiety, depression, insomnia, pain, headaches, and numerous addictions.

Individual psychotherapy, group therapy, marital therapy, and family therapy are offered under many different formats and methods. Throughout history, psychotherapy has been the backbone of the healing and restorative process in the lives of many patients. Without it, those who are angry continue to carry on destructive relationships. And, those that are medically impaired continue to live with ongoing limitations and disability.

The time, energy, and cost to produce healthy changes have generally been considered a worthy experience by those that enter into therapeutic relationships. Indeed, over recent years, therapists have gotten much better in bringing about mental, emotional, and cognitive change through major advances in technology, medications, and new therapeutic methodologies. Mood disorders, interpersonal relationship problems, forms of stress, and a host of other psychological and medical problems have been the arena in which therapists have worked in conjunction with other professionals such as physicians, ministers, and attorneys, to name a few. A collegial team approach has generally been preferred for the best results for the patient.

Part III includes forms, guidelines, rating scales, templates, and other tools to assist therapists in dealing with and conducting their therapeutic assignment with patients seeking their services for relief and lifestyle change regarding a variety of mental, emotional, and behavioral problems.

Chapter 18

Anxiety and Stress Relief with Relaxation Assessment and Exercises

Chapter Contents

Anxiety and stress have become earmarks of our society today. Therapy commonly begins with people experiencing overpowering and chronic stress, with anxiety being the major expression of the stress experience. Any existing and ongoing emotional or behavioral problems are generally exacerbated by stress, as are most medical problems. Therapists deal with anxiety and stress all the time. Intervention at the emotional, cognitive, behavioral, and physical levels of a person's life is essential to a comprehensive treatment plan.

This chapter consists of several forms, questionnaires, guidelines, and exercises to deal with these and related issues in therapy. Effective and long-lasting changes from therapy require that these issues be directly addressed.

16 WARNING SIGNS OF POST-TRAUMATIC STRESS

A Checklist

1. Recurrent and intrusive distressing memories
2. Recurrent nightmares
3. Acting or feeling as if the trauma were recurring
4. Intense emotional distress when exposed to reminders of the event
5. Intense physical reaction to said reminders
6. Avoidance of anything associated with the trauma
7. Memory loss of the trauma
8. Loss of interest in formerly enjoyed activities
9. Feeling apart from people
10. Unable to have loving feelings
11. Sense of having a foreshortened future
12. Difficulty falling or staying asleep
13. Irritability
14. Difficulty concentrating
15. Always on guard
16. Exaggerated nervousness

NOTE:

If any of these symptoms appear and do not subside in a reasonable period of time after a trauma, 2 to 4 months, please call to make an appointment with your physician and psychologist.

PERSONAL STRESS MANAGEMENT PROFILE

Personal Stress Profile: Part I

BALANCING YOUR PRIORITIES

First, indicate how much time you "Now" spend on each of these areas. Next, decide on the amount of time you would ideally spend – "Your Goal." Then decide how you can achieve your goal.

	Now	Your Goal	How will you move toward
	(Hours per week)		your goal?

WORK
Time on job/school
Bringing work home
Commuting

PERSONAL
Exercise
Television
Computer/video games
Hobby/recreation
Reading
Friends
Religious activities
Volunteering
Sleep (hours per night)

MARRIAGE (Couple)
At home together
Activities/dates
Discussions (minutes per day)

HOME
Cleaning
Cooking
Grocery shopping
Errands
Lawn/garden
Home maintenance

Cont.

FAMILY (if children at home)

Number of meals together	_____	_____	_____
Family activities	_____	_____	_____
Transporting children	_____	_____	_____
Helping with homework	_____	_____	_____
At home together	_____	_____	_____

COUPLE DISCUSSION

What areas feel out of balance to each of you?

What steps must you take in order for your goal to become reality?

Cont.

Personal Stress Profile: Part II

IDENTIFYING MOST CRITICAL ISSUES

Do you control stress in your life or does stress control you?

Stressors are events that cause an emotional and/or physical reaction. Stress can be positive (wedding, job promotion) or negative (loss of job, car accident, major illness). But what is important is to be able to manage the many stressors in your life.

One way to manage stress is to prioritize the issues that are most important to you. Another is to decide what issues can be changed or resolved and which ones cannot. This exercise will help you focus on the high priority issues and those that can be changed (Box 1 below).

COUPLE EXERCISE

1. You will each select four issues that are the most stressful for each of you from the Computer Report.
2. Review each issue and put it into one of the four cells below.
3. Box 1 contains the "Most Critical Issues."

High Priority

	Able to change	Difficult to change
	Box 1: Most Critical Issues *What changes can you each make?*	Box 2 *How do you plan to cope?*
	Box 3 *Are you spending too much time on low priority issues?*	Box 4: Least Critical Issues *Can you accept or forget about these issues?*

Low Priority

COUPLE DISCUSSION

Select one issue from Box 1 that you will work on together as a couple. Work together as a team to achieve your goals.

- Communicate about the issue.
- Use good conflict resolution skills.
- Be flexible with one another.

Cont.

Personal Stress Profile: Part III

ACHIEVING YOUR GOALS … TOGETHER

Clarify and define your personal, couple, and family goals for the next few years. Then share them with your partner. Remember your goals should be realistic and clearly stated. These goals also should be attainable within 3 to 6 months.

Partner 1 Goals

Personal Goals

1. _____
2. _____
3. _____

Couple Goals

1. _____
2. _____
3. _____

Family Goals

1. _____
2. _____
3. _____

Partner 2 Goals

Personal Goals

1. _____
2. _____
3. _____

Couple Goals

1. _____
2. _____
3. _____

Family Goals

1. _____
2. _____
3. _____

COUPLE DISCUSSION

- Were you surprised by any of your partner's goals?
- Which goals are most important to you right now?
- What are the current issues surrounding these goals?
- How do your partner's goals complement or compete with yours?
- How can you each contribute to achieving these goals?
- What will be the first step to make this goal become a reality?

PROGRESSIVE RELAXATION

1. Clench both <u>fists</u>, feel the tension. Relax slowly … feel the tension ease. Feel the difference now that the muscles are relaxed.

2. Make a muscle with both arms. Contract the <u>biceps</u> … now relax the arms slowly.

3. Curl the <u>toes downward</u> until the muscles are tight up through the thighs … now slowly relax … feel the tension ease.

4. Curl the <u>toes upward</u> until the muscles in the back of the legs are tight. Now relax slowly. Feel the tension ease.

5. Push the <u>stomach</u> muscles <u>out</u> as though you were going to be hit in the stomach and you are protecting yourself. Now slowly … relax. Your arms are relaxed … your legs are relaxed and your breathing is easy.

6. Pull your <u>stomach</u> in <u>up</u> until your diaphragm feels the pressure. Now … slowly relax … slowly. Feel the tension ease.

7. Pull your <u>shoulders</u> up to your ears. Feel the tension in your back and chest. Now … slowly relax. Let your arms relax. You are feeling good. Your breathing is easy.

8. Tilt your <u>head backwards</u> as far as you can. Stretch the muscles. Feel the tenseness. Now, slowly, relax. Let your head come to a comfortable position.

9. Put your <u>chin down</u> on your chest. Hold it. Feel the tension. Now, relax. Feel the tension go.

10. <u>Wrinkle your forehead</u>. Hold it. Now relax. Feel the tension go.

11. <u>Squint your eyes</u> as tight as you can. Hold it. Now … relax.

12. <u>Make a face</u> using all your face muscles. Hold it. Now relax … slowly. Your arms are relaxed … your breathing is easy and you feel good all over.

13. In a <u>state of perfect relaxation</u> you should feel unwilling to move a single muscle in your body. Now continue relaxing, and when you wish to get up, count backwards from four to one. You should then feel fine and refreshed, and wide-awake and calm.

INSTRUCTIONS FOR FOCUSED BREATHING

STRESS AND ANXIETY MANAGEMENT

To begin, take a long, slow, deep, relaxing, complete breath in through your nose and when you are ready exhale as slowly and as fully as you possibly can through your nose. Place all of your conscious awareness on your breathing. Turn off all unnecessary thoughts, tune out all distracting noises, and silence your internal voice.

Continue to breathe slowly, smoothly, and quietly. In your mind, picture fresh, clean, oxygen-rich air flowing through your nose and passing through your throat and chest until it reaches your lungs. Picture and feel your lungs expanding to their maximum capacity and then emptying totally like large pink balloons filling completely and then collapsing totally when empty.

When you inhale, feel your belly-button push out and your lower ribs separate. Feel your breath filling the bottom, the middle, and finally the top of your lungs. When you exhale, feel all the muscles in your body – from the top of your head to the tip of your toes, totally relax. Feel loose and limp, warm and heavy, deeply … deeply relaxed.

Now, think of nothing but the movement of air within yourself. Remember that each breath is nourishing your entire body with fresh oxygen-rich blood, and each exhalation is cleansing your body. If your thoughts stray from your breathing, bring them back and focus your entire awareness on your breathing. Continue to concentrate on your breathing until you hear my voice again. [*At this point in recording these instructions, let the recorder run for 5 to 10 minutes without speaking, then read the next sentence.*] When I count to three, you will open your eyes and feel much better than before; your eyesight will be improved, your reaction time quicker, your blood pressure lower, and your heart rate slowed down. You will feel totally refreshed and relaxed. One – Two – Three … Eyes open, but continue to be relaxed and calm.

NOW DO THIS EXERCISE DAILY ONCE OR TWICE FOR A TOTAL OF 10–20 TIMES TO LEARN IT WELL AND BE ABLE TO DO IT FROM MEMORY.

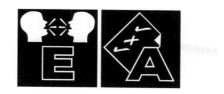

STRESSFUL LIFE EVENTS

Name: _____ Date: _____

The list below identifies the 20 most stressful events that come into our lives and affect us greatly. It is these events that we must learn to deal with and resolve if stress is to be well managed or reduced in our daily lives. Check those items in the list below that are now part of your life or have been an issue for you over the *past year* or more.

	Now	Past year
VERY HIGH STRESS LEVEL EVENTS:		
• The death of a spouse	_____	_____
• Divorce became final	_____	_____
• Marital separation for a lengthy time	_____	_____
• Held in jail or prison	_____	_____
• Death of a close family member	_____	_____
• Major illness or injury requiring care	_____	_____
• Marriage or remarriage	_____	_____
HIGH STRESS LEVEL EVENTS:		
• Fired from a job or work assignment	_____	_____
• Marital reconciliation with mate	_____	_____
• Retirement	_____	_____
• Major change in health or behavior status of a close family member	_____	_____
MODERATELY HIGH STRESS LEVEL EVENTS:		
• Pregnancy	_____	_____
• Sexual difficulties	_____	_____
• Gaining a new member to the family and household	_____	_____
• Major business change or readjustment	_____	_____
• Major change in financial status	_____	_____
• Changing to a new job or line of work	_____	_____
• An increase/decrease in the number of arguments with your spouse	_____	_____
• Purchase of a new home or business and taking on a mortgage to do it	_____	_____

Comments: The more of the above events that are now present in your life or have been for a year or more, the higher level of stress you are now experiencing. Also, if more of the events from the upper categories are part of your life, the greater your stress level. And, should you indicate a high stress level, be careful for illness, injury, accidents, mishaps, and other unfortunate events occurring in your life.

Source: Adapted from the Social Readjustment Rating Scale of Holmes and Rahe (1967).

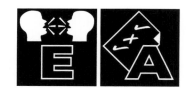

WELL-BEING SCALE

Our well-being is affected by a variety of situations and circumstances in our daily life. To a large extent we can influence how we feel and how we respond to daily events. Our well-being is largely in our own hands. Below are 10 situations or feelings for you to consider and note how often they occur in your life. Also, consider how you can alter your response to these feelings so your life is more enriched and stimulating.

HOW OFTEN DO YOU FEEL:	Never	Seldom	Sometimes	Often	Very Often
			CIRCLE YOUR ANSWER		
1. Particularly excited or interested in something?	0	1	2	3	4
*2. Feel bored much of the time?	0	1	2	3	4
*3. Very lonely or remote from other people?	0	1	2	3	4
4. On top of the world?	0	1	2	3	4
*5. Restless or impatient?	0	1	2	3	4
*6. Depressed or very unhappy?	0	1	2	3	4
7. Pleased about having accomplished something?	0	1	2	3	4
8. Like things are going your way?	0	1	2	3	4
*9. Upset because someone criticized you?	0	1	2	3	4
10. Proud because someone complimented you?	0	1	2	3	4

HOW I PLAN TO MAKE CHANGES IN MY WELL-BEING:

1.

2.

3.

4.

Note for the therapist:

*Score these items in the reverse order. Any patient obtaining scores above a two (2) on four of these items or more should be considered for a referral for individual or group psychotherapy.

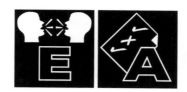

HOW WELL DO YOU COPE WITH LIFE'S CIRCUMSTANCES?

DIRECTIONS: For each question, check a box indicating **Yes** or **No** if at all possible. If you feel that you do not know the answer, or if it is one-half Yes and one-half No, check the **?** box.

Yes	?	No		
☐	☐	☐	1.	Do your friends think that you rarely get upset easily?
☐	☐	☐	2.	Do your friends think that you are easy-going and flexible?
☐	☐	☐	3.	Do your friends think you understand other people's points of view and accept them the way they are?
☐	☐	☐	4.	Do your friends think you get over being angry quickly?
☐	☐	☐	5.	Do your friends think you overcome problems easily?
☐	☐	☐	6.	Do your friends think you are reliable and responsible in meeting your obligations
☐	☐	☐	7.	Do you think the way you adjust to life can contribute to getting sick?
☐	☐	☐	8.	Do you think that changing your life in some way might make it easier to get well once you get sick?
☐	☐	☐	9.	Do you have good health?
☐	☐	☐	10.	Have you had a satisfying religious education?
☐	☐	☐	11.	Was your father supportive and understanding?
☐	☐	☐	12.	Was your mother supportive and understanding?
☐	☐	☐	13.	Do those close to you provide you the emotional support you need?
☐	☐	☐	14.	Have you set realistic goals for the future that satisfy you?

SCORING: Give yourself one point for every Yes response. In all items where your response was No, give yourself a minus one point. Give yourself zero points if you answered ? Total your score. It is possible to score from +14 to −14. Positive scores are indications of better coping skills and thought patterns.

Source: Adapted from Beatrice B. Berle's Coping Scale.

FEAR AND ITS MANAGEMENT

Fear is a potentially destructive emotion. It is self-defeating and can be self-destructive. We need to get a grip on our fears. Here is a start:

Consider the acrostic: FEAR

F Face your fear situation, person, or thing. Approach the fear object, but in gradual increments and with reasonableness.

E Expect you can change. Fear responses can be moderated if not eliminated. You can learn to develop a new set of responses to any fear situation.

A Assertive communication skills are a necessary component to fear management. Learn to be moderately confrontational and approachable. Use assertiveness towards a fear.

R Relaxation training is a vital component in learning how to engage in behavior that is the direct opposite of fear behavior. One cannot be relaxed and tense at the same time.

Reasons for having a fear of making a change or new directions in my life:

1. I fear what will happen to me if I change. I fear I will be endangered in some way. This is the Chicken Little Syndrome.
2. I fear that I will hurt you or someone if I change. I fear losing control over the changes; it will get out of control and I can't stop it.

THE MANAGEMENT OF STRESS, ANXIETY, AND PAIN

When you become aware of increased levels of stress, anxiety or pain sit down in a comfortable chair and read the statements below to yourself. Read them several times. Let your body and mind relax and experience the reduction of anxiety or pain.

ANXIETY CONTROL STATEMENTS

I can influence my own stress and anxiety.

I can reduce my stress and anxiety.

I can learn to better manage my stress and anxiety.

The feelings of anxiety should not be ignored. They provide important information which I need to learn from.

Anxiety feelings are not to be avoided; they are to be managed.

My anxiety can be viewed as though it were a wave coming in and going out, or a flowing river. Rather than fight against it, I will just lie back, relax, and float with it while slowly moving me in the direction of calmness.

PAIN CONTROL STATEMENTS

I can influence my own stress and pain.

I can reduce my stress, pain, and discomfort.

I can learn to better manage my stress and pain.

The feelings of pain should not be ignored. They provide important information which I need to learn from.

Painful feelings are not to be avoided; they are to be managed.

My pain can be viewed as though it were a wave coming in and going out, or a flowing river. Rather than fight against it, I will just lie back, relax, and float with it while it slowly moves me in the direction of comfort and calmness.

EMOTIONAL FITNESS

In the words of Scott Peck, "Life is difficult." We all encounter the daily heat of living – the pressures, the anxieties, the disappointments, and the deadlines – which can drain our emotional vitality unless we practice the **3 Rs** of emotional fitness:

1. **REMEMBER … a time to choose the best.** You may be saying, "In my circumstances, you've got to be kidding!" No, not really. Consider these questions:

   - In a shipwreck, can there be sunken treasure?
   - After a rainstorm, can there be a rainbow?
   - Even in the darkest night, is there the promise of a new morning?

2. **REST … a time to replenish.** Do you have a day in the week when activity and obligation are not synonymous? If not, consider this advice for emotional fitness:

   - Stop working for one day a week – enjoy a day of rest and relaxation.
   - During the day … highlight the positives – trash the negatives.
   - At bedtime … think on the best – forget the rest.

3. **REFRESH … a time to encourage.** Remember how good it feels to have someone give you an encouraging word when you really needed it? Why not:

   - Give a friend a call – with no agenda.
   - Give an associate a word of encouragement about their work.
   - Take the time to help someone who is not able to help themselves.
   - You'll feel good about yourself – and you'll help them to feel worthwhile. Both of you will be refreshed by the encounter.

Adapted from Dr Rick Warren, CBMC.

ADVICE FROM A FRIEND

Calm Down and Live in Peace

1. Meditate.
2. Go to bed on time.
3. Get up on time so you can start the day unrushed.
4. Say No to projects that won't fit into your time schedule or compromise your mental health.
5. Delegate tasks to capable others.
6. Simplify and "unclutter" your life.
7. Less is more. (Although one is often not enough, two are often too many.)
8. Allow extra time to do things and to get to places.
9. Pace yourself. Spread out big changes and difficult projects over time.
10. Take one day at a time.
11. Separate worries from concerns. If a situation is a concern, find out what seems to be the best option to do and let go of the anxiety. If you can't do anything about a situation, forget it.
12. Live within your budget; don't use credit cards for ordinary purchases.
13. Have backups; an extra car key in your wallet, an extra house key buried in the garden, extra stamps, etc.
14. K.M.S. (Keep Mouth Shut) ... This piece of advice can prevent an enormous amount of trouble.
15. Do something for the Kid in You everyday.
16. Carry a good book with you to read while waiting in line.
17. Get enough rest.
18. Eat well.
19. Get organized so everything has its place.
20. Listen to a tape/CD while driving that can help improve your quality of life.
21. Write down your thoughts and inspirations.
22. Every day, find time to be alone.
23. Having problems? Talk to someone and meditate on the spot. Try to nip problems in the bud.
24. Make friends with good people.
25. Keep a folder of favorite quotes, mottos, and verses on hand.
26. Laugh.
27. Laugh some more!
28. Take your work seriously, but not yourself at all.
29. Develop a forgiving attitude (most people are doing the best they can).
30. Be kind to unkind people (they probably need it the most).
31. Sit on your ego.
32. Talk less; listen more.
33. Slow down.
34. Remind yourself that you are not the general manager of the universe.
35. Every night before bed, think of one thing you're grateful for that you've never been grateful for before. TURNING THINGS AROUND FOR YOU IS POSSIBLE.
36. Add your own favorite actions that work for you.

Adapted from a paper by Roland Armstrong.

STRESS IS NOT A STOCKING STUFFER

The Holidays are to be a time of joy, sharing, contentment and a time to connect with our loved ones. Unfortunately, the storybook Holidays just do not come true for many of us. For some of us, the Holiday blues and depression can be a reality.

To prevent depression over the Holidays, it is important to take particular steps to be around others who care and provide positive, supportive companionship. Consider the following stress-reducing gifts, brought to us by the famous eight reindeer:

Reindeer 1: **Stress-proof yourself** by lightening your load and planning for times of fun in your schedule. Do not try to have a picture book perfection holiday. Be realistic.

Reindeer 2: **Limit spending** by sticking with a realistic budget for gifts, food, and travel. Do not over-use credit cards.

Reindeer 3: **Plan family time** by scheduling events such as a drive to see Holiday lights and decorations, watching a special television Holiday concert or program, taking a hike together or creating a new and unusual Holidays tradition for the family.

Reindeer 4: **Give "non-monetary" gifts** such as promising to do a favor for someone, doing chores for someone, and other many other random gifts of kindness.

Reindeer 5: **Create a meaningful gift attitude** by not giving gifts to impress but giving only to those who really need or will appreciate your gift. Cut your gift list to a reasonable and minimum number of names. You don't have to give a bigger gift than you received last year.

Reindeer 6: **Be a smart shopper** by finding something on sale and buying many of them to give to those on your list. Also, try to shop alone whenever possible. Farm the kids out so you can shop peacefully.

Reindeer 7: **Enjoy the true meaning of the Holidays** by expressing your love and gratitude in many ways other than gift giving. Express your feelings and thoughts in cards and personal notes to those for whom you are grateful.

Reindeer 8: **Read and reflect on Holiday stories.** Talk about them with others until they become meaningful to you and your family.

IDENTIFYING TRAUMATIC STRESS

Be aware of the following warning signs for traumatic stress:

1. Recurring thoughts about the event (intrusive thoughts)
2. Recurring nightmares about the event
3. Sleep disturbance/appetite disturbance
4. Acting or feeling as if traumatic event is recurring, changes in appetite
5. Experience of anxiety and fear, especially when exposed to event reminiscent of trauma
6. Being on edge
7. Hypervigilant
8. Feeling depressed/sad
9. Low energy/fatigue
10. Memory difficulty, including difficulty in remembering aspects of the trauma
11. Difficulty with attention and concentration, unable to focus on work tasks or daily activities
12. Difficulty making decisions
13. Low frustration tolerance, easily agitated, angry or resentful
14. Feeling numb and withdrawn
15. Feeling disconnected or different from others
16. Mood swings, crying without provocation, feeling a sense of despair and hopelessness
17. Restricted range of affect
18. Sense of foreshortened future
19. Feeling overly fearful and protective of the safety of loved ones
20. Avoidant behavior (avoiding people, places or activities that provoke thought of the event)
21. Flashbacks of the event

Therapist's Guide to Clinical Intervention, Second Edition by Sharon L. Johnson (© 2003 Elsevier Inc.)

WHAT MANAGEMENT CAN DO TO MINIMIZE EMPLOYEE STRESS

Stress in the workplace is all too common. It is the source of hurt and dissatisfaction. It is usually one of the main factors employees cite when leaving an employment for some other opportunity. Management is the primary source of change in the workplace to reduce stress and make the work environment a healthy place rather than a toxic place in which to earn a living. The list below will be helpful to management of any company to focus on the environment and turn the tables and become healthy and productive.

1. Be familiar with community resources and company resources available to employees.
2. Be sensitive to work demand and adequate support to get tasks done.
3. Make sure that employees are given advance notice of upcoming deadlines.
4. Keep employees informed of changes taking place in the organization or changes in philosophy so that they feel included in change.
5. Be respectful of general ongoing work demand when considering adding demands unless it is absolutely necessary, and be realistic, validating, and supportive:
   a. Acknowledge the extra stress and inconvenience
   b. Demonstrate appreciation
   c. When possible, reward for extra efforts.
6. Make sure that adequate training is offered.
7. Whenever possible, offer continuing education.
8. Maintain regular evaluations so that people are aware of how they are doing the job.
9. When employees request support or are in obvious need of support, offer it.
10. Reinforce positive efforts, contributions, and accomplishments.
11. Whenever possible, challenge employees with interesting work.
12. Promote employees who have earned advancement.
13. Clearly define employee roles, expectations, areas of responsibility, and limits of authority.
14. Encourage employees to take breaks and mealtime breaks.
15. Encourage good health behaviors in employees. Offer smoking cessation information, nutrition and exercise education, stress management, and so forth whenever possible. If your company is not large enough, then have available a list of community resources.
16. Recognize that work stress and personal stress mutually affect all areas of a person's life.
17. Educate management at all levels about the signs and symptoms of stress in employees.
18. Consult with a professional who specializes in workplace environments and employee issues to maintain an optimally positive work environment.
19. As management, be aware of your own level of stress, and be a role model in practicing stress management techniques yourself.
20. Recognize your own limits of responsibility and power in the workplace.

Therapist's Guide to Clinical Intervention, Second Edition by Sharon L. Johnson (© 2003 Elsevier Inc.)

Depression and Self-Esteem

Chapter Contents

The emotional state of depression in our general population is increasing at an alarming rate. It is a malady that has existed as long as man has populated the earth. It is considered the nation's number one emotional illness. It is considered to be one of the most difficult disorders with which to cope on a day-to-day basis.

Depression and low self-esteem correlate. They are both issues in the life of individuals that need to be addressed simultaneously in therapy. This chapter provides a number of guidelines, questionnaires, forms, and therapeutic methodologies to address these twin self-defeating issues with patients.

DEPRESSION MYTHS

The following myths of depression need to be addressed with all or most depressed patients as part of their treatment program. Patients express relief when the myths they consider to be true are confronted and dispelled.

MYTH 1:   People who become depressed have weak characters.

MYTH 2:   Depression is shared equally by both sexes.

MYTH 3:   Depression is always caused by emotional distress.

MYTH 4:   Depression is unpleasant, but it cannot make you physically sick.

MYTH 5:   Your age has nothing to do with your likelihood of becoming depressed.

MYTH 6:   Depression does not destroy your desire for sexual romance.

MYTH 7:   A person with depression will always feel better in time, even without therapy or medication.

MYTH 8:   Treatment of depression inevitably means years of psychotherapy.

MYTH 9:   The psychological trigger for a period of depression is always obvious.

MYTH 10:   You can be treated effectively for depression by the use of medication alone.

MYTH 11:   You can always help a person with depression with some old-fashioned pep talks, especially when using some well-known quotations.

MYTH 12:   An episode of depression is sure to leave scars.

MYTH 13:   Depression will always return in time if you have had one episode of depression.

What other myth does the patient have that needs to be addressed before therapy can proceed?

TRIPLE-COLUMN TECHNIQUE TO UNDERSTAND AND CHANGE MY DEPRESSION

1. Analyze your thoughts that are associated with depression by filling out the spaces below whenever a feeling of depression occurs in the course of the day.
2. Do this activity daily for at least 10 days on different occasions when depression occurs.
3. Be as specific as possible.

Events that seemed to trigger the depression	Depressive thought	Other ways of thinking of the depressive thought
1. Making a typing error.	I'm a failure.	A mistake is not equal to failure. I don't always make typing errors.
2.		
3.		
4.		
5.		
6.		
7.		
8.		
9.		
10.		

COMMENTS OR OBSERVATIONS:

BIPOLAR: HOW TO BE SELF-DEFEATING

1. Drink alcohol like a fish.

2. Don't get regular or long hours of sleep.

3. Stay isolated and reclusive.

4. Don't do what your therapist says.

5. Try to solve your problem with medication only, no therapy.

6. Be passive and do not learn assertive communication skills.

7. Seek no spiritual guidance, encouragement or support.

8. Do not read on the bipolar disorder; remain ignorant of its nature.

9. Don't take your prescribe medication and don't try to get a prescription.

10. Hang out with other bipolar people.

11. Blame your parents and heritage, not yourself.

12. Get mad at being bipolar and don't do anything to improve your status.

13. Treat yourself with street drugs; you know better.

14. Adopt an attitude of "I don't care."

15. Come to believe in fate, chance or luck as the way to get better.

16. Wait for some "Powerful Other Person" to come along and give you the answer.

17. Don't work or go to school.

18. Don't join an organization or club.

BIPOLAR DISORDER HYPERSEXUALITY

For individuals with bipolar disorder, the extreme behaviors associated with mania can be devastating. While there is a listing of potential extreme behaviors in the *DSM* indicative of manic episodes, the review of one of those behaviors serves to highlight the damaging results.

Hypersexuality is defined as an increased need or compulsion for sexual gratification. A person may be reluctant to expose his/her experience of hypersexuality in treatment because of the associated immense feelings of shame. With the decreased inhibition associated with hypersexuality, individuals find themself engaging in sexual behaviors that they may consider "deviant or forbidden" and that result in feelings of shame. For some, the frequency of their compulsion is at an addictive level. In addition to feelings of shame, hypersexuality can destroy a marriage or a committed relationship and increase the risk of sexually transmitted diseases.

Regarding the issue of the broad patterns of sexual addiction behavior, the Mayo Clinic defines sexual addiction as a loss of control with the focus on compulsion: "compulsive sexual behavior refers to spending inordinate amounts of time in sexual related activity, to the point that one neglects important social, occupational, or recreational activities in favor of sexual behavior." According to the National Council on Sexual Addiction and Compulsivity addiction is characterized as "loss of the ability to choose freely whether to stop or to continue ... continuation of the behavior despite adverse consequences, such as loss of health, job, marriage, or freedom ... obsession with the activity."

Examples of the specific behaviors that are common to those who struggle with hypersexuality's compulsive and reckless behaviors include the following:

1. Fantasy sex

2. Fetishes

3. Inappropriate sexual touching

4. Sexual abuse and sexual assault

5. Compulsive masturbation

6. Compulsive sex with prostitutes

7. Masochism

8. Patronizing sex-oriented establishments

9. Voyeurism

10. Exhibitionism

The range of consequences associated with hypersexuality include the following:

1. Shame

2. Low self-esteem

3. Fear

4. Financial distress (cost of prostitutes/phone sex and items or activities in sex-oriented establishments)

5. Destruction of relationships

6. Health risk, loss of job (pornography on the computer, inappropriate behavior, etc.)

While evaluating and treating someone with bipolar disorder, the aforementioned information should clarify the importance of fully understanding the manic experience of the individual because of the potential deep-seated emotional damage resulting from extreme personally unacceptable behavior. Education and validation are important interventions.

Therapist's Guide to Clinical Intervention, Second Edition by Sharon L. Johnson (© 2003 Elsevier Inc.)

FEELING OVERWHELMED AND DESPERATE

When a person is depressed they often lack the energy to resolve problems as they arise. As a result, all of the new problems pile up on top of the difficulties which originally contributed to the state of depression. When this happens a person becomes overwhelmed. Being overwhelmed feels like there is just too much to deal with. They feel desperate because it seems like no matter what they do they will be unable to accomplish all that they have to. It may feel like there are no choices that can really help them. When this happens it may appear that suicide is the only way to escape from the awful, trapped feeling that they are experiencing.

Unfortunately, they are considering a permanent solution to temporary problems. There is always another way no matter how difficult the problems may be. If a person is at the point where they feel desperate and unable to cope the thing to do is to ask for help. If they are feeling that bad then they know that they are not emotionally well and it may require that others who care (family members, friends, therapists, ministers, physicians) are needed to break this downward spiral. Reach out to the people in your support system. If you don't have a support system, tell your physician or call a hospital Emergency Room for help. Get whatever help is necessary to problem solve the solutions that will create the support and structure to stabilize and manage the potentially destructive behavior. Sometimes someone else can offer a solution that a person in a state of being overwhelmed would not even be able to see because they are focusing only on how to escape these awful feelings.

If you have ever felt overwhelmed and desperate describe how you felt:

_____

_____

_____

How did you resolve the situation?

_____

_____

_____

What did you learn that could help you now?

_____

_____

_____

Therapist's Guide to Clinical Intervention, Second Edition by Sharon L. Johnson (© 2003 Elsevier Inc.)

THE HAPPINESS FACTOR

Happiness comes as a result of many distinct factors from our family background and our daily living experience. We learn to be happy and stay happy. Happiness can change over time and as our life experiences change. Here is a simple formula to guide your understanding of this very important aspect of your life.

$$Happiness = G + S + C + A$$

G = Genetic history. What is your family history of happiness? How happy were your parents, grandparents, aunts and uncles, and your cousins?

S = Situation in life. What is your situation in life now? What has it been? Are your circumstances generally positive and pleasant?

C = Choice of giving to others. What is your pattern of giving to others as in volunteering, gift giving, and charity giving?

A = Appreciation for what you have. What are you thankful for and what do you have or have done that makes you grateful?

Based on the answers above, what is your estimated "happiness level?"

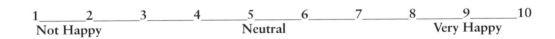

1_____2_____3_____4_____5_____6_____7_____8_____9_____10
Not Happy   Neutral   Very Happy

UNDERSTANDING SEASONAL AFFECTIVE DISORDER

Have you ever wondered why we associate light with love and happiness and why we associate darkness with emptiness and depression? Behavioral science research has discovered there is a relationship between light and mood. In some people a decrease in exposure to sunlight can cause symptoms of major depression. I experienced this with a family member who struggled with severe depression when she was living under the cloud cover of Seattle. When she moved to California she had almost a miraculous disappearance of depressive symptoms. Even in more sunny environments some people struggle with depressive symptoms during darker winter months.

The technical name for the depression produced by an absence of sunlight is Seasonal Affective Disorder (SAD). It is more common than you might think. It is estimated that 4 to 6 percent of the US population suffers from SAD. Ten to 20 percent of the population may suffer from a less severe form of sadness that we would call "winter-time blues."

WHO IS VULNERABLE TO SAD?

Because SAD is directly related to the absence of sunlight, people who live in northern climates with more cloud cover get SAD more often. One study found that about 10 percent of people in the northern USA, Finland, and Alaska suffer from SAD. Genetics also seem to be a factor. SAD is significantly higher in people who have close relatives who struggle with seasonal depression. Women comprise about 75 percent of the people with SAD. Most of the people who struggle with SAD are 20 to 40 years of age.

WHAT ARE THE SYMPTOMS OF SAD?

People who have the symptoms of SAD have a serious problem that can impair their ability to work and have healthy social relationships. Individuals with more severe symptoms of SAD have higher rate of suicide and substance abuse. The earlier SAD is treated the less likely it will be a problem in the future. Once the symptoms are recognized it is important to see a behavioral healthcare professional who can diagnose the problem. The symptoms of SAD include:

- Loss of interest in activities you once enjoyed
- Hopelessness
- Anxiety
- Loss of energy
- Social withdrawal
- Oversleeping
- Appetite changes, especially craving high carbohydrate foods
- Weight gain
- Difficulty concentrating

These symptoms may qualify you for diagnosis of depression whether of not your symptoms have a seasonal pattern. Many people struggle with depression that has no seasonal pattern.

A small number of people will actually have symptoms of reversed SAD during the summer months. These symptoms include:

- Persistently elevated mood
- Increased social activity
- Hyperactivity
- Abnormal enthusiasm

BIOLOGY OF SAD

The symptoms of SAD appear to be linked to the production of chemicals in the body that regulate mood. The mood regulating chemical that appears to be affected most by seasonal changes is serotonin. Drugs that allow more serotonin to get to the brain are effective in decreasing the symptoms of SAD. There is evidence that other hormones such as cortisol and thyroid may also play a part in the development of SAD symptoms.

DIAGNOSING SAD

If you think that you may have SAD it is important to see a mental health provider who can perform a psychological evaluation. They will ask you questions about seasonal changes in your mood, thoughts, lifestyle, work, and social situation. You may also be asked to fill out a depression questionnaire. Diagnosing SAD will depend on several factors such as:

- Whether you have experienced the symptoms of SAD at least two consecutive years in the same season.
- If the periods of depression have been followed by periods without depressive symptoms.
- If there are no other explanations for mood changes other than seasonal light.

TREATMENT OF SAD

Self-help
Mild seasonal mood changes that do not qualify for a diagnosis of SAD can often be managed without professional help. The things you can do that can improve your mood include:

- **Exercise:** Increase your exercise to improve your natural mood-regulating chemistry.
- **Get out:** Spend more time outdoors.
- **Vacation:** Take a annual winter vacation to a sunny location.
- **Move your desk:** If you can, move your desk or workstation to a window to get more sunlight.
- **Socialize:** Avoid isolation and keep connected with friends.
- **Manage stress:** Practice stress management during dark seasons.

Light Therapy

It is important to determine if you have SAD because light therapy may help decrease your symptoms. Light therapy uses bright lights that are designed to replicate sunlight. Controlled studies have found that 60 to 90 percent of people with SAD respond to light therapy. There are many different kinds of light devices on the market, which include the fluorescent light box, light visors, head-mounted units and small units that you can put on your desktop. The gold standard most-researched device is the fluorescent light box, which most people use in the privacy of their homes.

HOW MUCH LIGHT?

Getting a big enough "dose" of light is important. Average indoor lighting is about 500 lux while outdoor light can vary between 1000 and 50,000 lux. Most of the SAD research suggests that at least 2500 lux of light is requires for at least one to two hours a day. More recent research has found that 30 minutes a day with a light that produces 10,000 lux is also effective. Incandescent and fluorescent white light appear to be equally effective. Ultraviolet light is not necessary for the antidepressant response and should not be used due to long-term toxicity.

It takes at least one week of daily light therapy to see significant improvement in symptoms. Most people experience rapid recurrence of symptoms after discontinuing light therapy.

There are many types of devices on the market. The device you buy should meet government safety standards, have a filter for ultraviolet light, and have been tested in clinical trials.

SIDE EFFECTS

There are several side effects that people who use light therapy sometimes experience. These include eye strain or visual disturbances (19–27%), headache (13–21%), agitation or feeling "weird" (6–13%), nausea (7%), sweating (7%), and sedation (6–7%). These side effects are usually mild and tend to decrease over time.

You should get an ophthalmologic consultation before starting light therapy if you have any of the following risk factors for toxic light exposure:

- Retinal or eye disease
- Previous cataract surgery and lens removal

- Taking light-sensitive medications
- Phototherapy used for cancer or psoriasis
- Taking St John's Wort

Medication Treatment

Antidepressant medication has been found to decrease the symptoms of SAD in some cases. The medication that is right for you will depend on your individual biology. The Food and Drug Administration has approved several medications for the treatment of SAD. Consult with your physician to determine which medication is right for you.

Keep in mind that it normally takes several weeks to notice improvement when taking antidepressant medications. You may have to try several different antidepressants to find the one with the fewest side effects and best treatment response. Physicians often recommend that patients stay on antidepressants for a significant amount of time after the symptoms go into remission.

Psychotherapy

Most outcome studies have found that psychotherapy is as effective as medication in treating depression. With seasonal depression it may be wise to start psychotherapy before symptoms set in if you have a strong seasonal pattern. Cognitive behavioral psychotherapy has been found to be effective in helping people to change negative thought patterns that feed depressive symptoms.

If you struggle with recurrent depression having an established relationship with a therapist can be an invaluable resource. A professional who knows how you think and feel when you are slipping into depression can help you to more quickly make changes to avoid major problems. As with other health care, it is wise to check in several times a year to review how you are succeeding in your most important life areas.

Practicing spirituality

Having faith that your life has purpose is good medicine. Practicing spiritual disciplines can increase your capacity to focus your life in a positive direction. A great antidote for depression is connection. Many people have experienced that connection with others and with spiritual love decrease isolation and fear. Research has demonstrated that simply allowing yourself to feel love and gratitude during times of stress can improve your ability to think clearly and concentrate.

PURSUING PEACE IN THE MIDST OF A LOSS

A Personal Pursuit Exercise

Name: _____   Date: _____

Type of loss:
(Person, Thing,
Money, Identity, Image,
Possession, Trust)

Count my losses:
(What is the loss? What
will I miss? What will be no more?
Note prior losses)

Review my reactions:
(Initial reaction; Delayed
reaction; Emotions; Physical,
mental, and behavioral reactions)

Healthy response options:
(Actions with my support base;
Seeking out needed resources;
Drawing upon past experiences)

Future considerations:
(Skills I can draw on; People I
can depend on; How shall I
now live? My most likely option)

Recovery and resolution:
(I can make it; I want to live
beyond it; I forgive; I accept;
I can see benefits from it)

Other factors in finding my peace:

My next steps in my pursuit of peace:

THE SELF-ESTEEM REVIEW

DIRECTIONS: Review the following statements. Rate how much you believe each statement, from 1 to 5. The highest rating, 5, means that you think the statement is completely true; 0 means that you completely do not believe the statement.

RATING

1. I am a good and worthwhile person. _____

2. I am as valuable a person as anyone else. _____

3. I have good values that guide me in my life. _____

4. When I look at my eyes in the mirror, I feel good about myself. _____

5. I feel like I have done well in my life. _____

6. I can laugh at myself. _____

7. I like being me. _____

8. I like myself, even when others reject me. _____

9. Overall, I am pleased with how I am developing as a person. _____

10. I love and support myself, regardless of what happens. _____

11. I would rather be me than someone else. _____

12. I respect myself. _____

13. I continue to grow personally. _____

14. I feel confident about my abilities. _____

15. I have pride in who I am and what I do. _____

16. I am comfortable in expressing my thoughts and feelings. _____

17. I like my body. _____

18. I handle difficult situations well. _____

19. Overall, I make good decisions. _____

20. I am a good friend and people like to be with me. _____

Your score: _____

0 _____ 100

Total lack of self-esteem   **High self-esteem**

Therapist's Guide to Clinical Intervention, Second Edition by Sharon L. Johnson (© 2003 Elsevier Inc.)

10 SELF-ESTEEM BOOSTERS

1. Be realistic
   a. Do not compare yourself to others
   b. Be satisfied with doing your best

2. Focus on your accomplishments
   a. Each day review what you *have* done
   b. Give yourself credit for what you do

3. Use positive mental imagery
   a. Imagine success
   b. Mentally rehearse confidence

4. Look inside not outside
   a. Avoid being materialistic or identifying yourself by what you have
   b. Identify your sense of purpose

5. Actively live your life
   a. Set goals
   b. Think strategically

6. Be positive
   a. Substitute negative thoughts with realistic positive thoughts
   b. Acknowledge that how you think affects how you feel

7. Have genuine gratitude
   a. Be grateful for all that you have
   b. Appreciate your life as a gift

8. Meditate
   a. Think of peaceful, pleasant things
   b. Learn to relax and let go of stress
   c. Use positive affirmations

9. Develop positive self-care as a lifestyle
   a. Believe you are worthy of taking care of yourself
   b. Take care of your health

10. Appropriately get your needs met
    a. Identify what you need
    b. Identify your choices for getting those needs met

Positive self-esteem is an active process. Daily efforts will make a difference in your life experience.

Therapist's Guide to Clinical Intervention, Second Edition by Sharon L. Johnson (© 2003 Elsevier Inc.)

Insomnia and Sleep Therapy

Chapter Contents

Restful sleep is as crucial to mental health as it is to one's physical well-being. The lack of sleep and restless sleep are contributing factors to agitation, depression, learning impairments, relationship problems, and general ill health. It is not uncommon for patients to complain of chronic poor sleep habits and need professional help in this area of their life. While sleep impairment may be the basis for coming to therapy, it could be a secondary issue that emerges in the initial assessment and will need to be addressed before therapy can be completed.

The forms, questionnaires, exercises, logs, and guidelines in this chapter on sleep patterns will help the therapist deal with this problem area effectively and constructively.

10 TIPS FOR BETTER SLEEP

People suffer from insomnia for different reasons. Sleep disturbance can be related to physiological changes such as menopause, medical problems such as hyperthyroidism, emotional distress such as depression or anxiety, changes in lifestyle such as having a baby or any other changes that may influence daily patterns, and general life stressors. Take a few minutes to review what may possibly be related to the difficulty that you are experiencing with sleep.

If it has been some time since your last physical examination or you think that there may be a relationship between the sleep disturbance and physiological changes or a medical problem make an appointment with your physician to identify or rule out health-related issues. If health-related issues are definitely not a factor then consider the following ways to improve your sleep.

If you are not able to identify the exact symptoms of your insomnia keep a sleep journal for 2 weeks and write down your sleep–wake cycle, how many hours you sleep, and all the other details related to your sleep disturbance.

1. Establish a regular time for going to bed, and be consistent. This helps to cue you that it is time for sleep. Going to sleep at the same time and awakening at the same time daily helps stabilize your internal clock. Having a different sleep–wake schedule on the weekends can throw you off. For the best results be consistent.

2. Do not go to bed too early. Do not be tempted to try to go bed earlier than you would normally need to. If you have started doing this then identify the reason why (depression, stress, boredom, pressure from your partner). When people go to bed too early it contributes to the problem of fragmented sleep. Your body normally lets you sleep only the number of hours it needs. If you go to bed too early you will also be waking too early.

3. Determine how many hours of sleep you need for optimal functioning and feeling rested. Consider the following to determine the natural length of your sleep cycle.
   a. How many hours did you sleep on the average as a child?
   b. Before you began to experience sleep difficulty how many hours of sleep per night did you sleep on the average?
   c. How many hours of sleep do you need to awaken naturally, without an alarm?
   d. How many hours of sleep do you need in order not to feel sleepy or tired during the day?

4. Develop rituals that signal the end of the day. Rituals that signal closure for the day could be tucking the kids in, putting the dog out, and closing up the house for the night … then … it's time for you to wind down by watching the news, reading a book (not an exciting mystery), having a cup of calming herbal tea, evening prayers, or doing something like meditation, deep breathing exercises, or progressive muscle relaxation. All of these behaviors are targeted for shifting your thinking from the daily stressors to closure, that the day is over and it is time for rest so that you can start a new day tomorrow.

5. Keep the bedroom for sleeping and sex only. If you use your bedroom as an office or for other activities your mind will associate the bedroom with those activities, which is not conducive to sleep.

6. A normal pattern of sex can be helpful. However, it is only helpful if you are engaging in sex because you are interested in being close to your partner. Sexual stimulation releases endorphins that give you a mellow, relaxed feeling. Be careful to avoid trying to use sex to fall asleep. It can backfire because you are taking a pleasurable, ultimately relaxing behavior and putting expectations on it that can lead to pressure and feeling upset.

7. Avoid physical and mental stimulation just before sleep time. Exercising, working on projects, or house cleaning, watching something exciting on television, or reading something that has an exciting plot just prior to going to bed can energize you instead of helping you to have closure at the end of the day.

8. Be careful of naps. Some people are able to take naps and feel rejuvenated by them without interfering with their sleep–wake cycle. Other people may be overtired for various reasons and benefit from an hour nap early in the afternoon. However, for others it can be sabotaging. If you take naps, skip them for a week. If you find that you are sleeping better without the naps then stop napping.

Therapist's Guide to Clinical Intervention, Second Edition by Sharon L. Johnson (© 2003 Elsevier Inc.)

9. Get regular exercise. Regular aerobic exercise like walking can decrease body tension, alleviate stress, alleviate depressive symptoms, and contribute to an overall feeling of well-being. Less stress, better sleep.

10. Take a warm bath one to two hours before bedtime. Experiment with the time to determine what works best for you. A good 20-minute soaking in a warm bath (100–102 °F; 37–38 °C) is a great relaxer. It raises your core body temperature by several degrees which naturally induces drowsiness and sleep.

Be careful not to obsess about sleep. When someone is experiencing sleep disturbance they can become so focused on the issue of sleep that they nearly develop a phobia about not getting it, which creates a lot of stress and tension for them at the end of the day instead of relaxation which is necessary for the natural sleep rhythms to be initiated. Instead, try to relax and think about something pleasant. If, after 20 minutes, that does not work get up and go to another room to meditate, or engage in some other ritual that you find helpful to induce feelings of drowsiness so you can sleep.

INSOMNIA: WHAT IS IT AND WHAT DO WE DO ABOUT IT?

There is little question that insomnia is real. It is a significant problem for 37 million Americans over 55 years of age who do not get enough of deep restorative sleep they need to function well. Studies demonstrate that 13 percent of the male population and 26 percent of the female population complain of insomnia. Insomnia is no respecter of person or age. It is found among all ethnic groups. With increasing age, our need for sleep remains about the same but the quality of sleep slowly deteriorates. Insomnia is generally understood to be a significant sleep disorder if it occurs four or more times per week.

Sleep disorder researchers agree on six factors that contribute to insomnia. They are:

1. Underlying biological factors.
2. Underlying psychological factors.
3. The use of drugs and alcohol.
4. Disturbing environmental factors.
5. Negative learning experiences.
6. Pre-sleep and sleep habits.

WHAT DO YOU DO ABOUT IT

There have been many strategies proposed for the treatment of insomnia. For many people, the focus is placed on biological factors. For them medication therapies are thought to be the be-all and end-all of this problem. Unfortunately, medications to aid sleep are not the answer for most people. They can interact with other medications and create other problems. They can hide or cover up other medical conditions needing medical attention. They can impair motor and cognitive functioning if used over an extended period of time.

For others, insomnia is considered to be a result of learned behavior. For them there is a need to unlearn certain patterns of behavior associated with insomnia and learn new behavioral patterns associated with healthy sleep habits.

Others approach insomnia with a strong belief in the power of pre-sleep and sleep habits. Some specific home remedies or prohibitions are the answer for them. For example, coffee is not consumed after 6.00 p.m. Certain bedtime rituals must be followed obsessively.

There are as many answers for insomnia as there are people to be asked. We all think we know the answer. However, each sleeper must find his/her own answer and then stick with it. Research has indicated that there are some generally accepted strategies that help many people.

Whatever approach is adopted, it is important to start out with the selection of a mattress that fits the weight and frame of your body and your sleep style preference. Bed linens are also a strong consideration. For some, sleep is facilitated by the material of the sheets utilized. If a pad is utilized, it is important that the pad be stabilized and held in a smooth and comfortable position.

HELPFUL HINTS FOR EASING INTO SLEEP

1. Exercise in the morning or afternoon but not immediately before bedtime. However, a light evening stroll for relaxation purposes could be helpful.
2. Nap during the day, but restrict it to one hour and at the same time each day, preferably between noon and 4.00 p.m., as this is the body's natural down time.
3. Do not consume caffeine beverages such as coffee, chocolate, mocha, sodas, and tea after 6.00 p.m. Evening alcohol consumption and smoking is not recommended.
4. Use sleeping pills under a physician's directions and usually not for more than a month or two to break the cycle of insomnia.
5. Do not eat a large meal within an hour or two of bedtime. A light evening meal is recommended.

6. Develop a pre-sleeping routine such as proceeding through a series of relaxation exercises, listening to music, writing in a daily journal or taking a shower or bath. The use of the radio as part of pre-sleep routine may be helpful to distract interfering thoughts.

7. A bed is for sleeping so don't use it as a place for eating, watching television, reading or carrying out an argument.

8. If you do not fall asleep within 20 minutes, get out of bed and engage in some relaxing activity for 20 minutes. Return to bed and proceed through your pre-sleeping routine. However, if you are not sleeping within 20 minutes, get out of bed again and repeat the relaxing activity. After 20 minutes return back to bed and engage in your pre-sleeping routine. Repeat this procedure throughout the night until you fall asleep. Continue this routine for at least 30 days.

9. Room temperature and air quality may be important for sleep. Determine what is the best temperature for you and maintain that temperature in the bedroom all night.

10. Sleep the same hours each night of the week. Remember that while 7 or 8 hours of sleep is desirable, the body can function on 6 hours of sleep.

11. Some herbal teas have been found to be soothing. Some may have sedative qualities.

12. If you suspect sleep apnea such as heavy snoring, gasping for air while sleeping and have frequent brief sleep interruptions, consider consulting a medical sleep clinic.

13. If you are a person who worries and becomes stressed regarding problems in living, do not work on worrisome or stressful projects within an hour of bedtime.

14. Use imagery to your advantage. Select an image that you can focus on while falling asleep. Images commonly used are a burning candle, a favorite vacation scene, clouds, a pleasant fantasy, waterfalls, floating on or sinking into a mattress.

15. Use a muscle relaxation procedure in which five or six muscle groups are sequentially tensed and held tense for 5 seconds and then relaxed. Do this over a 10 to 15 minute period of time starting with the feet and legs and proceeding to the head.

16. Should you choose to have a late night snack, it would be best to select foods that are rich in L-tryptophane, an amino acid that may contribute to improve sleep patterns. A sample of such food products would be milk, eggs, cottage cheese, soy beans, tuna, and turkey.

17. Engage in a mental activity that exercises both sides of the brain simultaneously. The left brain processes a lineal sequence of information such as saying the alphabet, counting numbers or lining up objects from simple to complex or from small to large. The right brain processes the visual representation of an activity and creates the visual image of the activity. Hence, if you count backwards or say the alphabet backwards while visualizing numbers or letters being written on a large blackboard in your mind, both parts of the brain are active simultaneously and may serve to distract the brain from activity that would compete with sleep.

IS A MID-DAY NAP RECOMMENDED FOR INSOMNIA?

Some people find a mid-day nap helpful while others do not. It is important if you have insomnia to go to bed and wake up at the same time each night. It is also important if you do take a nap that you do so at the same time each day, such as mid afternoon, but only nap for one hour. This is called a "power nap." Do not sleep for lengthy periods of time. Be sure to program your day so that you will stay awake throughout the day other than at the time taken for the power nap and your regular bedtime.

IS PROFESSIONAL CONSULTATION INDICATED?

By all means. Genuine sleep disorders, such as insomnia, require professional evaluation and professional intervention should be seriously considered. As indicated above, there are many reasons for insomnia. There are also many alternative professional treatment approaches that can be utilized besides the informal approaches noted above.

A person with insomnia may benefit from different professional consultations and treatment approaches, such as, biofeedback training, acupuncture, chiropractic services, massage, and a referral to a medical sleep clinic. Whatever approach is utilized, it is important to pursue it for at least a few months before considering a different alternative.

IS SLEEP RELATED TO ANY KNOWN FACTORS?

Sleep patterns are enhanced by the general happiness level of an individual or group of people. In other words, the better the physical, mental, and emotional health of an individual, the better the quality of sleep. Times of unrest such as unemployment or worrisome situations interfere with quality sleep.

HOW CAN I LEARN MORE TO HELP ME SLEEP?

The following Internet websites would be good sources to consult:
www.talkaboutsleep.com After accessing the site, click on Sleep Basics.
www.sleepfoundation.org

SLEEP IMPROVEMENT PROGRAM

The instructions summarized here are designed to help you understand how to improve your sleep habits. Remember to follow them carefully. As you start your program, it may be somewhat difficult. After the first week or so, however, you will find that your efforts begin to pay off and these instructions will become easier to follow. In a short period of time, you should begin to sleep better and awake more refreshed.

1. Prepare for bed and go to sleep ONLY when you are actually sleepy.
2. Do not use your bed for anything except sleeping. That is, do not read, watch television, eat, or worry in bed. Sexual activity is the only exception to this rule. On such occasions, follow these instructions afterwards when you intend to go to sleep.
3. If you are unable to fall asleep, get up and go into another room. Stay up as long as you wish and then return to your bedroom to sleep. Remember, your goal is to associate your bed with falling asleep QUICKLY. So, if when you go to bed you are still awake after ten minutes or so, follow this instruction.
4. If you return to bed and still cannot sleep, repeat step 3 again. Do this as often as necessary until you fall asleep within about 10 minutes.
5. Set your alarm and get up at the same time every morning, regardless of how much sleep you got during the night. This will help your body develop a consistent sleep rhythm.
6. Do not take an extensive nap during the day. Keep it to 1 hour.
7. Prepare the sleeping area and bed in such a manner as to encourage sleeping. For example, if music helps, feel free to use it, if the door is best open or closed, arrange it accordingly.
   ALSO, REMEMBER TO:
8. Do your relaxation program exercises as you go to bed, besides your usual daily practice sessions. Fill out your sleeping log improvement each morning.
9. Fill out your Sleep Diary each morning upon getting up.

FOLLOW THESE SAME INSTRUCTIONS IF YOU AWAKEN AND CANNOT FALL BACK TO SLEEP.

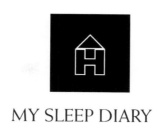

MY SLEEP DIARY

NAME: _____

This diary is designed to help you identify your particular sleep patterns and follow your progress in changing it. Remember to fill the form out regularly each morning upon awakening. Do not be discouraged if your problem does not improve every night. Remember that you are learning an important new skill. This takes time, effort, and patience. Separately, state what strategy you are using to improve your sleep problem, e.g.: "As of today, I am going to do the following to help me sleep better (i.e., bell-alarm program, daily record keeping system, a pre-sleep routine).

	I WENT TO BED AT ____ (time)	I AWOKE ____ TIMES IN THE NIGHT	I SLEPT A TOTAL OF ____ HOURS	WHEN I GOT UP THIS MORNING, I FELT _____ (circle one)	OVERALL, MY SLEEP LAST NIGHT WAS _____ (circle one)
Night 1				<u>Exhausted Refreshed</u> –3 –2 –1 0 +1 +2 +3	<u>Very Restless Very Sound</u> –3 –2 –1 0 +1 +2 +3
Night 2				–3 –2 –1 0 +1 +2 +3	–3 –2 –1 0 +1 +2 +3
Night 3				–3 –2 –1 0 +1 +2 +3	–3 –2 –1 0 +1 +2 +3
Night 4				–3 –2 –1 0 +1 +2 +3	–3 –2 –1 0 +1 +2 +3
Night 5				–3 –2 –1 0 +1 +2 +3	–3 –2 –1 0 +1 +2 +3
Night 6				–3 –2 –1 0 +1 +2 +3	–3 –2 –1 0 +1 +2 +3
Night 7				–3 –2 –1 0 +1 +2 +3	–3 –2 –1 0 +1 +2 +3

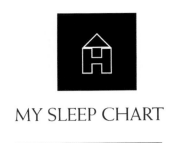

MY SLEEP CHART

NAME: _____

To help change my sleep pattern, I will engage in a relaxation program to reduce the tension and level of arousal of my body. I will commit to one or more relaxation times during my day and before I end my day and go to bed. I will also keep records of my sleep patterns for the next 20 days.

Day	5-minute brief relaxation today	10-minute evening relaxation before bed	Number of times of night-time awakening	Degree of restful sleep (Very Poor, Poor, Fair, Good, Very Good)
1				
2				
3				
4				
5				
6				
7				
8				
9				
10				
11				
12				
13				
14				
15				
16				
17				
18				
19				
20				

SLEEPING IMPROVEMENT LOG

Day	Did I do my brief relaxation exercises today?	Did I do my 10 minute relaxation pre-bedtime routine?	Number of night-time awakenings	Degree of restful sleep (Poor, Fair, Good)	Other
1					
2					
3					
4					
5					
6					
7					
8					
9					
10					
11					
12					
13					
14					

COMMENTS AND NOTES:

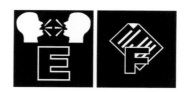

HELPING SLEEP THROUGH USE OF MEDICATION

MEDICATION ISSUES:

☐   The patient is on medication for sleep assistance.

☐   The risks and benefits have been reviewed in the past three months.

☐   The patient's Responsible Party and physician have been consulted and agree with the ongoing use of this medication.

☐   The factors for which the medication is being used have been reviewed.

☐   All other factors that may be contributing to poor sleep have been reviewed.

☐   The side effects of this medication have been reviewed and addressed.

☐   A dosage reduction of the medication has been considered and it was determined that a reduction or discontinuance of the medication is not warranted.

☐   The ongoing use of this medication is in the best interest of the patient and results in a positive quality of life.

☐   The use of the medication is being monitored closely for side effects, possible dosage reduction, and relative benefits.

☐   A change of medication has been considered or is under consideration.

☐   Other _____

Therapist signature: _____ Date: _____

IMPORTANCE OF GOOD SLEEP HABITS

Over 60 million Americans suffer from some type of sleep disorder to the degree to which their health and daily functioning is impaired. Many more have generally poor sleep habits. As a step in the process of developing a positive sleep pattern, one needs to know the consequences of chronic sleep disturbance.

- Poor sleep tends to break good eating habits resulting in weight gain.
- Poor sleep habits contribute to death at an earlier age.
- Poor sleep habits lead to the onset of diabetes.
- Poor sleep habits are associated with heart disorder risks.
- Poor sleep habits are associated with states of depression and low self-esteem.
- Poor sleep habits contribute to increased alcohol intake and associated addiction.
- Poor sleep habits are related to increased auto accidents and injuries at work and in the home.
- Poor sleep habits lead to blood pressure increases.
- Poor sleep habits contribute to poor decision making and choices.
- Poor sleep habits are likely to promote falls and balance problems.

COMMENTS:

1. Which of the above factors are relevant to your sleep patterns?

2. What help do you need to get started on changing your current sleep habits?

3. What needs to be done to assure that you stay with a new sleep pattern for the next 30 days?

Addictive Behavior

Chapter Contents

The addiction to alcohol, drugs, medication, pornography, gambling, sexual activity, computer gaming, jogging, and a variety of other activities can be the downfall of anyone. Such individuals show up in the office of a therapist at the time of a crisis. Generally, when a patient has lost or is about to lose everything, a referral for counseling is activated. Of all self-defeating behavior, addiction may be of the worst kind. It often takes years of therapy and concerted effort on the part of the patient's support system before a patient can be addiction free.

The forms in this chapter will assist the therapist aggressively help addicted patients and start them out on a new path of personal, cognitive, and emotional freedom. Success requires the participation of the family as the primary support system. Forms are also provided to help with family intervention.

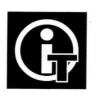

SIGNS OF ALCOHOLISM

Red Flag #1: Physiological Detection

- Genetic predisposition
- Liver problems
- Diabetes
- High blood pressure
- Weight fluctuations
- Rhinorrhea
- Lip and finger burns
- Dilated or pinned pupils
- Excess perspiration

Red Flag #2: Psychological Detection

- Past history of psychiatric problems or treatment
- Chronic pain problems
- Depression
- Anxiety
- Attention deficit disorder
- Avid psychopharmacologic interest
- Excessive mood swings
- Loss of interest in friends and activities

Red Flag #3: Behavioral Detection

- Past history of drug and/or alcohol problems
- Legal problems
- Poor work history
- Financial problems
- Extremely talkative
- Poor judgment
- Chronic relationship problems
- Erratic behavior

Red Flag #4: Style of Alcohol Consumption

- Early problematic use
  - Relief drinking
  - Surreptitious drinking
  - Anticipatory drinking
  - Gulping drinks
  - Tendency to never leave unconsumed alcohol
- Signs of great problem severity
  - Rationalizing drinking
  - Protecting the supply
  - Geographic escapes to facilitate drinking
  - Regular morning drinking
  - Attempts to set control points

Red Flag #5: On-the-Job Signs

- AOD excessive use
  - Late (after lunch)
  - Leaves job early
  - Occasionally absent
  - Fellow workers complain
  - Overreacts to real or imagined criticism
  - Complains of not feeling well
  - Shades the truth
  - Misses deadlines
  - Mistakes through inattention or poor judgment
  - Decreased efficiency

Red Flag #6: On-the-Job Signs

- AOD abuse
  - Frequent days off for vague ailments or implausible reasons
  - Statements become undependable
  - Begins to avoid associates
  - Borrows money from co-workers
  - Exaggerates work accomplishments
  - Hospitalized more than average
  - Repeated minor injuries on and off job
  - Unreasonable resentment
  - General deterioration
  - Spasmodic work pace
  - Attention wanders, lack of concentration

Cont.

Red Flag #7: On-the-Job Signs
- AOD severe abuse
  - Frequent time off, sometimes for several days
  - Fails to return from lunch
  - Domestic problems interfere with work
  - Apparent loss of ethical values
  - Money problems – garnishment of salary
  - Increased hospitalizations
  - Refusal to discuss problems
  - Trouble with the law
  - Performance far below normal

Red Flag #8: On-the-Job Signs
- AOD dependence
  - Prolonged
  - Unpredictable absences
  - Drinking on the job
  - Totally undependable
  - Repeated hospitalizations
  - Visible physical deterioration
  - Money problems increase
  - Serious family problems and/or divorce
  - General incompetence
  - Work interferes with drinking
  - Compulsive attempts to store alcohol for future needs

Adapted from Matrix Institute on Addictions, UCLA Alcoholism and Addiction Medicine Service.

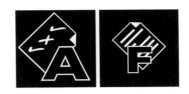

ALCOHOL ADDICTION QUESTIONNAIRE

Name: _____ Date: _____

The following three questionnaires are used to assess alcohol addictive behavior. The scores on all three questionnaires should be considered, especially if the scores are internally consistent. A plan of action needs to be developed from these results.

CAGE

1. Have you ever felt you should *Cut down* on your drinking or drug use?   Y   N
2. Have people *Annoyed* you by criticizing your drinking or drug use?   Y   N
3. Have you ever felt bad or *Guilty* about your drinking or drug use?   Y   N
4. Have you ever had a drink or used drugs first thing in the morning to steady your nerves or to get rid of a hangover or withdrawal state (*Eye-opener*)?   Y   N

FOY

1. Does anyone in your *Family* think you drink or use too much?   Y   N
2. Do any *Others* think you drink or use too much?   Y   N
3. Do *You* think you drink or use too much?   Y   N

TWEAK

1. How many drinks can you hold? (3+ suggests *Tolerance*)   Y   N
2. Have close friends or relatives *Worried* about your drinking in the past year?   Y   N
3. Do you sometimes take a drink in the morning when you awaken (*Eye-opener*)?   Y   N
4. Have friends or relatives ever told you something you said or did while you were drinking that you could not recall (*Amnesia*)?   Y   N
5. Do you ever feel the need to *(K)cut* down on your drinking?   Y   N

COMMENTS OR PLAN OF ACTION:

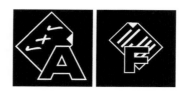

ALCOHOL INVOLVEMENT SCALE

Name: _____ Date: _____

PLEASE RATE EACH DRINKING BEHAVIOR ON THE SCALE AS INDICATED:

0 = never   1 = rarely or infrequently   2 = half the time   3 = usually/mostly   4 = always

1. Stops drinking when effects felt _____
2. Eats when drinking _____
3. Drinks to safe limit _____
4. Drinks as part of other activity _____
5. Enjoys social occasions where few drinks _____
6. Drinks before party _____
7. Annoyed by a low drinking _____
8. Continues to drink after party _____
9. Drinks more than intends _____
10. Unable to control drinking _____
11. Enjoys social occasions only if drinking _____
12. Sneaks drinks _____
13. Extravagant when drinking _____
14. Drinks whatever available _____
15. Attends non-drinking party _____
16. Leaves non-drinking party _____
17. Drinks when upset _____
18. Buys enough alcohol for Holidays _____
19. Suffers loss of memory _____
20. Suffers hangovers _____
21. Treats hangover with drink _____
22. Uneasy with talk of drinking _____
23. Worries about drinking _____
24. Drinking part of doing _____
25. Goes on binges _____
26. People disapprove of drinking _____
27. Gets drunk without intending to _____
28. Drinks regardless of consequences _____
29. Drinks in morning _____
30. Drinks alone _____
31. Needs days to recuperate from drink _____
32. Drunk steadily _____
33. Ashamed of habit _____
34. Drinks to relieve depression _____
Total Score _____

CIRCLE THE FIVE ITEMS THAT REPRESENT A SIGNIFICANT PROBLEM FOR YOU OR YOUR FAMILY OR OTHERS

AM I ABUSING ALCOHOL AND AT RISK?

QUESTIONS TO BE ASKED AND CONSIDERED

1. Have you ever felt like you need to reduce the amount of alcohol consumed?
2. Have you ever felt like you need to stop drinking altogether?
3. Have your friends, family or physician ever expressed concern for your drinking?
4. Have you ever used alcohol to prevent "the shakes" or as a morning eye-opener?
5. Have you ever felt guilty and/or shameful about your use of alcohol?
6. Do you drink to remove feelings of sadness and loneliness?
7. Do you drink to stop negative thinking or painful thoughts?
8. Have you consumed alcohol to excess after experiencing a loss/death in your life?
9. Does your drinking put others at risk for their own safety?
10. Has your drinking been associated with an accident, a seizure or suicide ideas?

If you answer yes to more than one of the above questions, it is time to change your drinking behavior

OTHER CONSIDERATIONS

Researchers from the University of Montreal and the University of Western Ontario have found evidence for limited or moderate drinking to be set at one drink per occasion. A drink is defined as:

- 5 ounces of wine
- 1.5 ounces of liquor
- 12 ounces of beer or cooler
- 3 ounces of port, sherry or vermouth

Additionally, they warn against drinking for the festive feeling. Further, they warn against the tendency to drink increasing amounts of alcohol over time, which is the natural tendency and a sure sign of addictive patterns being established.

If you have a problem with any one of these drinking styles, it is time to change your drinking behavior.

MY PLANS FOR CHANGING MY DRINKING BEHAVIOR:

1.
2.
3.
4.
5.

GUIDELINES FOR MODERATE DRINKING

Moderate drinking, also known as controlled drinking, is possible for some people to achieve, but the risk of excessive and out-of-control drinking is always present. Some people want to try to achieve moderate drinking. Some have to try it before they will be convinced it is not possible for them to consume alcohol in a controlled manner. For those that desire to try a period of moderate drinking, here is a set of guidelines that might yield positive results. If it fails, abstinence is the next alternative.

WHEN, WHAT

1. Drink only in social settings, with other people – avoid drinking alone.
2. Wait until after 5:00 p.m. before having a drink; never drink in the morning.
3. Drink only at mealtime or in the evening at parties.
4. During a meal, a glass of beer or wine is better than distilled liquor.
5. Distilled liquor is drunk only before a meal, or at a party.
6. Drink only beer, wine or mixed drinks – avoid straight drinks.
7. Avoid drinking when you are upset, anxious, worried or angry. Find someone to talk to instead.

HOW, HOW MUCH

1. Take at least 20–30 minutes to finish a drink.
2. Make a drink last for at least 6–8 sips, even more, if possible.
3. Pause for a while between sips and try to increase the length of the pause.
4. When you finish a drink, wait 5–15 minutes before starting another.
5. Limit yourself to 2 drinks at a meal.
6. Limit yourself to 2 drinks per hour at a party, and less if it is a long party – say, 5 drinks per 3 hours, or 6 drinks per 4 hours.
7. At parties, eat something along with drinking.
8. Avoid drinking at parties more than 2 or 3 nights per week.
9. Learn how to say "no" when offered a drink, or when someone really tries to talk you into drinking. Think of 5 possible answers you can give --- be ready with an answer.
10. If you are partying, drink an occasional glass of water or soda; it gives you something to sip while helping to space out your drinks.

SCREEN FOR GAMBLING ADDICTION

When conducting an intake there are many different types of problems and addiction to be queried. The addiction to gambling is one of them these days, with a huge number of casinos now available in most states. This is not to overlook the more traditional gambling experiences of people. As a screening strategy, Johnson and his colleagues (*Psychological Reports*, 80, 83–8, 1988) formulated two questions that can be asked in the initial diagnostic interview.

If the person answers "Yes" to one or both questions, further inquiry is in order. A problem may exist. The therapist is then encouraged to pursue it, as the indications of an addiction or problem are present. If the person answers "No" to both questions, no further inquiry would seem necessary.

TWO QUESTIONS ON GAMBLING

1. Have you ever felt the need to bet more and more money?
2. Have you ever had to lie to people important to you about how much you gambled?

While these questions were designed to assess gambling problems, there may be some face value reason to employ these questions when assessing other addictions, such as alcoholism, pornography, drug addiction, and compulsive eating. In such cases use the results with caution. Further assessment may be indicated. Independent verification is always a good avenue to undertake.

DO I HAVE A GAMBLING PROBLEM?

A. In the past 12 months:

1. Have you needed to gamble with increasing amounts of money or with larger bets than before in order to get the same feeling of excitement?

   Yes ☐   No ☐

2. Have you continued to gamble in spite of adverse consequences that have affected your finances, family relationships, work, or other parts of your life?

   Yes ☐   No ☐

3. Have you lied to family members, friends, or others about how much you gamble?

   Yes ☐   No ☐

4. Have there been periods lasting 2 weeks or longer when you spent a lot of time thinking about your gambling experiences or planning out future gambling ventures or bets?

   Yes ☐   No ☐

5. Have you tried but not succeeded in stopping, cutting, down, or controlling your gambling behavior?

   Yes ☐   No ☐

B. In the past 12 months:

1. Have you contemplated or attempted suicide?

   Yes ☐   No ☐

2. Have you contemplated or attempted to do physical harm to another person?

   Yes ☐   No ☐

C. In the past 30 days, how many days have you played and gambled?

Bingo ☐
Bowling, pool, golf, or other games of skill ☐
Card games (non-casino) ☐
Casino table games ☐
Dice games, dominoes ☐
Horses, dogs, roosters ☐
Gambling more than you can afford ☐
Gambling and substance use in the same day ☐
Internet gambling ☐
Lottery, numbers, instant tickets, scratch offs ☐
Other forms of gambling ☐
Play slots, poker machines, and video lottery terminals ☐
Various sports (Professional) ☐
Various sports (Semi-Professional) ☐
Various sports (College) ☐
Stock options, commodities ☐
Other ☐

D. In the past 30 days:

1. How much money would you say you spent per week on gambling and all associated expenses? $_____
2. Number of gambling episodes per week _____

E. What do you need to do to totally stop gambling forever?

1.

2.

3.

4.

5.

Name: _____ Date: _____

MY GAMBLING PATTERN IN THE PAST YEAR

Name: _____

Date: _____

	Yes	No
1. Have you often found yourself thinking about gambling (e.g., reliving past gambling experiences, planning the next time you will play or thinking of ways to get money to gamble)?	☐	☐
2. Have you needed to gamble with more and more money to get the amount of excitement you are looking for?	☐	☐
3. Have you become restless or irritable when trying to cut down or stop gambling?	☐	☐
4. Have you gambled to escape from problems or when you are feeling depressed, anxious or bad about yourself?	☐	☐
5. After losing money gambling, have you returned another day in order to get even?	☐	☐
6. Have you lied to your family or others to hide the extent of your gambling?	☐	☐
7. Have you made repeated unsuccessful attempts to control, cut back or stop gambling?	☐	☐
8. Have you been forced to go beyond what is strictly legal in order to finance gambling or to pay gambling debts?	☐	☐
9. Have you risked or lost a significant relationship, job, educational or career opportunity because of gambling?	☐	☐
10. Have you sought help from others to provide the money to relieve a desperate financial situation caused by gambling?	☐	☐

Comment:
5 or more "Yes" answers indicates a likely diagnosis finding for Pathological Gambling. Less than 5 "Yes" answers indicates a potential problem and/or a risk indicator which may warrant further support, education, and treatment services.

Adapted from the American Psychiatric Association Diagnostic Manual *DSM IV*, 1994.

GAMBLERS ANONYMOUS – 20 QUESTIONS

Are you Living with a Compulsive Gambler?

If there is a gambling problem in your home, the Gam-Anon family group may be able to help you cope with it. If you are living with a compulsive gambler, you will answer "Yes" to at least 6 of the following questions. To indicate a "Yes" answer, circle the items that best describe your situation.

1. Do you find yourself constantly bothered by bill collectors?
2. Is the person in question often away from home for long, unexplained periods of time?
3. Does this person ever lose time from work due to gambling?
4. Do you feel that this person cannot be trusted with money?
5. Does the person in question faithfully promise that he/she will stop gambling; beg, plead, for another chance, yet gamble again and again?
6. Does this person ever gamble longer than he/she intended to, until the last dollar is gone?
7. Does this person immediately return to gambling to try to recover losses, or to win more?
8. Does this person ever gamble to get money to solve financial difficulties or have unrealistic expectations that gambling will bring the family material comfort and wealth?
9. Does this person borrow money to gamble with or to pay gambling debts?
10. Has this person's reputation ever suffered due to gambling, even to the extent of committing illegal acts to finance gambling?
11. Have you come to the point of hiding money needed for living expenses, knowing that you and the rest of the family may go without food and clothing if you do not?
12. Do you search this person's clothing or go through his/her wallet when the opportunity presents itself, or otherwise check on his/her activities?
13. Does the person in question hide his/her money?
14. Have you noticed a personality change in the gambler as his/her gambling progresses?
15. Does the person in question consistently lie to cover up or deny his/her gambling activities?
16. Does this person use guilt induction as a method of shifting responsibilities for his/her gambling upon you?
17. Do you attempt to anticipate this person's moods, or try to control his/her life?
18. Does this person ever suffer from remorse or depression due to gambling, sometimes to the point of self-destruction?
19. Has the gambling ever brought you to the point of threatening to break up the family unit?
20. Do you feel that your life together is a nightmare?

WHAT STEPS I NEED TO TAKE NOW:

CAFFEINE CONSUMPTION QUESTIONNAIRE

		Average number of drinks/doses/tablets per day	Average total per day
BEVERAGE			
Coffee (6 oz.)	125 mg x	_____ =	_____
Decaf Coffee (6 oz.)	5 mg x	_____ =	_____
Tea (6 oz.)	50 mg x	_____ =	_____
Hot cocoa (6 oz.)	15 mg x	_____ =	_____
Caffeinated soft drinks (12 oz.)	40-60 mg x	_____ =	_____
Chocolate candy bar	20 mg x	_____ =	_____
OVER-THE-COUNTER MEDICATIONS			
Anacin	32 mg x	_____ =	_____
Appetite-control pills	100-200 mg x	_____ =	_____
Dristan	16 mg x	_____ =	_____
Excedrin	65 mg x	_____ =	_____
Extra Strength Excedrin	100 mg x	_____ =	_____
Midol	132 mg x	_____ =	_____
NoDoz	100 mg x	_____ =	_____
Triaminicin	30 mg x	_____ =	_____
Vanquish	33 mg x	_____ =	_____
Vivarin	200 mg x	_____ =	_____
PRESCRIPTION MEDICATIONS			
Cafergot	100 mg x	_____ =	_____
Darvon compound	32 mg x	_____ =	_____
Fiorinal	40 mg x	_____ =	_____

Total mg caffeine per day _____

NOTE:

- Greater than 250 milligrams per day *may* interfere with deep sleep.
- To cut down, do so gradually.
- Consultation with your physician may be a wise thing to do.

REASONS TO QUIT SMOKING

Smokers generally desire to quit smoking, but can't seem to do it. The power of addiction is great. Every smoker that does quit does so for a different reason. Health care concerns are not strong factors in the decision making process.

A decision to quit smoking is a personal and individual decision. The timing of the decision is vital to the eventual success level achieved. Each person must come to a point in his/her life when it is time to quit. Success is more likely to occur when quitting is carried out when the time is right. Here are a few factors to consider in making the decision to quit.

1. Smoking hurts and weakens the bones.
2. Smoking dulls the vision.
3. Smoking may jeopardize sex life.
4. Smoking speeds the process of menopause.
5. Smoking increases the likelihood of diabetes.
6. Smoking facilitates infections.
7. Smokers are more prone to heart disease, cancer, dementia, and a variety of other diseases.
8. Smoking clouds the mind and advances the signs of dementia.
9. Smoking impairs sleeping.
10. Smoking advances the aging process of the skin.
11. Smoking discolors the skin.
12. Smoking impairs social relationship with nonsmokers.
13. Smokers live with a distasteful odor in their clothing, hair, homes, and cars.
14. Smokers feel less confident and less proud of themselves because of their smoking.

Suicidal Behavior

Chapter Contents

Almost 100,000 people commit suicide each year. Many more attempt suicide but do not succeed. The potential for suicide requires the therapist to be actively observant, intentionally responsive, caringly supportive, and decisively proactive. Proactive and timely intervention is the key element in suicide prevention. Treatment of any patient in which suicide is a possibility or has been attempted in the past must be addressed carefully and supportively.

This chapter provides information, guidelines, assessment tools, and sample contracts to utilize when providing services to this very distressed and tender population.

THE INTERVENTION PERSPECTIVE OF SUICIDE

A Therapist's Guide

Suicide is a real event for many people. It is the fourth leading cause of death for those over 18 and younger than 65 years of age. It is the third leading cause of death among teens and young adults. Treatment with an experienced and forthright therapist is essential for a good outcome and long-term resolution. Below are several areas of this topic that need to be understood and accepted as a guideline for effective intervention when it is needed.

SUICIDE DETECTION

- Giving away of personal possessions.
- Sudden purchase of a gun, poison, insurance policy or quantities of medication.
- Increased anger or mood change.
- Talk of suicide or stating he/she wants to die.
- Isolation, loss of interest, and refusal to participate in preferred activities.
- Increased drug use or alcohol consumption.
- Intolerable pain, irresolvable stress situation, or hopeless medical condition.
- Person speaks of an inner storm that cannot be quelled.

SUICIDE INTERVENTION

- Ask the person if he/she is planning to commit suicide.
- Ask about the plan to be utilized.
- Empathically, express your concern and ask for a change in plans.
- Stay with the person and be sure others do so also.
- Go with the person for professional consultation and support.
- Remove lethal objects from the environment.
- Propose a realistic solution to the presumed problem.
- Call 911 if necessary or take the person to the hospital or Crisis Unit.

SUICIDE PREVENTION

- Be aware of the signs of possible high-risk behavior and suicide.
- Be comfortable in confronting the person with your concerns and suspicion.
- Be ready to intervene by your action and taking charge of a situation of high risk.
- Give up your time and stay with the distressed person at the time you feel needed.
- Seek professional consultation early and be prepared to go along as support.
- Urge hospitalization if the risk is great and other forms of help are rejected.
- Be a source of encouragement and hope at all times.

SUICIDE RECOVERY FOR FAMILY

- Talk to the family with compassion, empathy, and understanding, not platitudes.
- Actively listen and hear the family's grief, loss, anger, self-blame, and despair.
- Connect them with others that have gone through similar situations for support.

- Avoid sermons, pep talks, stories, and don't pretend you know how they feel.
- Encourage them to tell their story and be cautiously open with others.
- Be a connection with local support grief groups and offer to go along with them.
- Be in contact with the survivor around the time of holidays and anniversaries.
- Be thoughtful of the person's own faith and spiritual foundations; don't preach.
- Give permission to grieve, cry, laugh, socialize, and heal when ready.
- Help bring closure and finality.

RISK FACTORS

- Previous unsuccessful attempts
- Family history of suicide
- Substance abuse
- Mental illness
- Elderly white men
- Artistic prone people
- Come from highly dysfunctional families

DANGEROUSNESS: WARNING FACTORS

A Guideline for Detecting Dangerousness

Dangerousness is a risk factor to be assessed when evaluating patients with known histories of aggressiveness or explosiveness. Those without a positive anger management program may be at risk and may need to be assessed periodically. Here are the main risk factors, as outlined by Dr Ansar Haroun, on which to focus in such situations.

1. Is the family home atmosphere in a chronic state of discord and distress? Does aggressiveness prevail as a primary means to make things happen? Is it a bully-based home life?
2. Is the family relationship between parent and child void of a close bond? Is a bond missing with both parents? Is a rejection or alienation pattern felt within the family?
3. Is criminality a history of one or both parents? Is it a criminal history associated with hurt imposed on others?
4. Is the family known for harsh and abusive discipline and punishment?
5. Is the family absent in attention and void of activities that create togetherness? Does a "lone ranger" feeling or pattern prevail?
6. Is the father absent from the home? Is he absent from the lives and experiences of the children?
7. Is the family pattern all male? Is it mostly male? Is it a domineering male profile?
8. Is there a history of running away by family members?

COMMENTS AND OBSERVATIONS

How many of the eight points are true for the family member being evaluated?

What are the main three or four problems in this family? How serious are they?

What action steps need to be taken now to reduce the risk factors now prevailing?

Other?

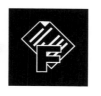

NO HARM AGREEMENT

_____

I, _____ commit to Dr _____ not to harm myself at any time.

I further commit to remove from my house any possession or item that makes me think of harming myself and by which I could harm myself.

I will keep myself socially engaged with people who would help me and prevent me from harming myself. I will choose to be with those who are good for me to be around.

If I should give thought to harming myself, I will call Dr _____ (phone _____); call my friend, _____ (phone _____); or I will call 911 and ask for help.

I will continue in therapy to address the things, people, and experiences that make me think of self-harmful urges and acts. I do want to be rid of my self-harm thoughts, urges, and acts as soon as possible.

Signature of patient: _____ Date: _____

Signature of therapist: _____ Date: _____

Chapter 23

Pain Management and Coping with Medical Disorders

Chapter Contents

Therapists bring to their community a health care expertise that, when combined with the expertise of those in the medical profession, achieves health benefits for the patient that could not have been achieved apart from each other. Patients with psychological problems commonly seek help from physicians. Likewise, those with medical problems present to therapists for help. A team approach is often the best care modality and the most cost-effective. A systems approach is an excellent way to deal with most medical problems, including the therapeutic input of therapists who have health care training, experience, and interest.

The forms in this chapter include checklists, exercises, templates, and homework assignments. They are designed to help a therapist address in a direct and coordinated manner the psychological overlay of the physical disorders of their patients. Confidence on the part of the patient in the applied treatment applications is essential to healing and wellness.

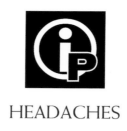

HEADACHES

Headaches are caused by many different problems. Most commonly, headaches are caused by muscle tension from an injury, fatigue, or emotional upset. Excessive muscle contractions, voluntary or involuntary, in the scalp and neck result in a headache that often feels like a tight band around the head. Tension headaches often have areas of tenderness over the scalp and the back of the neck. Tension headaches may last for days or longer, and some may build up into migraines.

Migraines usually cause a throbbing headache, which is made worse by activity and stress. Sometimes only one side of the head hurts. Nausea, vomiting, and sinus pain or stuffiness are common with migraines. Visual symptoms such as light sensitivity, blind spots, or flashing lights may also occur. Loud noises may worsen migraine headaches. Many factors may cause migraine headaches:

- Emotional stress, lack of sleep, and menstrual periods
- Alcohol and some drugs (such as birth control pills)
- Diet factors (fasting, caffeine, food preservatives, chocolate)
- Environmental factors (weather changes, bright lights, odors, smoke)

Other causes of headaches include minor injuries to the head. Arthritis in the neck, problems of tension in the jaw, eyes, ears, or nose are also causes of headaches. Allergies, drugs, alcohol, and exposure to smoke can also cause moderate headaches. Rebound headaches can occur from excessive use of pain medications. Nervous system infections, brain tumors, strokes, and other blood vessel problems could also cause bad headaches.

Treatment of headaches includes medicines for pain and relaxation. Ice packs or heat applied to the back of the head and neck help some people. Massaging the shoulders, neck, and scalp are often very useful. Relaxation techniques and stretching can help prevent these headaches. Avoid alcohol and cigarette smoking as these tend to make headaches worse. Please see your doctor if your headache isn't better in a few days. For persistent headaches, psychological treatment (Behavior Therapy) should be considered.

SEEK IMMEDIATE MEDICAL CARE IF ...

- You develop a high fever, chills, or repeated vomiting.
- You pass out or have difficulty with vision.
- You develop unusual numbness or weakness of your arms or legs.
- You develop severe pain despite medication.
- You develop confusion, or neck stiffness.
- You have a worsening of a headache or do not obtain relief.

TREATMENT OF CHRONIC PAIN

Chronic pain, be it nocioceptive, neuropathic or deep visceral, is usually accompanied by a distressing emotional response. These clients are often angry, depressed, or feel cursed. Often these problems do not show up on X-rays or lab tests, and so the client may be told "Nothing is wrong." So it is understandable that they would be angry or display painful emotions. Poorly trained clinicians may therefore assume the pain is psychogenic, or worse, "drug-seeking." Once patients are so labeled, adequate care is sometimes denied them, and patients are told their pain is "all in their head."

The bodily pain is often about only one-third of the client's experience. Co-morbid major depression and anxiety are often the other two-thirds of the pain experience. Simply palliating the bodily pain is not enough.

WHAT TO DO?

- Psychologists need to have more education about chronic pain; whether the clinician chooses to treat pain or not, it is still there.
- Learn about chemical dependency, and how to assess for it.
- Basic psychopharmacological training is essential. Though therapists are not prescribers, this training increases their credibility with physicians, making the psychologist a better advocate for the client.
- Encourage rational treatment planning, including an exit strategy. These ideas are discussed in detail at PainEDU.org.
- Clients need a better way to describe their pain experience. The "1–10 scale" is inadequate. Work with clients to determine the level of pain experienced, and the interventions needed for relief.

SUCCESSFUL TREATMENT

Treatment success means an active client engaged in life. There is increased activity and good concentration. Thus, the client is better able to manage flare-ups and co-morbid problems are also better addressed. Pain will continue to be an unfortunate part of life, but need not consume the life and thoughts of the patient.

Adapted from *The California Psychologist* (California Psychological Association).

ASSESSMENT OF CHRONIC PAIN

Everyone suffers from acute pain when injured, but acute pain abates quickly. Chronic pain is defined as pain that has not gone away or reoccurs often, even after 6 months have passed. The management of chronic pain is so difficult because traditional methods of pain management frequently fail to bring relief.

The most common types of chronic pain are back pain, headaches, and pain associated with arthritis. However, there are many other origins of chronic pain. Unfortunately, in many of these cases, the underlying cause of the pain is not identified.

The most common pain syndrome is *myofascial pain*, which refers to pain in the muscles or connective tissue. This pain tends to be diffuse and described as "achy," and is often associated with the muscles of the head, neck, shoulders, and lower back. The onset can be rapid or gradual, and generally will diminish on its own. There can be a cycle with myofascial pain which: (1) originates with muscle tension that produces pain; (2) focuses attention on the pain; (3) increases muscle tension; and (4) results in more pain. When an individual is not focusing on the pain, but instead doing other things and thinking about other things the distraction acts to minimize the experience and a normal alleviation or subsiding of the pain occurs.

Another pain syndrome, *neuralgia*, is similar to myofascial pain in that there appears to be a lack of tissue damage. The primary sign of neuralgia experienced by people is a severe sharp pain along a nerve pathway. This pain can occur suddenly with or without stimulation. It is transient and brief, but can reoccur and at times be intense enough to be incapacitating.

FACTORS AFFECTING THE EXPERIENCE OF PAIN

1. *Cultural.* Varying cultures offer different explanations of origin or meaning and expectation. However, there are few differences in sensation thresholds cross-culturally.

2. *Cognitive Response.* The thoughts and beliefs that an individual has are one of the strongest influences on the perception of pain. Cognitive distortions such as excessive worrying, catastrophizing, negative self-fulfilling prophecy, overgeneralization, and personalization are common to individuals who suffer chronic pain. This type of thinking can play a role in the exacerbation of depression, requiring a thorough assessment of mood disturbance issues. The interpretation of pain will determine the overall experience of it, as well as feelings of control and self-efficacy in pain management.

3. *Affect and Stress.* As stress increases there is also an increase in the perception of pain. Psychogenic pain is chronic pain that lacks any physical etiology, and is believed to be a response to psychological need or disturbance. Often, people with depression or other emotional distress will manifest their distress in pain.

4. *Prior Experiences of Pain.* Even though the reaction to pain is autonomic, earlier experiences influence pain perception. There is no cure for pain; it is a survival mechanism to prevent harm and death.

CLINICAL INTERVIEW

Individuals with pain often present with additional coping difficulties. Chronic pain is exhausting, physically limiting, and challenges an individual's identity and sense of control. Be sensitive not to minimize or invalidate the patient's experience of pain.

The assessment interview might be structured as follows:

1. Identifying information
2. Relationship history
3. Work/academic history
4. Relevant background information and developmental history

Therapist's Guide to Clinical Intervention, Second Edition by Sharon L. Johnson (© 2003 Elsevier Inc.)

5. History of pain (intensity, frequency, quality)
6. Medical history (injuries, hospitalization/surgery, medication, etc.)
7. Psychiatric history (therapy, biofeedback, hospitalization, medication)
8. Mental status
9. Coping mechanisms and problem-solving ability
10. Strength and weakness
11. Diagnosis
12. Tentative treatment plan listing planned collateral contacts for further information and case management

MMPI (Minnesota Multiphasic Personality Inventory) scales can be very helpful when used as predictors of pain-coping strategies likely to be preferred by individuals with chronic pain.

ASSESSMENT AND MEASURING PAIN

1. *Behavioral Observation.* Observed outward manifestations of pain may be offered by any significant person in the individual's life and by the therapist. These observations may include distorted posture, distorted ambulation, negative affect (irritable, fatigue, etc.), avoidance of activity, verbal complaints, and distressed facial expressions.
2. *Subjective Reports.* The accuracy of subjective reports of pain are highly variable. It can be helpful to offer a conceptual range of pain from no experience of pain to pain that is intolerable (can't be any worse). This information can be clarified by using:

   A. A basic anatomical chart for identifying location/points of pain and type of pain.
   B. The initiation of a journal for a brief period of time if clarification is necessary. Note: There is a concern that this activity may create increased focus on the pain. However, information that can be gathered includes location, frequency, intensity, time of day when pain is worse, pain management techniques (what is helpful), etc.

Cont.

Patient Pain Assessment

Use the pain chart on the next page to show where you experience pain. There are different symbols you can use for the types of pain that can be experienced.

Every area that you mark as a location where pain is experienced should also be numbered between 0 and 10 to indicate the intensity of the pain experienced. For example, if a location had the symbols and numbers:

//// 4

it would mean that at the location marked there is an experience of stabbing pain with a low–moderate intensity.

Please answer the following questions about your experience of pain:

1. About how often do you get the pain?

☐ more than once every day
☐ once a day
☐ at least once per week
☐ at least once per month
☐ less than once per month
☐ only during specific activities (if Yes, please explain)

_____

_____

_____

_____

2. How do other people try to help you when you have pain?

_____

_____

_____

_____

3. How does the pain interfere in your life? What activities does it prevent you from doing?

_____

_____

_____

_____

Pain Identification Chart

_____

Name: _____ Date: _____

Mark the areas on your body where you feel the described sensations. Use the appropriate symbol. Mark areas of radiation. Include all affected areas.

LOCATION AND TYPE OF PAIN

Numbness: = = = =   Pins and Needles: + + + +
                   = = = =   + + + +

Burning: OOOO   Stabbing: ////
                 OOOO   ////

Please rate the average pain intensity for each location on a 10-point scale:

0 = no pain   10 = very intense pain

FRONT   BACK

COMMENTS:

_____

_____

_____

_____

CHARTING PERCEIVED PAIN

Name: _____ Date: _____

Rate your daily and hourly level of perceived pain on the chart below using the scale of 1 to 10. 1 is the lowest level of pain and 10 is the highest level of pain. At the end of the day draw a line connecting the marks to make a graph.

Hour of the day	Level of perceived pain									
	1	2	3	4	5	6	7	8	9	10
1 am										
2 am										
3 am										
4 am										
5 am										
6 am										
7 am										
8 am										
9 am										
10 am										
11 am										
12 noon										
1 pm										
2 pm										
3 pm										
4 pm										
5 pm										
6 pm										
7 pm										
8 pm										
9 pm										
10 pm										
11 pm										
12 midnight										

COMMENTS AND OBSERVATIONS:

PHYSICAL DISORDERS ASSOCIATED WITH PSYCHOLOGICAL DISTRESS

Therapists need to be alert to a number of physical disorders and conditions that have known psychological corollaries. In the treatment plan, it is necessary to take into account any such disorders and manage them appropriately to improve the patient's coping skills and self-management skills, secondary to the primary reason for psychotherapy being undertaken.

- Brain decline and dysfunction
- Peripheral artery disease
- Osteoporosis
- Sexual dysfunction
- Bowel and bladder incontinence
- Muscle loss and general bodily weakness
- Chronic pain
- Osteoarthritis
- Visual and hearing loss
- Cancer
- Wrinkles and other body image factors
- Varicose veins
- Obesity
- Diabetes
- Physical deformity
- Dry or damp palms
- Hand tremors
- Sexual dysfunction
- Insomnia
- Headaches
- Asthma/Bronchitis
- Epilepsy
- Alcohol problems
- Arthritis
- Anxiety
- Depression
- Heart problems
- Thyroid problems
- _____
- _____
- _____

PATIENT REPORT OF ILLNESSES AND MEDICAL PROBLEMS

Please mark with an **X** any of the following illnesses and medical problems you have had and indicate the year when each started. If you are not certain when a illness started, write down an approximate number of years ago it occurred.

ILLNESS	X	YEAR	ILLNESS	X	YEAR
Eye or Eyelid Infection			Venereal Disease		
Glaucoma			Genital Herpes		
Other Eye Problems			Breast Disease		
Ear Condition			Nipple Drainage		
Deafness or Decreased Hearing			Headaches		
Thyroid Problems			Head Injury		
Strep Throat			Stroke		
Bronchitis			Convulsions/Seizures		
Emphysema			Black Outs		
Pneumonia			Dizziness		
Allergies, Asthma, or Hayfever			Mental Problems		
Nose Bleeds			Arthritis		
Tuberculosis			Gout		
Other Lung Problems			Cancer or Tumors		
Difficulty Breathing			Bleeding Tendency		
High Blood Pressure			Diabetes		
High Cholesterol			Measles/Rubeola		
Arteriosclerosis (hardening of arteries) .			German Measles/Rubella		
Heart Attack			Polio		
Chest Pain			Mumps		
Irregular Heart Beat			Scarlet Fever		
Heart Murmur			Chicken Pox		
Other Heart Conditions			Mononucleosis		
Stomach/Duodenal Ulcer			Eczema		
Nausea			Psoriasis		
Vomiting			Skin Rash		
Weight Loss			Open Wounds		
Weight Gain			Infection		
Difficulty Swallowing			Muscle Stiffness		
Diverticulosis			Muscle Weakness		
Colitis			Muscle Pain		
Other Bowel Problems			Bone Fracture		

Therapist's Guide to Clinical Intervention, Second Edition by Sharon L. Johnson (© 2003 Elsevier Inc.)

ILLNESS	X	YEAR	ILLNESS	X	YEAR
Blood in Stools			Bone Stiffness		
Diarrhea			Others		
Hemorrhoids			. . . .		
Easily Fatigued			. . . .		
Hepatitis			. . . .		
Liver Problems			. . . .		
Gallbladder Problems			. . . .		
Hernia			. . . .		
Kidney or Bladder Disease			. . . .		
Prostate Problem (male only)			. . . .		
Ovarian Problem (female only)			. . . .		
Last Menstrual Period			. . . .		
Last Pregnancy			. . . .		
Menstrual Flow Pattern			. . . .		

PSYCHOLOGICAL FACTORS AFFECTING PHYSICAL CONDITION

When initially assessing an individual in whom physical symptoms are present, note if there appears to be a significant relationship between the individual's coping mechanisms and the physical complaint(s). This information will be helpful in treatment planning if the primary care physician clarifies that there is no organic basis for the symptom presentation or that the physical symptoms are exacerbated by the individual's coping mechanisms.

GOALS

1. To educate and increase awareness
2. To promote appropriate adjustment to changes
3. To improve coping skills
4. To improve stress-management skills
5. To improve self-esteem

TREATMENT FOCUS AND OBJECTIVES

1. *Lack of Sufficient Information*
   a. Consult with physician regarding tests that have been made and their results.
   b. Explore feelings of fear and anxiety related to physical functioning. Unless contraindicated, the person should be given the information related to his/her state of health and treatment issues.
   c. Educate person regarding the mind–body connection. How they think, believe, and interpret things will have an impact on how they experience something.
   d. Encourage venting of thoughts and feelings.
   e. Facilitate development of questions that the person can use with the physician to clarify his/her own understanding and to clarify with the physician if there is any symptomatology that would be important for the person to monitor and to report to the physician.
   f. Recommend that the person keep a journal to vent thoughts and feelings, to clarify, and problem-solve issues. It may help the person identify dysfunctional patterns.
   g. Recommend that the person keep a daily log of appearance, duration, and density of physical symptoms.
   h. Increase awareness and understanding for the relationship between emotional distress and exacerbation of symptomatology.
   i. Facilitate identification of primary and secondary gains. The person must identify needs that are being met through sick role to develop more appropriate and effective methods for fulfilling these needs.
   j. Facilitate development of assertive communication so that the person can express self honestly and effectively.
   k. Facilitate development of stress-management skills.

2. *Change in Self-perception and Role Due to Physical Functioning*
   a. Consult with physician to understand the extent of change in physical functioning, if the problem is progressive, or if there is expected progress to be made with return to prior level of functioning:
      • Necessary for appropriate treatment planning.
   b. Encourage venting of thoughts and feelings associated with physical functioning.
   c. Facilitate identification of stressors that negatively influence functioning.
   d. Facilitate increased awareness for the relationship between physical symptoms and emotional functioning.
   e. Facilitate identification of maladaptive responses.

Therapist's Guide to Clinical Intervention, Second Edition by Sharon L. Johnson (© 2003 Elsevier Inc.)

f. Facilitate identification of family's response to the situation and its effect on the person.

g. Encourage family participation as necessary in treatment. Educate them regarding prognosis, identify dysfunctional patterns, and in enlisting their support.

h. Facilitate development of appropriate responses to situations.

i. Model and role-play appropriate responses with the person.

j. Facilitate identification of desired changes that the person would like to make.

k. Positive feedback and reinforcement for efforts and accomplishments.

3. *Ineffective Coping*

a. Consult with physician to obtain thorough picture of what the person has experienced and what the prognosis is.

b. Facilitate identification of goals.

c. Facilitate development of problem-solving skills.

d. Encourage the person to take appropriate risks and challenge irrational thinking.

e. Encourage the person to take responsibility by making decisions, following through, and being prepared with a contingency plan.

f. Encourage venting of thoughts and feelings (such as powerlessness and lack of control, appearance, etc. associated with physical condition).

g. Facilitate identification of how the person can maintain a feeling of control.

h. Facilitate increased awareness for the relationship between physical symptoms and emotional functioning.

i. Facilitate increased awareness for learned behavior and secondary gains.

j. Facilitate increased awareness for primary or secondary gains that may be present.

k. Refer the person to appropriate community resources.

l. Journal writing to increase awareness and self-monitor positive efforts.

m. Positive feedback and reinforcement for efforts and accomplishments.

4. *Ineffective Stress Management*

a. Teach relaxation techniques:
   • Progressive muscle relaxation
   • Visual imagery/meditation
   • Deep breathing.

b. Self-care (exercise, nutrition, utilization of resources).

c. Educate regarding the role of negative self-talk.

5. *Low Self-Esteem*

a. Facilitate identification of realistic goals.

b. Facilitate identification of strengths.

c. Minimize focus on physical symptoms.

d. Focus on strengths, positives, efforts, and accomplishments.

e. Facilitate development of problem-solving skills.

f. Facilitate identification of appropriate responses to variety of situations to increase feelings of ability and capability.

g. Break down goals into manageable steps. If the person experiences difficulty, work with him/her to break down steps of change further. Prepare the person that this is an expected experience in behavior modification and that no step is too small.

h. Promote feelings of control by encouraging the person to participate in decision making regarding treatment planning.

i. Positive feedback and reinforcement for efforts and accomplishments.

DIZZINESS QUESTIONNAIRE

Name: _____ DOB: _____ Date: _____

I. Your dizziness
Please circle Yes or No and fill in the blank spaces.

1. When did dizziness first occur?_____
2. My dizziness is: Constant   In attacks   (Please circle one)
3. If in attacks, how often?_____

    How long do they last?_____
    Do you have any warning that the attack is about to start?   Yes   No
    If Yes, what kind of warning? _____
4. Are you completely free of dizziness between attacks?   Yes   No
5. Does change of position make you dizzy?   Yes   No
6. Do you have trouble walking in the dark?   Yes   No
7. When you are dizzy, must you support yourself when standing?   Yes   No
8. Do you know of any possible cause of your dizziness?   Yes   No

    If Yes, what?_____
9. Do you know of anything that will:
    Stop your dizziness? _____
    Make it better?_____
10. Were you exposed to any irritating fumes, paints, etc., at the onset of dizziness?   Yes   No
11. If Yes, what? _____
12. Have you ever had a severe head injury?   Yes   No
13. If Yes, were you unconscious? _____ How long for?_____

II. When you are "dizzy" do you experience any of the following sensations?
Please read the entire list first then circle Yes or No to describe your feelings most accurately.

1. Lightheadedness   Yes   No
2. Swimming sensation in the head   Yes   No
3. Blacking out   Yes   No
4. Loss of consciousness   Yes   No
5. Tendency to fall: To the right?   Yes   No
                        To the left?   Yes   No
                        Forward?   Yes   No
                        Backward?   Yes   No
6. Objects spinning or turning around you   Yes   No
7. Sensation that you are turning or spinning inside, with outside objects remaining stationary   Yes   No
8. Loss of balance when walking:
                        Veering to the right?   Yes   No
                        Veering to the left?   Yes   No
9. Headache   Yes   No
10. Nausea or vomiting   Yes   No
11. Pressure in the head   Yes   No

III. Do you have any of the following symptoms?
Please circle the appropriate answer.

1. Difficulty in hearing?

     Both ears   Right   Left   None

2. Noise in your ears?

     Both ears   Right   Left   None

3. Describe the noise _____

4. Does noise change your dizziness?   Yes   No

5. If so, how?_____

6. Pain in your ears?

     Both ears   Right   Left   None

7. Discharge from your ears?

     Both ears   Right   Left   None

IV. Have you experienced any of the following symptoms?
Please circle Yes or No and circle if Constant or In episodes:

1. Double vision.	Yes	No	Constant	In episodes
2. Blurred vision or blindness.	Yes	No	Constant	In episodes
3. Numbness of face or extremities.	Yes	No	Constant	In episodes
4. Weakness in arms or legs.	Yes	No	Constant	In episodes
5. Clumsiness in arms or legs.	Yes	No	Constant	In episodes
6. Confusion or loss of consciousness.	Yes	No	Constant	In episodes
7. Difficulty with speech.	Yes	No	Constant	In episodes
8. Difficulty with swallowing.	Yes	No	Constant	In episodes

V. Further information
Please circle either Yes or No.

1. Do you get dizzy after exertion or overwork?   Yes   No
2. Are you a nervous person?   Yes   No
3. Do you tend to get upset easily?   Yes   No
4. Have you had any recent emotional trauma?   Yes   No
5. Are you under a great deal of stress or tension at home or at work?   Yes   No
6. Do you get dizzy when you have not eaten for a long time?   Yes   No
7. Is your dizziness connected with your menstrual period?   Yes   No
8. Have you ever had a neck injury?   Yes   No

     If Yes, when? _____

9. If you have had a head injury, did you injure your neck at the same time or was your neck sore at the time?   Yes   No

_____

TO BE COMPLETED BY THE THERAPIST:

PATTERNS AND TRENDS NOTED:

MEDICATIONS BEING TAKEN BY PATIENT

Name of patient: _____ Date: _____

Name of patient's physician: _____

Medication and Purpose	**Dosage**
1. _____	_____
2. _____	_____
3. _____	_____
4. _____	_____
5. _____	_____
6. _____	_____
7. _____	_____
8. _____	_____

COMMENTS AND SUGGESTED CHANGES FOR THE PHYSICIAN'S CONSIDERATION:

Therapist's signature: _____ Date: _____

GASTROESOPHAGEAL REFLUX DISEASE (GERD)

Reflux means that the stomach acids and juices flow up from the stomach back into the tube that leads from the throat to the stomach. This is called the esophagus. This causes heartburn. When you experience heartburn at least two times a week, it is called gastroesophageal reflux disease, or GERD.

To minimize the discomfort of the reflux reaction and the associated heartburn, the following eating behaviors and lifestyle changes are recommended:

Eating Behaviors to Control GERD Symptoms

- Do not eat too much at each meal.
- Do not bend forward after eating.
- After eating, wait 2 to 3 hours before lying down.
- Eat smaller meals more often
- Do not drink milk or eat milk-based products containing calcium and fat within 2 hours of bedtime.

Lifestyle Changes to Manage GERD Symptoms

- Lose weight.
- Quit smoking or using tobacco.
- Raise the head of your bed 6 to 8 inches by putting blocks under the frame or a foam wedge under the head of the mattress. You may also use extra pillows.
- Wear loose-fitting clothing around your waist and mid-section to put less pressure on the stomach.
- Sleep on the left side to reduce night-time reflux episodes.

Foods to Avoid to Manage GERD Symptoms

- Avoid chocolate and peppermint.
- Avoid carbonated soft drinks, with or without sugar.
- Avoid onions, spinach, cabbage, cauliflower, broccoli, Brussels sprouts.
- Avoid tomatoes and tomato-based preparations, citrus fruits, and citrus juices.
- Avoid coffee, alcohol, and excessive amounts of Vitamin C supplements, especially before bedtime.
- Avoid foods that are high in fats as fat delays stomach emptying.
- Avoid all foods that you recognize make you feel worse.

Things to Do or Take to Manage GERD Symptoms

- Use chewing gum or hard candies to increase the amount of saliva your mouth produces. Saliva washes stomach juices out of the esophagus into the stomach and can control stomach acid.
- Use over-the-counter anti-acid medication. If this does not work sufficiently, consult your physician for a prescriptive medication.

PARKINSON'S DISEASE

Winning Over Depression

- Be knowledgeable in your understanding of PD
- Be accepting and wise in your thinking about your own PD

DEPRESSION AND ME:

- I'm one of 500,000 PD patients
- I could be one of the 50% with depression

PLANNING MY LIFE-MAP:

- Plan A   The way it was supposed to be
- Plan B   The way it is
- Plan C   The changes to which I must accommodate
- Plan D   The great depression I must confront and defeat

WHERE DOES IT COME FROM?

- Brain changes
- Family history
- Life events: past, present, future
- Losses and impairments

WINNING OVER DEPRESSION:

- Embrace tragic optimism
- Stop "stinkin' thinkin'"
- Enjoy graduated accomplishments
- Get into the bright light daily
- Reward yourself for accomplishments
- Listen to historic and relaxing music
- Gather your support team
- Be a blessing, an encouragement to others
- Utilize antidepressants
- Consider the use of herbal medicines
- Remember, friends make good medicine
- Associate with encouraging people
- Reduce exposure to hurtful people and events

Anger and Violent Behavior

Chapter Contents

Anger and violence are part of the human experience. Unfortunately, these two emotional and behavioral patterns occur far too often. These problems are not uncommon referral issues. They represent one of the tougher issues that face and challenge a therapist. Lengthy therapy is often required. Generally, the roots of anger and violence are deep in the life history of many patients. Prevention of ongoing hurt and pain is of utmost importance. Helping patients learn new responses to old anger triggers is the key to effective therapy.

The forms in this chapter are designed to assist the therapist in confronting anger and violent behavior habits and start the change process. Checklists, guidelines, inventories, and questionnaires are included to help the therapist take assertive action and be effective.

HOW TO HANDLE ANGRY PEOPLE

The acronym "BULLETS" is useful when dealing with people who are angry:

Be seated. Place yourself in a relaxed position sitting down and ask the other person to also sit down. This could slow behavioral reactiveness as well as maintain a measure of distance for personal space.

Use the person's name. Speak directly to someone who is angry in a calm and low tone of voice addressing them by name.

Lower your voice. With awareness of the tension that is present, systematically lower your voice and do not verbally react.

Listen. Listen and be validating about what the person has to say. Remember, validation does not mean agreement; it is only acknowledgment for the other person's thoughts or feelings. Listen thoroughly to what the person has to say and do not try to rush him/her out the door and minimize the anger that the person is experiencing.

Eliminate humor. Do not try to make light of the situation when someone is upset. Such a response feels disrespectful and minimizing. It immediately conveys that the person is not being taken seriously, which would escalate anger.

Talk, don't argue. Arguing increases tension and escalates feelings of anger. When things have calmed down, then share your ideas if you have points to share that you feel are important. Discussing things rationally requires people to be relatively calm and prepared to validate and problem-solve.

Slow down. Slowing the rate of speech is a way to initiate calm and role-model to the other person the manner in which to speak, without addressing it directly.

From *Assertiveness: Get What You Want Without Being Pushy* (Inc. National Press Publications, 1990)

Therapist's Guide to Clinical Intervention, Second Edition by Sharon L. Johnson (© 2003 Elsevier Inc.)

ANGER AND HOW TO DEAL WITH IT

Anger is one of the strongest emotions known to man. Mild degrees can cause us to act and address a situation that needs resolution or change. It can motivate and direct our actions to accomplish good.

On the other hand, strong anger can be destructive and self-defeating. It can lead us to act in hurtful ways towards others and even act against the wrong person. This is called misplaced aggression. Strong anger produces no good thing, generally.

Below are 10 attitudes to help control anger actions when we feel angry in some situation. It is not anger that is self-defeating; it is our anger reaction or loss of control when angry. Consider the following:

1. Be tolerant of the shortcomings of others. You may even share their shortcomings.

2. Do not provoke anger in others. You would not like to be provoked into anger either.

3. Do not knowingly put yourself in a situation where you know it is likely that you will become angry. Stay clear of anger-producing situations.

4. Stop a quarrel with others before it goes too far and gets out of control. You can always walk away or change the topic.

5. Do not talk behind the back of another person. You would not like it either.

6. Give yourself time to think before you talk, especially when you are dealing with a point of disagreement. Thinking and listening time is more important than talking time.

7. Do remember to lower your voice when speaking with someone with whom you have a disagreement. Speaking slower and softer will reap you respect and moral credit.

8. Be quick to seek forgiveness from others and be quick to forgive, even if not asked. Forgiveness can be carried out quickly, but forgetting is very long term.

9. Do give thought to the needs of the other person as being more important than your own. Self-help is not always the first book to buy.

10. Act kindly towards others as kindness will overcome evil with good. Speak kindly and act kindly at all times. Defeat anger with acts of love and kindness.

HOSTILITY DISCOMFORT SCALE

For each item below, circle T (True) or F (False) as your best answer.

1. I have felt disturbed during the times I have been about to yell or swear at someone because of what others would think of me.   T   F

2. I usually try to avoid becoming angry because it upsets me afterwards.   T   F

3. If I ever got mad enough to break things, I would feel badly afterwards.   T   F

4. Everyone gets mad sometimes and I for one rarely regret it later since it's often unavoidable.   T   F

5. I am often concerned over what people would think of me if I ever struck someone in public.   T   F

6. I become upset watching movies on war and killing.   T   F

7. I enjoy good heated arguments because it sharpens my thinking.   T   F

8. If I ever felt that I hated someone, the awareness of the feeling would be upsetting.   T   F

9. When I get over being angry I generally become upset at having been angry.   T   F

10. Watching people doing physical violence to each other upsets me.   T   F

11. Knowing that I would regret it later is generally enough reason to prevent me from yelling or swearing at persons who provoke me.   T   F

12. I am afterwards ashamed of myself when I threaten someone for reasons that seem important at the time.   T   F

13. I get into arguments although at the time I regret my participation in them.   T   F

14. I try not to get grouchy and irritable because I only punish myself later by feeling remorseful.   T   F

NOTE FOR THE THERAPIST: Score 1 point for each T marked, except for items 4 and 7. On these two items, score a point if the F is marked. Those with high scores (above 6) are uncomfortable in anger or hostility situations and may not cope well in such situations. A referral for counseling in conflict resolution, assertive communication training, and/or anger management training may be helpful for such patients.

BEHAVIORAL ANGER SCALE

For each item below, circle T (True) or F (False) as your best answer. Consider how *you generally behave* when angry.

1.	When arguing I tend to raise my voice.	T	F
2.	I am often so annoyed when someone tries to get ahead of me in a line of people that I speak to him/her about it.	T	F
3.	I seldom strike back even if someone hits me first.	T	F
4.	I never get mad enough to throw things.	T	F
5.	I sometimes show my anger by banging on the table.	T	F
6.	When people yell at me, I yell back.	T	F
7.	When I really lose my temper, I am capable of slapping someone.	T	F
8.	If someone hits me first, I let him have it.	T	F
9.	When I am mad, I sometimes slam doors.	T	F
10.	Even when my anger is aroused, I don't use "strong language."	T	F
11.	I often make threats I don't mean to carry out.	T	F
12.	If I have to resort to physical violence to defend my rights, I will.	T	F
13.	I have had several bitter arguments with my mother/father.	T	F
14.	When I get mad, I say nasty things.	T	F
15.	I can remember being so angry that I picked up the nearest thing and broke it.	T	F

NOTE FOR THE THERAPIST: Score 1 point for each T marked, except for items 3, 4, and 10. On these two items, score a point if the F is marked. Those scoring greater than 6 might be appropriately referred for anger management counseling, assertiveness training, conflict resolution training or psychotherapy.

ANGER INVENTORY

For each of the 10 items below, indicate the extent of your agreement. The general question is "How do I feel about anger?"

For each item, mark *your best answer* in the space provided. Mark

SA   If you strongly agree with the statement
A   If you agree but not as strongly
N   If you are neutral or undecided
D   If you disagree but not too strongly
SD   If you strongly disagree with the statement

1. If I am provoked to anger it means I have failed somewhere. _____

2. My view is that angry feelings should be avoided if at all possible. _____

3. If I should get angry, I feel it is generally better to avoid letting other people know about it. _____

4. I see people who often are angry as less mature than people who seldom are angry. _____

5. It is my opinion that the ideal person very seldom is angry. _____

6. I think that the most effective person is one who never blows his/her cool. _____

7. I go to considerable lengths to avoid provoking people to anger. _____

8. I would say that angry feelings are generally undesirable. _____

9. I would rather become angry myself than have another person become angry. _____

10. I generally seek to avoid responding with anger to a person who is angry. _____

NOTE FOR THE THERAPIST: The more SA and A answers, the more the person is uncomfortable with anger feelings. High scoring persons (above 4 points) would benefit from anger management classes, assertive communication training, and conflict resolution training.

BEHAVIORAL HOSTILITY CHECKLIST

For each of the following statements, circle T (True) or F (False).

1. I don't blame anyone for trying to grab everything they can get in this world.　　　T　　　F

2. It is safer to trust nobody.　　　T　　　F

3. When someone does me a wrong, I feel I should pay them back if I can, just for the principle of the thing.　　　T　　　F

4. I like to make fun of people.　　　T　　　F

5. Someone has it in for me.　　　T　　　F

6. I like to play practical jokes on others.　　　T　　　F

7. I do not try to cover up my poor opinion of a person or pity for them so that they won't know how I feel.　　　T　　　F

8. I am often said to be hot-headed.　　　T　　　F

9. I commonly wonder what hidden reason another person may have for doing something nice for me.　　　T　　　F

10. At times, I feel like picking a fist fight with someone.　　　T　　　F

11. Sometimes I enjoy hurting persons I love.　　　T　　　F

12. I can easily make other people afraid of me, and sometimes do it for the fun of it.　　　T　　　F

13. Horses that don't pull should be beaten or kicked.　　　T　　　F

14. There are certain people I dislike so much that I am inwardly pleased that they are catching it for something they have done.　　　T　　　F

NOTE FOR THE THERAPIST: Score all True checks +1; score all False checks −1.

Sum for total score _____ (add negative and positives scores).

For those whose score falls between +5 and +14, the person should be referred for therapy and anger management classes. For those whose scores fall between +5 and −5, the person should be referred for therapy.

MY ANGER STORY... About Which I Am Not Proud

In the space below, write out your Anger Story using the following outline: childhood years, adolescent years, adult years, and past month. Tell of the losses you underwent due to your anger. Tell good and bad things. Then state how you have changed and tell how and why. Then tell how you plan to live in the future without angry behavior as a lifestyle. Be specific. Go back into history as needed. <u>Do it all on one page.</u>

My Childhood Years:

My Adolescent Years:

My Adult Years:

This Past Month:

How Have You Changed, If You Have?

How Do You Plan to Live in the Future Without Angry Behavior?

Name: _____ Date your story was written: _____

MY DIAGNOSTIC ANGER MAP

Please indicate your *angry behavior today* on the chart below. Note when in the day you got mad and acted in an angry manner, and what it was that defined your mad behavior for the day. Do this for a week.

Mad behaviors	Mornings	Afternoons	Day's-end
Raised voice in anger			
Pushed someone			
Felt like hitting someone			
Acted in a rude and abrupt manner			
Hit wall			
Tossed things on floor			
Hit, kicked or threw objects			
Rage or road rage			
Other			
Other			

What I notice about my anger:

1.

2.

3.

4.

FIVE STEPS OF ANGER CONTROL

The control and management of anger is vital to effective relationships. All relationships. While anger is a strong emotion and is often associated with a corresponding strong reaction pattern, it need not get out of control and hurt others. It is vital to learn a simple and brief system of anger control. Here goes …

When feeling a tinge of anger or being faced with an anger-producing situation, do the following:

1. Stop and think about the current cause of your anger. What is going on?
2. Take five deep breaths by counting to 5 on inhalation and to 5 on exhalation.
3. Count or say a series of words, numbers or verse of some type.
4. Walk away or get distance between you and the source of your anger.
5. Say out loud five or six statements that will help you calm down and refrain from acting out in anger. Say words, such as "chill," "calm down," "cool it," relax," "easy does it," and "I can handle this." What are your words or phrases?

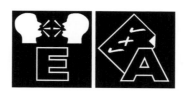

DANGEROUS PROPENSITIES OF A MINOR

The following is what we know regarding known and/or suspected dangerous propensities of a minor (*check appropriate box for each item*):

- Violence towards others: Physically threatening and/or assaultive behaviors; property destruction or damage; cruelty to animals; robbing/stealing with use of force of weapons; and/or gang involvement.

  ☐ No known history   ☐ Yes, known or suspected history. Specify and describe below:

- Violence towards self: Suicide attempts/ideation; deliberate harm to self and/or drug overdose.

  ☐ No known history   ☐ Yes, known or suspected history. Specify and describe below:

- Sexual, maladjustment problems: Sexual molestation of others and/or sexually acting out/rape.

  ☐ No known history   ☐ Yes, known or suspected history. Specify and describe below:

- Arsonist behavior: History of fire-setting.

  ☐ No known history   ☐ Yes, known or suspected history. Specify and describe below:

Name of minor: _____

ON THE BASIS OF THIS QUESTIONNAIRE, I ESTIMATE THIS MINOR'S LEVEL OF DANGEROUSNESS AT THIS TIME TO BE:

I FURTHER RECOMMEND THE FOLLOWING COURSE OF ACTION BASED ON THE RESULTS OF THIS QUESTIONNAIRE:

Signature of therapist: _____ Date: _____

RISK FOR RE-OFFENDING AS A SEX OFFENDER

The probability that a sex offender will be re-arrested or will commit a new sex offense depends upon a number of risk factors operating in the person's life at the present time, as well as historical behavior patterns and traits. No one instrument can fully and accurately predict the probability of re-offending. However, there are a number of factors that do need to be considered and assessed when making such a prediction. The more high-risk factors are present, the more likely it is that a re-offense could occur.

   To assist in evaluating adult male sex offenders, the Static-99 questionnaire designed by Drs R. Karl Hanson and David Thornton as an actuarial assessment instrument, gives a fairly well thought out informal interview format. Below are listed a series of issues modified and adapted from the Static-99 to provide a reasonably good understanding of a sex offender being evaluated. Training and practice in the use of the updated form of the original Static-99 is recommended if the form is to be used for forensic purposes. (www.Static-99.org).

HISTORICAL RISK FACTORS   Yes/No

1. Young age   _____
2. A pattern of living with a female while unmarried   _____
3. Conviction for a non-sexual act of violence   _____
4. Conviction for a sexual act of violence   _____
5. Conviction for non-contact sex offenses   _____
6. History of unrelated victims   _____
7. History of stranger victims   _____
8. History of male victims   _____

GENERAL CRIMINALITY AND LIFESTYLE   Yes/No

1. Childhood maladjustment as defined by two or more of the following
   instances: history of grade failure, psychiatric treatment, group home
   placement or running away from home   _____
2. Meets the criteria for conduct disorder   _____
3. Psychopathic traits   _____
4. Violation of conditional release or a new offense while on probation   _____
5. Frequent and prolonged unemployment   _____

SEXUAL SELF-REGULATION IMPAIRMENT   Yes/No

1. Sexual preoccupation   _____
2. Uses sex as a coping mechanism   _____
3. Deviant sexual interests   _____

GENERAL SELF-REGULATION IMPAIRMENT   Yes/No

1. Impulsive acts   _____
2. Poor cognitive problem solving skills   _____
3. Negative emotionality/hostility   _____

ATTITUDES THAT ARE TOLERANT OF SEXUAL ASSAULT   YES/NO

1. Holds attitudes or values that excuse, permit or condone deviant sexual behavior   _____

SEXUAL DEVIANCE VARIABLES   YES/NO

1. Prior sexual offenses against two or more children under the age of 12, one of which was an unrelated child victim   _____
2. Sexual offenses as a juvenile (under the age of 18) and as an adult   _____

PERSONALITY DISORDERS (CLUSTER B)   YES/NO

The following disorders are generally associated with a higher level of risk: antisocial personality disorder, borderline personality disorder, histrionic personality disorder, and/or narcissistic personality disorder (Underline the relevant disorders)   _____

HISTORY OF FAILED TREATMENT PARTICIPATION   YES/NO

1. Dropping out of a recent attempt at a specific sex offender treatment program   _____
2. Not cooperating with probation/parole supervision   _____

MITIGATING FACTORS TO BE CONSIDERED   YES/NO

1. Lengthy period of time in the community free of any offense, but particularly free of any sexual offense   _____
2. Elderly status, 65 years or older   _____
3. Pattern and history of poor health   _____
4. Successful participation and completion of a behavioral treatment program for sex offenders   _____
5. Significant but stable lifestyle changes due to successful completion of a comprehensive rehabilitation treatment program, renewed religious faith, or a major change in marital and family relationships (for example)   _____
6. Cooperating with supervision   _____

Skill Building Strategies and Tools for Personal Growth and Life Improvement

It is not uncommon for patients to present themselves to a therapist and in the initial session say, "We need to learn how to communicate better." Others will say, "My child has an anger problem and he needs to learn how to control his anger." And others may say, "We are always in conflict and we need to learn how to change."

In other words, skill building is a common request of patients. Therapists need to be ready to teach the basics in many areas of interpersonal relationships and have ready a series of homework exercises to advance the skills being taught during the therapy session.

In skill building, the therapist changes from a more passive role to a very active role, from a listening role to a teaching role, from one of guidance and counseling to that of a didactic interchange focusing on new skills and problem-solving strategies.

As a result of the teaching role assumed by a therapist, patients experience personal growth and become very aware of areas of their life that need to be improved. Teaching patients how to handle one kind of problem can then be utilized for changing other problem areas in their life. It is the hope that a patient learns strategies and gains tools for their own personal growth and then applies them in many areas of their daily life experience.

Part IV provides an array of forms, guidelines, checklists, and handouts for the therapist to use in their educational role with patients. Indeed, the therapist becomes a professional educator based on the needs of patients for certain skills that will help them live productively and effectively in their homes, with their families, and in their work environment.

Chapter 25

Strategies and Tools for Personal Growth and Health Awareness

Chapter Contents

Personal growth does not just happen. Personal growth and development is a result of an intentional and systematic learning process. It is the outcome of planned change and the benefit of a new and more effective lifestyle.

Therapists generally play a critical role in the personal growth experiences of their patients. Besides focusing on a particular presenting problem, therapy produces significant personal benefits in many areas of a patient's life. These areas include relationships, decision making, classroom learning, emotional intelligence, work performance, and learning to live life with personal meaning.

This chapter contains many forms, templates, guidelines, questionnaires, and homework exercises to assist the therapist in bringing about personal growth and personal development in their patients. This may be an intentional focus of therapy or it may come about as a by-product of therapy that has focused on some other specific problem.

MY DEVELOPMENTAL EXPERIENCES OF PERSONAL GROWTH AND DEVELOPMENT

Development and personal growth proceeds systematically and experientially. We grow physically as we are nourished and exposed to exercise, for example. So we undergo growth cognitively, spiritually, socially, and interpersonally. Each area has several specific influences that help us maximize or stunt the learning and growing process from early life to our later years in life.

The list below is your opportunity to assess the influences on your life and how they have contributed to the person you have become (or are becoming). At each stage in development, we can direct some of the influences on us, but not all of them. Some experiences we must accept and adapt to, while others we can shape, minimize or encourage more of them.

In the spaces below, jot down the major experiences or events that shaped your life and contributed to your personality and the person you have become at this time in your life. Put some comment in each specific area. This will then be discussed in our upcoming therapy sessions together. Feel free to discuss your answers with the family.

AREAS OF INFLUENCE

Educational experiences:

Biblical/spiritual teachings:

Cultural patterns:

Activities, sports, toys:

TV/Video program and personalities:

Peer influences:

Parental influences:

Sex typing and patterns:

Basic family genetics:

Traumatic events:

Special people in my life:

Books read and their characters:

Health and wellness patterns:

Self-defeating influences from others:

Other:

MY SELF-ANALYSIS

List at least 5 to 7 personal characteristics you view as assets or strengths of your personality or lifestyle. Then list 5 to 7 weaknesses, or deficits you see in your personality and lifestyle. Include any of the things you like about yourself and the things you dislike about yourself.

ASSETS/STRENGTHS	DEFICITS/WEAKNESSES
1.	1.
2.	2.
3.	3.
4.	4.
5.	5.
6.	6.
7.	7.
8.	8.
9.	9.
10.	10.

QUESTIONS:

1. What excess baggage (weaknesses) do I need to get rid of and how will I do it?

2. Which of my qualities (strengths) do I need to display more often and how will I do it?

3. Which trait am I most proud of and willing to exercise and which one am I most ashamed of and need to address?

4. Other:

CONSIDERATIONS IN SELF-IMAGE BUILDING

We build our self-image by drawing upon many other people in our life and how we feel and think about them. We take from some and not others. We take much from some and little from others. We learn the way we come to think of ourselves by our associations and how we imitate those we admire. Here is a self-examination exercise.

1. Who are my role models in life?

2. What are their strengths and what do I admire in them?

3. Who in my life experience has made me feel and want to do better?

4. What are their strengths and what do I admire in them?

5. Am I willing to learn the strengths and lifestyle of those I have identified above, and become a more positive person and try to help others do likewise?

MY PLAN TO IMPROVE MY SELF-IMAGE:

MY FRIENDSHIP CIRCLE

Please name 10 or more of your friends. Select them because they are the persons that influence you, and you influence them in some way.

Now from your list of friends, select those that serve in the role of a COACH and help you go forward and succeed in school, work and in all areas of your personal live. They help you make the right choices and do the good things in your daily life.

Secondly, select those that serve in the role as a HELPER to you in some way and you need them in your life right now. They help keep you from engaging in self-defeating behavior and choices.

Thirdly, select those that serve like an ANCHOR on you and hold you down and prevent you from being successful and from experiencing positive accomplishments and passing grades.

Lastly, note that some friends play more than one role in our life. At different times they play a different role.

COACHES	HELPERS	ANCHORS
1.	1.	1.
2.	2.	2.
3.	3.	3.
4.	4.	4.
5.	5.	5.

OTHER FRIENDS AND THEIR ROLE IN MY LIFE:

MY LIFE'S JOURNEY OF GROWTH EXPERIENCES

While physical growth proceeds by age in a fairly predictable manner, psychological growth proceeds by experiences. Positive and negative experiences are the basis of our growth emotionally. Such experiences are very personal and subjective. No two people are the same. One particular experience may affect two people very differently. One person may have been affected profoundly, while another to a much lesser degree.

Review the questions below and respond to them as your experiences dictate. Learn from your answers as you reflect on your history of growth experiences.

1. Name one event by which you grew and gained maturity:

_____

_____

_____

2. Name one event that had a stagnation influence on you. It made you unmotivated and discouraged:

_____

_____

_____

3. Name one event that caused you to become happy, encouraged and hopeful:

_____

_____

_____

4. Name one event that taught you one important lesson in life:

_____

_____

_____

COMMENTS AND ANY OTHER EXPERIENCES TO MENTION:

LEARNING TO LIVE A LIFE OF MASTERY

The famous New York psychiatrist Dr Ari Kiev, first-ever psychiatric coach to America's Olympians, said that mastery "is ultimately about taking a leap of faith and stepping into the abyss of uncertainty. We need to be ready to commit to an out-sized goal and then do what it takes by way of work, analysis, coaching, asking for help and, among other things, to be able to stay on top of the goal in the face of difficulties that cannot be predicted at the time of the initial conversation." He further states, "Simply put, you will need a self-awareness that allows you to change." And, "Once you have a vision, you set in motion a whole train of events based on nothing but your decision to act. In this way, you carve out an opening for action simply by committing, with no certainty about the outcome, only a sense of what it is that you are going to do and what it is that you want to happen."

Dr Kiev says you are approaching mastery when you:

1. Are able to endure high levels of tension.
2. Are able to monitor your anxiety and control it.
3. Are comfortable about expressing aggression and being venturesome, bold, and uninhibited.
4. Are realistic about your abilities.
5. Can overcome obstacles of fear, self-doubt and lack of confidence when they interfere with the accomplishment of the goal.
6. Are able to tune out distractions and focus on one thing at a time.
7. Can establish and stick to goals and set priorities and have the capacity to mentally visualize your mission so as to formulate a game plan to respond to events.
8. Feel imbalance within yourself with immediate awareness or controlled spontaneity.
9. Rely on a minimization of defensiveness, concealment, blocking, and "passing the buck."

EXERCISE

What can I do to improve or develop my mastery seeking behavior?

MASTERING MOTIVATIONAL LIVING

Getting and Staying Motivated by Following Your Personal Plan

Every one of us, at one point or another, could use an extra dose of motivation. The keys to staying motivated are as follows: write goals that tap into your passions; review those goals regularly; measure and compare your progress toward your goals periodically; and lastly, surround yourself with people who are goal-directed.

GET CONNECTED TO YOUR GOALS

What do you really want? What are you working toward in your work, family, physical and spiritual life? Think big. Choose one area you want to grow in and work on that. Take short-term "sprints" toward long-term objectives.

Most professional marathoners don't think about their race as 26.2 mile runs, they think of them as an accumulation of similar sprints, with a spurt for the finish at the end. By breaking down your objectives into smaller goals, or sprints, you make them more psychologically attainable, as well as less monumental and massive.

MEASURE AND COMPARE

You can't improve what you don't measure, so make sure your spirits are specific and measurable. You can control activities, but not results.

Sometimes, no matter how closely you have followed your action plan, you still miss the mark. Why is this? Since your goals are often a long stretch, it is difficult to envision the exact outcome. Times like these are when it is most important to adhere to your plan. If you do, and are consistent, you'll eventually experience your desired growth, but in a deeper and more powerful way.

MAKE MOTIVATION YOUR LIFESTYLE

What are you reading, listening to, and watching? Everything that you choose to surround yourself with is an influence on your behavior, so consider your lifestyle and keep it goal-directed.

CALENDAR EVENTS

Plan now to attend positive, goal-affirming events. By putting goal-oriented events on your calendar in advance, you'll be able to evaluate last minute invitations much better and won't be tempted by every random invitation.

JOURNAL

Journaling is key to keeping your life plan in perspective. In addition to providing time for you to reflect on each day, it is an invaluable opportunity to gain a true perspective on yourself. After a year or two, you'll be able to look back at your writing as an objective observer and see how far your motivational planning has taken you.

The Motivation Worksheet

A. What is my driving force, my passion? Why do I get up every morning?

B. What do I plan to do for the next 30 days to put my passion into a set of goals?

C. My goals are as follows:

1.

2.

3.

D. I plan to build my action plan in the following way to achieve my goal(s).

E. The motivation lifestyle I will engage in will be known for the following activities.

1.

2.

3.

4.

Adapted from 'Master of Motivation', Buffini & Co.

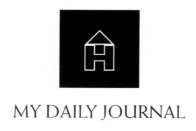

MY DAILY JOURNAL

A daily or weekly journal can play a vital role in the therapy program of most people. It is a good way to chart progress, record significant events, notice change taking place, monitor feelings, thoughts, and behavior patterns as well as keeping a historical record of your life experiences to be brought to therapy for further consideration and interpretation.

To help you get started in writing a journal, write a two- or three-sentence statement on this form for the next 9 days. Make any comments you would like. They may be kept personal and private or can be shared with others along with your therapist. The benefit comes from the whole process, writing down an experience, re-reading it from time to time, and from the discussions you have with others about what you wrote and experienced. Enjoy the journey of journaling.

Day 1

Day 2

Day 3

Day 4

Day 5

Day 6

Day 7

Day 8

Day 9

Keep going and change the process and procedure as you so desire. Make it a meaningful experience for yourself. It's your life and your growth to experience and share. If you decide to keep up the journaling exercise, daily, weekly or as needed, you might want to buy a booklet or notebook to carry with you and write in it as experiences take place.

TEST OF PERSONAL MEANING

The purpose of this questionnaire is to measure the meanings of certain things to various people by having them judge concepts against a series of descriptive scales. In taking this test, please make your judgments on the basis of what the named concept means to you. Rate the concept on each of these scales. If you feel that the concept at the top of the page is **very closely** related to one end of the scale, or the other end, place a check mark that best describes your feeling or assessment. Do not try to remember how you checked earlier items. Make each item a separate and independent judgment. Work at a fast speed. Give your first impressions.

Person or thing to be rated

Sincere	____:____:____:____:____:____:____	Insincere
Unpredictable	____:____:____:____:____:____:____	Predictable
Weak	____:____:____:____:____:____:____	Strong
Slow	____:____:____:____:____:____:____	Fast
Delicate	____:____:____:____:____:____:____	Rugged
Cold	____:____:____:____:____:____:____	Warm
Dangerous	____:____:____:____:____:____:____	Safe
Tense	____:____:____:____:____:____:____	Relaxed
Worthless	____:____:____:____:____:____:____	Valuable
Ineffective	____:____:____:____:____:____:____	Effective
Complicated	____:____:____:____:____:____:____	Simple
Colorless	____:____:____:____:____:____:____	Colorful
Undependable	____:____:____:____:____:____:____	Dependable
Feminine	____:____:____:____:____:____:____	Masculine
Excitable	____:____:____:____:____:____:____	Calm
Boring	____:____:____:____:____:____:____	Interesting
Weak-willed	____:____:____:____:____:____:____	Strong-willed
Unemotional	____:____:____:____:____:____:____	Emotional
Twisted	____:____:____:____:____:____:____	Straight

Adapted from the SDS, Osgood.

THE INTERACTIVE COGNITIVE MODEL OF EMOTIONAL INTELLIGENCE

THE MODEL

How we behave in any given situation is a result of certain thought patterns and certain emotional patterns we have acquired based on historical experiences. Likewise, behavior patterns in turn influence our emotional and thought patterns. We can change feelings by changing how we behave in a situation or changing how we think on some topic, issue or about someone. We can change both in the positive and negative directions.

The Interactive Cognitive Model is a potent educational exercise for patients in therapy to undergo significant lifestyle changes. The Model is easy for patients to understand and tends to make sense for a wide variety of presenting problems.

$$\leftarrow \textbf{THOUGHTS}(+/-) \rightarrow \leftarrow \textbf{EMOTIONS}(+/-) \rightarrow \leftarrow \textbf{BEHAVIORS}(+/-) \rightarrow$$

THE MODEL APPLIED TO THE COMPONENTS OF EMOTIONAL INTELLIGENCE (EI)

The components of EI noted below represent areas of personal change and improved lifestyle effectiveness. The above model will help explain how we can achieve these components of EI.

It is vital that I am able to ...

1. ... fully appreciate my emotions.
2. ... fully manage my emotions.
3. ... fully resist my impulses.
4. ... fully motivate myself to engage in focused action.
5. ... fully maintain an alert social awareness.
6. ... fully connect with others empathically.
7. ... fully feel and express sympathy for others.
8. ... fully manage my interpersonal relationships.

EXERCISE

Draw the model and describe for the patient how the above model explains the patient's current problem and how the use of the model can help bring about the desired changes in the life of the patient.

HAPPINESS AND OPTIMISM EXERCISES

Happiness and optimism are two key mind states for effective living and human excellence. They influence one's level of achievement, and the level of contentment attained. Together, they toughen our resolve to excel and live a healthy lifestyle. Practice the following exercises until you learn to make happiness and optimism part of your regular routine of daily life. As you practice these exercises, they will soon become part of your attitudinal system.

The Optimist vs. the Pessimist
1. The Optimist describes good things as permanent and pervasive, and describes bad things as temporary and narrowly focused. Thus, he/she may feel hopeful and energized.
2. The Pessimist describes good things as temporary and narrowly focused, and describes bad things as permanent and pervasive. Thus, he/she may feel despair and hopeless.

Happiness Exercises
1. Express your gratitude to somebody who has touched and enriched your life at some point in the past. Do this in a verbal or in written format.
2. Increase positive meaning in your life by engaging in something you believe in that is larger than you, such as volunteering or being part of a community-based charity project.
3. Be friendly to someone each day; as you continue, you may in turn gain a friend.
4. Become associated with a challenging situation and work to make that situation better and successful.
5. Write a gratitude journal each day by writing down 3 to 5 things for which you were thankful during the day.
6. Let go of anger and resentment by writing a letter of forgiveness to a person who has hurt or wronged you in the past.
7. Identify what you consider to be your top 5 strengths. Then make use of one of the top 5 strengths in a new and different way each day for the next week. Then repeat the process with strength.

Optimism Exercises
1. Look for something of value in each and every person and circumstance in your life today. Repeat this for the next week or two.
2. Express optimistic statements daily to your children, colleagues, family, and others.
3. When something goes wrong or sour, examine it to see if the situation could have been avoided or changed had you been more optimistic from the start.
4. Develop optimistic strategies for coping with stress and hardship. For example, quote axioms to yourself, such as, "This too shall pass," or, "That which doesn't kill me makes me stronger."
5. When experiencing some type of trauma or tragedy, consider what could be optimistic about the situation and how it may impact your future positively.
6. When you want something you cannot have, think about 5 things you do have.
7. The next time you write a note or letter or send an e-mail message, look it over before you send it and change the wording to reflect a more optimistic view.

ACTION PLAN: In the lists above, circle the items that you need to work on and will do so over the next month.

GOOD HABITS FOR HEALTHY LIVING

Good habits encourage others to be attracted to us and to see us as a role model for their lives. Our children, family members, neighbors, and work colleagues are a few such people that may see us as their role model. How then shall we live? How do we shape our daily behavior pattern so others will be drawn to us and see us as their preferred role model? Below are a few suggested behavior patterns that most of us would acknowledge as good habits.

1. Live honestly and blamelessly so your conscience is clear and without guilt.
2. Practice a peaceful lifestyle and encourage peace among those around you.
3. Live a life of generosity; give cheerfully and reap happiness.
4. Do the best you can in each situation and be adequate for each task you undertake.
5. Respond to criticism with openness and a non-defensive, learning attitude.
6. Take time to meditate and reflect on your day's experiences and lofty thoughts.
7. Daily decisions reflect wisdom if they are based on a mix of emotional factors.
8. Start many projects, but finish what you start with diligence and determination.
9. Keep the faith, utmost; expect something good to happen in your day.
10. Clear the record regularly through offering and accepting forgiveness of wrongs and hurts.
11. Engage regularly in a mind-stretching activity to learn skills and expand your knowledge base.
12. Social friendships need to be fostered and strengthened through regular contact and meaningful engagement.
13. Be a communicator in all areas of your life; initiate conversation and respond to those that engage you in dialogue.
14. Overcome hurts and attacks with good.

COMMENTS AND MY PLANS TO IMPROVE MY LIFE:

COMPONENTS OF BRAIN FUNCTIONING

The brain is the engine that drives the body and mind to perform their daily functions and help us live effectively and efficiently. If the brain is healthy, so is our body.

What are the factors that contribute to a healthy brain? Ask yourself if you are doing these nine things each week or regularly.

1. I feed and nourish my brain.
2. I protect my brain from trauma and impairment.
3. I engage my brain in meaningful and challenging tasks.
4. I keep my brain from experiencing stress.
5. I deal with and treat problems soon after onset.
6. I reduce the aging speed and process of my brain.
7. I push my brain by exercise and graduated activity.
8. I am sure to provide the proper medication and nutritional supplements.
9. I provide my brain with strategies of wisdom.

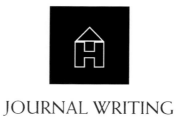

JOURNAL WRITING

Sometime changes can occur just through recognizing the source of the problem. However, most changes come from an accumulation of changes in beliefs, priorities, and behaviors over a period of time. Consistency and an investment in yourself is necessary. Journal writing can be useful for keeping track of a wide variety of things that can help you achieve your goals.

Use your journal to record your thoughts and feelings. "Just doing it" can make a difference. Acknowledging underlying thoughts and feelings and writing about them can help increase self-understanding, and self-awareness which can make it easier to change old patterns of behavior and to start new ones. Consistently keeping a journal is a strong message to yourself that you want to change and that you are committed to making it happen.

People often experience greater successes when they have established goals. Unpredictable situations do occur, which can cause setbacks, but they can also allow for a re-evaluation of your problems and can offer an opportunity. However, when goals are defined and the unexpected happens, you are more likely to reach them even if you are initially thrown off course.

Most people don't clearly establish their goals, let alone write them down and think about what it will take to accomplish them.

STEP 1
Write down the goals you want to accomplish in the next 12 months. Make them as specific as possible. They should be realistic, but also challenging.

STEP 2
Write down 10 goals you want to accomplish this month. These should help you move toward some of your goals for the year. The monthly goals should be smaller and more detailed than the yearly goals.

STEP 3
Write down 3 goals you want to accomplish today. Goals need to be accompanied by plans to make them happen. If your goals are too large, you are likely to stop before you start. Better to start small and build upward. Small successes build big successes.

STEP 4
Self-monitoring: Keep track of where you are now. Create realistic plans that can get you to your goals.

STEP 5
Begin observing which self-talk has been maintaining the old patterns you want to change. List at least 5 to 10 negative self-statements that feed into your old patterns.

STEP 6
List 5 to 10 positive statements that are likely to help create the new patterns you want to create.

STEP 7
Create challenges that will replace the negative self-talk you listed in Step 5.

STEP 8
Programming new healthy self-talk. Each day, say at least 10 positive self-statements to yourself.

STEP 9
Imagination and visualization: Five times each day, take one minute to visualize a positive image.

Therapist's Guide to Clinical Intervention, Second Edition by Sharon L. Johnson (© 2003 Elsevier Inc.)

STEP 10
Building self-esteem: Use your journal to list good things about yourself. Be supportive to yourself.

STEP 11
Each day record 3 of the day's successes – big or small. Praise yourself. Plan small rewards for some accomplishment each week.

STEP 12
In your journal, frequently ask what parts of yourself you are involved with. The various issues you face (e.g., the needy child, the rebellious adolescent, etc.).

STEP 13
Each day, forgive yourself for something you have done. Like self-esteem, forgiveness is one of the keys to successful change. Forgiving yourself for past actions allows you to take responsibility for what happens in the future.

STEP 14
List the fears of success that the different parts of you may have. Work on making success safe.

STEP 15
Be willing to do things differently. If you don't, nothing is going to change.

Chapter 26

Communication Tips and Exercises

Chapter Contents

Communication is the art of human relationships. Through communication we solve problems, learn new dimensions of life, expand our social circle, reduce conflict and stress, teach others new skills and navigate life to its fullest extent. Communication is a skill we learn during early childhood. We keep on improving our communication and relational skills as we proceed from one grade to the next. We learn to better communicate as we study it and apply it to everyday problems. Therapy is one format in which we learn the communication skills that were not learned in the home and school during childhood.

This chapter contains forms, guidelines, informational documents, questionnaires, and templates to help the therapist teach and guide patients in their new pursuit of learning to communicate. As a result, the future of patients will be different and much more impactful.

COMMUNICATION TIPS FROM THE TENNIS COURT

Tennis is an excellent model by which to learn communication skills. As in tennis, the aim is to keep the ball in the air and moving. Some of the best tennis matches are when two individuals are equally matched and/or play respectfully. The fun is in the game of back and forth, not in the winning.

MY COMMUNICATION SCORE (1–10)

TENNIS ANYONE?

AT HOME   AT WORK

THE WARMUP: The skill of initiating conversation, such as small talk.

THE SERVE: The skill of asking questions to get others involved and participating.

THE SERVER: The skill of taking the lead in a social situation and reaching out to others that are not talking.

THE VOLLEY: The skill of idea exchange and developing a topic into a full discussion.

THE TENNIS BALL: The skill of selecting topics others will be interested in and will discuss.

THE GAME PLAN: The skill of thinking ahead of time and planning a conversation with someone.

THE NET: The skill of avoiding various conversation-stoppers and keeping the discussion going.

THE HANDICAP: The skill of not letting an impairment or disability stop you from talking and being part of the conversation.

THE SLAM: The skill of hurting or beating your partner by finding his/her weakness. A skill not to be encouraged in interpersonal communication.

THE REVIEW OR DEBRIEFING TIME: The skill of learning from your mistakes and using the situation to help others learn to communicate better in the future.

WHAT KIND OF LISTENER AM I?

	I'm Good	I'm Fair	I Need to Improve
1. Do I prepare myself physically by facing the speaker, and making sure that I can hear?	_____	_____	_____
2. Do I maintain eye contact as well as listen?	_____	_____	_____
3. Do I avoid deciding from the speaker's appearance and delivery whether or not what he/she has to say is worthwhile?	_____	_____	_____
4. Do I listen primarily for ideas and underlying feelings?	_____	_____	_____
5. Do I determine my own bias and try to allow for it?	_____	_____	_____
6. Do I keep my mind on what the speaker is saying?	_____	_____	_____
7. Do I avoid interrupting if I hear an incorrect or stupid statement?	_____	_____	_____
8. Before answering, have I taken in the other person's point-of-view?	_____	_____	_____
9. Do I make a conscious effort to evaluate the logic and credibility of what I hear?	_____	_____	_____
10. Do I avoid trying to have the last word?	_____	_____	_____
11. Do I avoid the use of status (e.g., allowing people to interrupt meetings to get your approval, signature, etc.)?	_____	_____	_____
12. Do I avoid glancing at my watch or papers on my desk?	_____	_____	_____

COMMENTS/MY PLAN TO IMPROVE:

COMMUNICATION EXERCISES IN THE PERCEPTION OF FEELINGS

Please complete each sentence with a "feeling" or "emotional" statement. In so doing, you will become more aware of the feelings of others and more attuned to them. Sensitivity to the feelings of others is a prime attribute of a highly functioning person.

1. "Life just doesn't seem worth struggling with any more. I don't think I can make it. I just can't go on any more." I feel

_____

_____

2. "I wrote Fred a special tune for his birthday, and he never said anything about it, whether he appreciated it or didn't like it." I felt

_____

_____

3. "I don't shower comfortably. I'm embarrassed about my body, about being overweight." I feel

_____

_____

4. "It's my job to give a brief talk at the anniversary party this weekend." Every time I think about it I feel

_____

_____

5. "My husband loves his job as a bus driver, but I wish he'd consider working at something else. When he's gone for five days on a trip, the house seems so big and empty I can hardly stand it." For the five days of his absence I feel like

_____

_____

6. "I really got into a battle with my wife last night. I was an hour later than usual because I had to go to an AA meeting after work. She got on my back because I didn't call to tell her I'd be late. I don't feel like I should have to check in with her like I'm one of the kids." She makes me feel

_____

_____

7. "I know we talked last time I saw you about my not losing my temper with the kids. But what do you do when they don't seem to learn. Just before I left home today my 4-year-old ran out in the street twice after I'd warned him. It made me feel

_____

_____

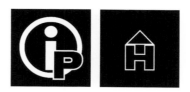

MODEL OF COMMUNICATION PATTERNS

Find your style of communication and develop plans to make the necessary improvements so your social relationships will be more honorable and effective. Move towards Excellent Communication as your goal. Commit to improved social relationships over the coming week by speaking more directly and honestly. Ask for any help you might need to achieve this goal.

	HONEST	**DISHONEST**
DIRECT	Excellent Communication	Deceptive Communication
INDIRECT	Inadequate Communication	Confusing Communication

MY PLAN TO IMPROVE MY COMMUNICATION STYLE:

STYLES OF COMMUNICATION

A Guideline for Self-Evaluation

Good communication facilitates the development of confidence, feelings of self-worth, and effective relationships with others. It makes life with those around us more pleasant and helps others develop good feelings about themselves and towards those with whom they associate in daily life. Below are two styles of communication. Which one is more like you and which specific styles of communication do you need to address and correct?

FACILITATIVE STYLES OF COMMUNICATION

1. Listens in an alert, attentive manner.
2. Assertively "speaks out."
3. Self-discloses.
4. States feelings and opinions in the "here and now."
5. When sending a message, seeks feedback.
6. When receiving a message, gives feedback.
7. Checks out perceptions and interpretations.
8. Explicitly tells what is wanted.
9. Takes responsibility for self.
10. Listens for free information and uses it to build a conversation.

OBSTRUCTIVE STYLES OF COMMUNICATION

1. Talks over others and is not receptive.
2. Speaks indirectly to others.
3. Gives contradictory, incongruent, or double messages.
4. Distorts reality.
5. Encourages misunderstanding by vague messages and incomplete sentences.
6. Avoids or evades questions.
7. Assumes he/she knows others' motivations, thoughts, feelings or wants.
8. Intellectualizes and neglects to express feelings.
9. Directs or tells others what to do and what not to do.
10. Does not provide words of encouragement, support, and acceptance.

THE LISTENING SKILLS LADDER

The following actions are the basic steps in effective listening. The mnemonic of a LADDER will help fix these steps in your memory.

L   Look at the person speaking to you

A   Ask open-ended questions for more information

D   Don't interrupt; listen patiently

D   Don't change the topic or shift the topic to one of your choosing

E   Empathize with the speaker and show some feeling about the subject

R   Respond both verbally and nonverbally to the speaker

THE STINGS AND THORNS OF COMMUNICATION

People communicate in a variety of ways. Unfortunately, some people are hostile, harsh, and hurtful in the way they communicate. We do have to be prepared to deal effectively with such communication patterns when we face them, often without warning. Here are a few examples of hostile communication and how you can deal with such situations with reason and calmness. The main point is not to be taken into the dark world of hostile and harsh communication when faced with it in your daily interchanges of life.

1. **Hostile communication:** Attempt to establish points of agreement, even if you must dig to uncover an area of common ground and understanding. Make use of "I" statements and minimize the use of "you" statements. When you use an "I" statement, it clarifies what you think and feel and minimizes criticism. Keep calm and do not speak in a manner that challenges, argues, or rejects statements being made. Stay in the neutral zone, emotionally and verbally. Let the hostile person speak their entire story while you listen attentively. Respond in a non-argumentative manner, such as using phrases like, "I understand."

2. **Those who "know it all":** Do not adopt a contrary or adversarial stance in the conversation. Ask questions. Introduce alternative ideas to be considered. Give facts or ideas that might expand the discussion taking place. Hopefully, the "know it all" person will incorporate your ideas and thoughts on the topic.

3. **Absolute statements:** Do not get drawn into absolute statements yourself. Remain non-absolute. Use phrases that suggest tentativeness, caution, possibilities. Be sure that you interpose a way out of any discussion and alternative ways of looking at things. Be a voice of moderation.

4. **Negative and discouraging words:** Do not go to the opposite extreme, but do introduce compliments, reasons for hope and affirmation. Express graciousness. Look for reasons to be courageous regarding the future. Be compassionate, caring, and understanding.

5. **Distracting gestures:** Do not imitate the same gestures. Keep relaxed, open, and friendly. Be non-threatening and do not attack. Perhaps there will be an opportunity to comment on the gestures being made and how they are distracting. Only say this if you can do so graciously and non-critically. Do not over-use gestures yourself.

6. **"NO" is the answer:** Be prepared to accept and live with the "NO" answer. Introduce exceptions and alternatives and the possibility of a change or variation in the future. Seek opportunity to introduce additional and new information for consideration.

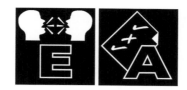

NONVERBAL COMMUNICATION CHECKLIST

The checklist below provides the therapist a structured format by which to assess a patient's nonverbal communication habits and patterns. Once assessed, the therapist is in a good position to help the patient unlearn improper nonverbal communication habits and learn new or more effective nonverbal communication skills. These can then be practiced in a session and given as a homework assignment.

Behaviors observed (check all observed) _____

	Yes	No
A. EYE CONTACT		
1. Spontaneous eye contact and eye movements	☐	☐
2. Breaking eye contact	☐	☐
3. Staring too intensely	☐	☐
4. Looking down	☐	☐
5. Looking directly at helper when speaking	☐	☐
6. Looking directly at helper when listening	☐	☐
7. Looking away	☐	☐
8. Staring blankly	☐	☐
B. BODY POSTURE		
1. Slight forward lean	☐	☐
2. Body facing helper	☐	☐
3. Relaxed posture	☐	☐
4. Relaxed hand position	☐	☐
5. Spontaneous hand and arm movements	☐	☐
6. Gestures for emphasis	☐	☐
7. Touching helper	☐	☐
8. Relaxed leg position	☐	☐
9. Slouching	☐	☐
10. Fixed, rigid position	☐	☐
11. Physically distant from helper	☐	☐
12. Physically too close to helper	☐	☐
13. Arms across chest	☐	☐
14. Body turned sideways	☐	☐
C. HEAD AND FACIAL MOVEMENTS		
1. Affirmative head nods	☐	☐
2. Calm, expressive facial movements	☐	☐
3. Appropriate smiling	☐	☐
4. Expressions matching helper mood	☐	☐
5. Face rigid	☐	☐
6. Continual nodding	☐	☐
7. Extraneous facial movements	☐	☐
8. Continual smiling	☐	☐
9. Little smiling	☐	☐
10. Cold, distant expression	☐	☐
11. Frowning	☐	☐
12. Overly emotional expression	☐	☐

Cont.

Therapist's Guide to Clinical Intervention, Second Edition by Sharon L. Johnson (© 2003 Elsevier Inc.)

D. VOCAL QUALITY
    1. Pleasant intonation ☐ ☐
    2. Appropriate loudness ☐ ☐
    3. Moderate rate of speech ☐ ☐
    4. Simple, precise language ☐ ☐
    5. Fluid speech ☐ ☐
    6. Monotone ☐ ☐
    7. Too much affect ☐ ☐
    8. Too loud ☐ ☐
    9. Too soft ☐ ☐
  10. Use of jargon ☐ ☐
  11. Use of slang ☐ ☐
  12. Too fast ☐ ☐
  13. Too slow ☐ ☐
  14. Use of "you know" ☐ ☐
  15. Use of "um," "ah" ☐ ☐
  16. Voice quiver ☐ ☐

E. DISTRACTING PERSONAL HABITS
    1. Playing with hair ☐ ☐
    2. Fiddling with pen or pencil ☐ ☐
    3. Chewing gum ☐ ☐
    4. Smoking ☐ ☐
    5. Drinking ☐ ☐
    6. Tapping fingers or feet ☐ ☐
    7. Other

ASSERTIVENESS INVENTORY

The following questions will help determine how passive, assertive, or aggressive you are.

Answer the questions honestly and write out how you would handle each of these situations:

1. Do you say something when you think someone is unfair?
2. Do you find it difficult to make decisions?
3. Do you openly criticize the ideas, opinions, and behavior of others?
4. If someone takes your place in line do you speak up?
5. Do you avoid people or events for fear of embarrassment?
6. Do you have confidence in your own ability to make decisions?
7. Do you insist that the people you live with share chores?
8. Do you have a tendency to "fly off the handle?"
9. Are you able to say "no" when someone is pressuring you to buy or to do something?
10. When someone comes in after you at a restaurant and is waited on first do you say something?
11. Are you reluctant to express your thoughts or feelings during a discussion or debate?
12. If a person is overdue in returning something that they have borrowed from you do you bring it up?
13. Do you continue to argue with someone after they have had enough?
14. Do you generally express what you think and feel?
15. Does it bother you to be observed doing your job?
16. If someone's behavior is bothering you in a theater or lecture, do you say something?
17. Is it difficult for you to maintain eye contact while talking with someone?
18. If you are not pleased with your meal at a restaurant, do you talk to the waitress about correcting the situation?
19. When you purchase something that is flawed or broken do you return it?
20. When you are angry do you yell, name-call, or use obscene language?
21. Do you step in and make decisions for others?
22. Are you able to ask for small favors?
23. Do you shout or use bullying tactics to get your way?
24. Are you able to openly express love and concern?
25. Do you respond respectfully when there is a difference of opinion?

You can tell by your pattern of responses if you generally fall within the descriptor of being passive, assertive, or aggressive. Use this exercise to better understand yourself and to help you set a goal for change if necessary. Share the results with your therapist.

Cont.

Therapist's Guide to Clinical Intervention, Second Edition by Sharon L. Johnson (© 2003 Elsevier Inc.)

To further clarify what style of communication and behavior you use, explore how you would handle the following situations:

1. You are standing in line and someone cuts in front of you, or it is your turn and the clerk waits on someone else.
2. Your doctor keeps you waiting for half an hour for your appointment.
3. You are not served something that you ordered at a restaurant.
4. Your neighbors are keeping you awake with loud music.
5. Your teenager is playing the stereo too loud.
6. Your friend borrowed some money from you. It is past the date that they promised to pay you back.
7. You receive a bill and it looks like there is an error on it.
8. You purchased something and decide that you want to return it to the store for a refund.
9. The people behind you at the theater are talking during the movie or show.
10. You realize that the person that you are talking to is not listening to you.
11. You are displeased by your partner's behavior.
12. The dry cleaners did a poor job on several articles of clothing.

This exercise will help you better understand yourself, and help you determine appropriate and effective responses to normal, everyday experiences.

Passive: Failing to stand up for yourself or standing up for yourself ineffectively, which can lead to a violation of your rights.

Assertive: Standing up for yourself in a way that does not violate the rights of others. It is a direct, appropriate expression of thoughts and feelings.

Aggressive: Standing up for yourself in a way that violates the rights of another person. They may feel humiliated or put down by your response.

Adapted from R. Alberti &M. Emmons, *Stand Up, Speak Out, Talk Back*, Pocket Books, 1975.

Eating and Exercise Logs

Chapter Contents

Keeping a log of food intake and exercise is basic to weight control, body shape, and general health. A healthy lifestyle is the general goal or objective of most patients and very important to some. Keeping logs helps to focus a patient's attention on the intentional purpose and goal of a healthy lifestyle being achieved.

This chapter provides the therapist with forms, logs, record keeping forms, and guidelines. The therapist will be appreciated by those patients for whom the logs contained in this chapter are utilized.

PERSONAL EXERCISE RECORD

Make a weekly record of gross energy expenditure and do so in 5-minute intervals. Each tick you make represents 5 minutes of exercise. Record only the exercise beyond your normal activity.

(Cut out and carry with you)

✂

PERSONAL EXERCISE RECORD

Week commencing: _____

EASY (Golf, Walking, Dancing, Sailing)
Place a tick on the dotted line for each 5 minutes of exercise this week. Then enter the total number of ticks in the space below and multiply by 20 to get the total of EASY exercise.

– –
– – – – – – – – – – – – – – – – – – – –

CALORIES BURNED = _____ x 20 = _____

MODERATE (Cycling, Tennis, Swimming)
Place a tick on the dotted line for each 5 minutes of exercise this week. Then enter the total number of ticks in the space below and multiply by 35 to get the total of MODERATE exercise.

– –
– – – – – – – – – – – – – – – – – – – –

CALORIES BURNED = _____ x 35 = _____

VIGOROUS   (Jump Rope, Jogging, Handball)
Place a tick on the dotted line for each 5 minutes of exercise this week. Then enter the total number of ticks in the space below and multiply by 50 to get the total of VIGOROUS exercise.

– –
– – – – – – – – – – – – – – – – – – – –

CALORIES BURNED = _____ x 50 = _____

TOTAL CALORIES BURNED THIS WEEK = _____

Add the subtotals of the three types of exercise to calculate the total calories burned this week by exercise. GOAL = 3500 calories burned.

✂

3500 calories = 1 lb of stored fat burned up by exercise. **If you have burned over 3500 calories, reward yourself!** Keep this chart going for 6 weeks to start a pattern of exercise

WEEKLY HOME EXERCISE PROGRAM

Week commencing: _____

Much research has demonstrated that exercise is not only good for the heart, but also good for the health of the brain and its functioning. A strong brain combats depression, anxiety, and one's general mental health. A healthy brain is also vital to the delay of dementia and to the prevention of a variety of health disorders, such as Parkinson's disease. Weight management is another benefit of intentional exercise. In general, what is good for the heart is good for the brain.

The spaces below are provided for the tracking of a weekly exercise program. Also note the reason for the exercise in which you engage during the week. For example, exercising for weight loss purposes, becoming physically fit, body shape refinement or even going to a gym for exercise and social engagement and friendship development.

EXERCISE	REASON	WHEN
1. _____	_____	_____
2. _____	_____	_____
3. _____	_____	_____
4. _____	_____	_____
5. _____	_____	_____
6. _____	_____	_____
7. _____	_____	_____
8. _____	_____	_____
9. _____	_____	_____
10. _____	_____	_____
11. _____	_____	_____
12. _____	_____	_____

COMMENTS AND OBSERVATIONS:

REWARDS FOR CONSISTENCY AND PROGRESS:

EATING BEHAVIOR SCHEDULE

As part of my eating and weight management program this chart will be kept and analyzed periodically to see if I have any bad habits to be changed.

Name: _____   Week commencing: _____

Day	Eating time	Duration of eating	Location of eating	Body position (sitting, standing, reclining)	Other activity during eating	Mood during eating	Hunger rating at the start of eating time	Type and amount of food consumed (meal = M; snack = S)	Calories (est.)
1									
2									
3									
4									
5									
6									
7									

HELPING PATIENTS LIVE AN ACTIVE LIFESTYLE

Living a lifestyle that is active and healthy is in the best interest of every individual. It is especially important for those, like us, that work in sedentary jobs. The following guidelines will help make the process reasonably safe when a client is undertaking a program of exercise and increased activity. Consider the following long-term guidelines for creating a healthy lifestyle.

1. Look to yourself first and engage in an exercise-based lifestyle. Be an example and model, not just a director that sends out orders.

2. Refer a client to someone that is considered an expert or coach. Don't try to be both therapist and coach. Keep your role clear.

3. Conduct an exercise assessment at the time of the initial evaluation. Help clients develop a plan of exercise and lifestyle that will result in good mental health and positive general health.

4. Start clients out by taking small steps to begin the process, and then taking on larger and more demanding tasks and exercises.

5. Assign a series of homework assignments or tasks to help a client find an exercise program that they will stay with and undertake conscientiously.

6. Ask the client to keep a journal or record of the exercises selected and note how they affect the person's energy level, thinking patterns, and health.

7. Potential problems need to be identified and confronted so the client will not drop out due to discouragement or some complex problem.

8. Plan ways to introduce rewards at specific achievement levels to maintain motivation, goal attainment, and create a healthy lifestyle.

9. Take the client out to a site, such as a local track, to encourage better compliance and interest. Use *in vivo* procedures to help the client feel more committed and involved.

10. Schedule regular discussions and review points to assess the client's progress.

TIPS TO MANAGE WEIGHT LOSS

The following tips have been found helpful by many people who are seriously and actively engaged in a weight loss program. Each person finds some of these tips particularly helpful. It is suggested you try all or most of them and then utilize the specific tips you find more helpful.

1. Develop a realistic body image. If necessary, use pictures of yourself or a model at an ideal healthy weight.
2. Set a goal, a concrete one, for yourself, such as buying a dress, or an outfit two sizes smaller than your present size, and hang it in a visible place.
3. Set a cue-weight, such as losing a pound a week.
4. Keep a record, log, diary or journal of your emotions and thoughts as you are losing weight.
5. Learn simple techniques in behavior management for self-regulation, including self-reinforcement, self-punishment, and behavioral rehearsal.
6. Use stimulus narrowing pertaining to food and eating.
7. Develop cognitive aversion to foods you are not to have; foods that are high in fat, sugar and salt.
8. Enjoy your meals, eat slowly, and roll your food in your mouth to get every bit of taste out of it.
9. Put your fork down between bites.
10. Set up a series of consequences if you do not attain your goal or follow your eating plan.
11. Focus on internal cues from your body signaling hunger and fullness; learn to ignore external cues for eating.
12. Slow down your eating and reduce the number of places you eat; restrict your eating to only the kitchen or dining room.
13. Avoid eating in front of the television or while reading.
14. Avoid eating when you are upset or depressed, or in response to any other emotion.
15. Recruit social support for your project of self-improvement.
16. Engage in relaxation and guided imagery exercises to improve your "will power."
17. Become more assertive by practicing assertiveness (learn to say NO when it is necessary for self-improvement).
18. Increase your usual physical activity level and engage in regular physical exercise.
19. Think thin and imagine yourself as thinning.

Chapter 28

Cultural Diversity Appreciation Exercises

Chapter Contents

Most therapists have had extensive training and education in cultural diversity. Social Psychology, Sociology, Anthropology, and courses in Individual Differences are fields of study common to the professional training of most therapists. Cultural factors are generally taken into account in the therapy sessions when they are relevant. Helping patients with their cultural and ethnic awareness and sensitivity is a task often brought to the attention of a therapist during therapy. It is vitally important for a therapist to be aware of this issue and address its relevance to the goals of the therapy plan.

The forms in this chapter were selected to aid the therapist in working with patients needing to confront their own issues of intolerance and bias. Homework assignments and exercises are provided to help patients make the changes needed in their human perspective and social relationships.

MOVIES AND VIDEOS FOCUSING ON DIVERSE POPULATIONS

African American
Autobiography of Miss Jane Pittman
Boyz N the Hood
White Man's Burden
Colors
The Color Purple
Remember the Titans
Do the Right Thing
Driving Miss Daisy
The Power of One
Eye on the Prize
Mississippi Masala
Sounder
Jungle Fever
Long Walk Home
Malcolm X
Guess Who's Coming to Dinner
To Kill a Mockingbird
American History X
I Know Why the Caged Bird Sings
In the Still of the Night
Matewan
Mo-Better Blues
Raisin in the Sun
The Human Stain
Amistad
Roots I & II

Asian American
Dim Sum
Double Happiness
Farewell to Manzanar
Joy Luck Club
Come See the Paradise
The Wash
Wedding Banquet
Eat Drink Man Woman

Latino/Latina
American Me
Ballad of Gregorio Cortez
Born in East L.A.
El Norte
Like Water for Chocolate
Mi Familia
Milagro Beanfield War

Romero
Tortilla Soup

People with Disabilities
Born on the 4th of July
Coming Home
If You Can See What I Hear
My Left Foot
One Flew Over the Cuckoo's Nest
Waterdance
I Am Sam
Children of a Lesser God
Frankie Starlight
Miracle Worker
The Other Side of the Mountain
A Patch of Blue
What's Eating Gilbert Grape

Native American
Dances with Wolves
The Last of the Mohicans
The Mission
Never Cry Wolf
Pow Wow Highway
Thunderheart
Pocohontas
Smoke Signals

Elderly
Cocoon
Driving Miss Daisy
Foxfire
Fried Green Tomatoes
Nobody's Fool
On Golden Pond

Others
Not Without My Daughter
A Walk in the Clouds
City of Joy
Monsoon Wedding
My Big Fat Greek Wedding
What's Cooking?
The Color of Paradise
Children of Heaven
Songcatcher

Cont.

Q & A

1. What were your personal reactions, feelings, and thoughts to the film?
2. In the film viewed, what were the life barriers and hurdles for the minority group focused on?
3. In viewing the film, what did you learn about yourself and your style of relationship building?
4. What new learning did you acquire about the minority group who were the subject of this film?
5. What were you able to learn from this film about other people and how can you use this new knowledge as you relate to those of a different background?
6. What was the one main "take away" from this film that will have a lasting impact on you and influence how you relate to others that are similar and different from you?
7. Other thoughts …

PERSONAL IDENTITY PROFILE

RATIONALE

This assignment is based on the assumption that awareness of your own perspective will better your understanding of others. It is difficult to understand let alone respect others' cultural orientations unless you know something about your own frames of reference. When your own system of rules and meanings can be understood as simply "another voice heard from," a foundation is laid for the mutual respect that is necessary for constructive intercultural communication.

PROCEDURE

Write a word or phrase that describes you, in response to each of the following categories:

1. Age/Age group/Generation: _____

2. Gender: _____

3. Gender identity: _____

4. "Race": _____

5. Heritage/Ethnicity: _____

6. Nationality: _____

7. If American, what region: _____

8. Rural/Suburban/Urban: _____

9. Religious orientation: _____

10. Affectional (sexual) orientation: _____

11. Class: _____

12. Language(s): _____

13. Current family: _____

14. Family background (family of origin): _____

15. Vocation (job): _____

16. Avocation (hobby): _____

17. Others: (e.g., traumatic events, physical challenges, chronic health issues): _____

After you have responded to each item, **put a mark by the 3 or 4 that play the most significant role in your everyday life.** They may be significant because they are meaningful to you, or because of the time they take up, or because you keep "bumping into them", etc. These key categories can be said to make up a cultural profile. They are the critical elements in your "identity." Summarize your profile below.

MY PERSONAL IDENTITY PROFILE

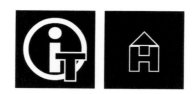

THE CULTURAL GENOGRAM

Therapists must be prepared to facilitate improved relationships with people coming from a range of cultures and ethnic origins. First, a therapist needs to have a good grasp of his/her own cultural significance and sensitivity. Then, a therapist will be in a stronger position to interact in a meaningful and helpful way with those of other cultures.

The following questions will help a therapist come to terms with his/her own background and the issues of racial and cultural influences.

QUESTIONS FOR THE THERAPIST TO CONSIDER AND DISCUSS

- Under what conditions did your family enter the United States (e.g., immigrant, refugee)?
- What significance do race, skin color, and hair play within your culture?
- How are gender roles defined within your culture? How is social class defined?
- What occupational rules are valued and devalued?
- What prejudices and stereotypes does your culture have about itself?
- What prejudices and stereotypes do other cultures have about your culture?
- What prejudices and stereotypes do you have about other cultures?
- What are the ways in which pride/shame issues are manifested in your family system?
- What impact will these pride/shame issues have on your work and with those associates and friends from both similar and dissimilar cultural backgrounds?
- If more than one culture comprises your family makeup, how are these differences negotiated in your family?
- What are the intergenerational consequences of a mixed family culture? How has this impacted you personally as a friend, neighbor or work colleague?

OBSERVATIONS, CONCLUSIONS, AND FUTURE STEPS

Chapter 29

Conflict Resolution and Problem Solving

Chapter Contents

We live in a world that is increasingly conflictual at all strata of society. It is not uncommon for patients coming for therapy to be enmeshed in conflict with someone. Unfortunately, conflict resolution skills are not often learned in the home during the formative years nor taught in the schools. We have a societal dearth of problem solving and conflict management skills. In the face of widespread conflict and increasing domestic and interpersonal violence, therapists need to be ready and prepared to help their patients prevent and process conflict in positive and healthy terms.

This chapter contains forms, guidelines, templates, questionnaires, and exercises to teach conflict resolution as a central part of therapy. This chapter will be of help to many therapists as they attempt to deal constructively with conflict and violence.

WALKING AROUND THE EDGES OF CONFLICT

The following steps will help you deal effectively with conflict. Learn them well so you are ready to deal with those that create conflict or bring it into your life.

1. **Present** the "issue" in terms that are specific and non-accusatory. Use "I" statements such as, "I understand that …," "I had it presented to me…," "I received a message stating that … ."

2. **Listen** carefully to the person's initial response. Restate it, as you understand it.

3. **Ask** for information or documentation in a declarative but reasonable and gracious manner. Do not demand.

4. **Listen** carefully to the reply. Be sure you understand any objections raised or any conditional terms of acceptance of your request.

5. **Restate** your interpretation or perception of what was said rather than assume you understood the objection or conditional terms.

6. **Propose** alternative or compromised actions or press for your original request should an impasse develop. Be reasonable and always propose something that you feel could be the starting point. Should a counter-request be offered, let them know your limitations and use this to begin the process of brainstorming to find a helpful way to resolve the impasse or the voiced objection.

7. **Veto** unacceptable proposed solutions. Be clear and direct.

8. **Summarize** the full discussion up to this point. Restate the pros and cons or limitations of the possible options. Ask if your summary concurs with their understanding of the conversation up to this point. Keep the focus on your initial request.

9. **Accept** one of the proposed solutions or a compromise that offers a starting point. Begin to act on it immediately.

10. **Remember,** you have options "outside the box" to propose or to implement if you are up against a brick wall. Be firm, but try to be accommodating.

11. **Follow-up** in a timely manner and monitor any agreements, points of compromise or action steps to be taken.

12. **Implement** the strategy of RID to help you debrief the experience:

    Recognize your anger signals.

    Identify a positive way to think about the situation.

    Do something constructive to calm down.

THE FIVE STEPS TO PROBLEM SOLVING

Use the mnemonic "I COPE" to develop your problem solving skills.

I   **Identify** the problem and state it in specific terms

C   Determine whether the problem is **Changeable**:

Am I able to change the problem or not?
Is the potential for change under my control?
If no change is possible, do I express my feelings on the topic or change my thinking?

O   **Options** for solving the problem must be explored. What are the:

Advantages of each option?
Disadvantages of each option?

P   Choose the best option and **Plan** how to implement it. Determine what specific steps need to be undertaken.

E   **Evaluate** the action undertaken. Did the plan work? If not, go back to "O."

CONFLICT RESOLUTION AND PROBLEM SOLVING

The way we resolve conflict and solve problems can be systematic and non-violent. We can conduct ourselves in a peaceful manner and exhibit a sense of respect for the other person. The diagram below illustrates the process and suggests we do all we can to avoid an argument. What is worse is to leave the field and engage in abusive and hurtful or violent behavior. As the second diagram shows, in such cases we go from an argument to abuse and then we have great difficulty getting back on track and into the problem solving.

NON-VIOLENT PROBLEM SOLVING

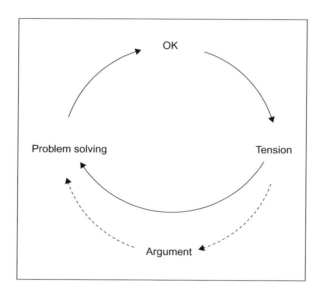

In non-violent behavior:
- There is no physical violence, intimidation, or attempt to control the other person.
- There is no verbal abuse, such as name-calling, humiliation, or verbal threats.
- There is no attempt to hurt the other person.
- You take personal responsibility for controlling your own anger.
- The goal is to communicate, not to hurt or bully.

VIOLENT PROBLEM SOLVING

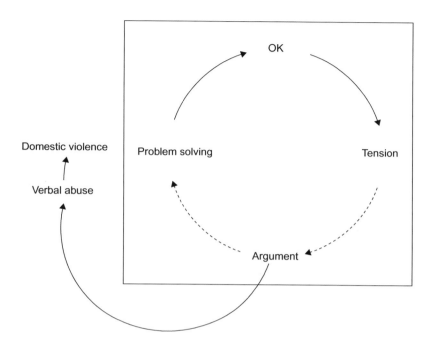

In verbally abuse behavior:
* There is name calling, such as "bitch, whore, idiot" or any other derogatory names.
* You make threats to hurt the other person, leave her/him, or harm her/him if the person doesn't do what you want.
* There is shouting and yelling.
* There is cursing and swearing.
* You use language that belittles or demeans the other person.

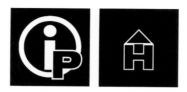

PROBLEM SOLVING DIAGRAM

Take a few minutes to focus on yourself. Are you (1) a person who generally copes well but is having current difficulties associated with a specific situation or (2) a person who experiences difficulty coping? If you identified yourself as generally experiencing difficulty coping, be prepared to be patient as you learn to improve your problem solving skills, and use the necessary resources for reaching this important goal.

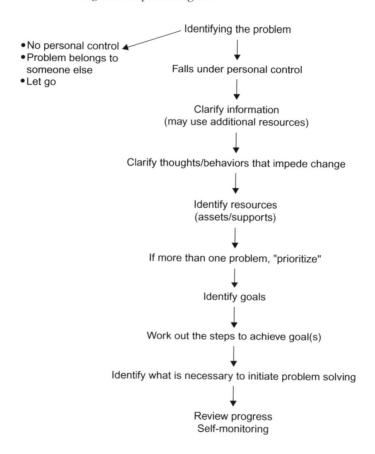

- No personal control
- Problem belongs to someone else
- Let go

Identifying the problem
↓
Falls under personal control
↓
Clarify information
(may use additional resources)
↓
Clarify thoughts/behaviors that impede change
↓
Identify resources
(assets/supports)
↓
If more than one problem, "prioritize"
↓
Identify goals
↓
Work out the steps to achieve goal(s)
↓
Identify what is necessary to initiate problem solving
↓
Review progress
Self-monitoring

THE PROBLEM SOLVING WORKSHEET

Problem solving is both a science and an art. An orderly sequence of steps is usually followed to get to a solution and resolve a conflict or issue of uncertainty. Most people follow the steps outlined below as they have been found to be an excellent systematic process of getting to a workable solution after identifying a problem. Learn the sequence and become better skilled in problem solving in all areas of your life.

1. What is <u>the</u> <u>problem</u> and its scope?

2. What do you consider to be the <u>possible</u> <u>causes</u> for the problem (there may be many)?

3. What might be some <u>possible</u> <u>solutions</u> to the problem?

4. Considering the various <u>probable</u> <u>solutions.</u> What might be the likely consequences associated with the various solutions under consideration?

5. Select the <u>most</u> <u>likely</u> <u>solution</u> and implement it over the next 1–3 months.

6. Did the solution you selected <u>work</u> and does it need to be modified for greater satisfaction?

PROBLEM SOLVING AND CHANGING VIOLENT BEHAVIOR PATTERNS

A Therapy Work Sheet

Please complete the work sheet on how you go about solving problems. Complete both parts if they are relevant to your situation. Do both parts to learn how to better engage in problem solving methods in all your relationships.

VIOLENT MODEL:

We were doing well until:

_____

_____

_____

Tension then developed; we have a difference of opinion:

_____

_____

_____

Our talking broke down; we then argue, accuse, blame, attack, and fight:

_____

_____

_____

We agree to try other ways to work out the difference and solve the problem:

_____

_____

_____

We resume our life but are not doing very well:

_____

_____

_____

NON-VIOLENT MODEL:

We have been doing well:

_____

_____

_____

Tension then developed; we have a difference of opinion:

_____

_____

_____

We talk and reach an agreement; our problem is solved:

_____

_____

_____

We resume our activities and life goes on better; we did learn from it:

_____

_____

_____

NON-VIOLENT PROBLEM SOLVING TIPS

- No physical violence, pushing, finger pointing, grabbing, or bullying behavior to gain control over the other person.
- No name calling, verbal abuse, yelling, cussing or use of a threat to intimidate the other person into accepting your way.
- No attempt to hurt the other person, physically, emotionally or mentally.
- Take personal responsibility for the control of your own anger and your expressions of anger.
- Keep the goal of problem solving in mind; communicate, reach some type of agreement and learn from each situation how to get along better.
- After a little time has passed, sit down and debrief the way you improved and how you did better than the last time you had a disagreement.
- Plan how to do it better next time.

COMMENTS AND SUGGESTIONS:

Chapter 30

Thinking Distortions: Information and Patient Exercises

Chapter Contents

Patients come to therapy with a host of predetermined thinking distortions. Most patients do not know that their thoughts are abnormal thought patters as they are so second-nature to them. Therapy, essentially, is a process of exposing distortions of thought and correcting such distortions as a means of changing their destructive behavior patterns. Mood and behavior are both a direct result of one's style of thinking. This issue needs assertive attention paid to it in therapy.

The forms and guidelines in this chapter will be most helpful to therapists as they work with patients in changing their distorted and unhealthy thought patterns.

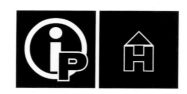

THE BANE OF PERFECTIONISM: AN OBSESSIVE COMPULSIVE DISORDER

WHAT IS IT?

Obsessive compulsive disorders (OCD) are expressed in many ways. Perfectionism is just one way. There are three basic components of OCD: Obsessions, Compulsions, and Avoidance patterns of behavior. It is the preoccupation in thought and ritualistic behavior patterns to avoid feelings of anxiety or distress. These actions are engaged in at the expense of flexibility, openness, and efficiency. Some are preoccupied with rules and order, others with strict standards and expectations, while others struggle with rigidity, stubbornness, over-conscientiousness, or routine, meaningless actions.

WHAT CAN YOU DO ABOUT IT?

1. Relinquish your extreme behavior and move to the middle range on a 10-point scale.
2. Set reasonable expectations of yourself and others.
3. Admit you have limitations and inadequacies.
4. Learn to be flexible when responding to some event.
5. Make a list of priorities by which to live.
6. Know that you can escape the past for the sake of a better future.
7. Identify your destructive attitudes and begin to change them.
8. Select better mottoes and say them to yourself and to others.
9. Some things need to be done well; some things just need to be done.
10. Help others with their nitpicking and bothersome behaviors.
11. Confront your fears that underlie the perfectionism.

HOW TO STOP IT: AN EXERCISE TO BRING ABOUT CHANGE

Name an OBSESSION and state how you will go about changing its intensity:

1.

2.

3.

Name a COMPULSION and state how you will go about changing its intensity:

1.

2.

3.

Name an AVOIDANCE behavior and state how you will go about changing its intensity:

1.

2.

3.

THINKING DISTORTIONS

1. **All-or-Nothing Thinking.** You see things in black and white categories. If your performance falls short of perfect, you see yourself as a total failure.

2. **Overgeneralization.** You see a single negative event as a never-ending pattern of defeat.

3. **Mental Filter.** You pick a single negative detail and dwell on it exclusively so that your vision of all reality becomes darkened, like the drop of ink that discolors the entire beaker of water.

4. **Disqualifying the Positive.** You reject positive experiences by insisting that they don't count for some reason or other. In this way you can maintain a negative belief that is contradicted by your everyday experiences.

5. **Jumping to Conclusions.** You make a negative interpretation even though there are no definite facts that convincingly support your conclusion.

   a. Mind Reading. You arbitrarily conclude that someone is reacting negatively to you, and you don't bother to check it out.

   b. The Fortune Telling Error. You anticipate that things will turn out badly, and you will feel convinced that your prediction is an already established fact.

6. **Magnification, Catastrophizing, or Minimization.** You exaggerate the importance of things (such as failure, falling short of the mark, or someone else's achievement), or you inappropriately shrink things until they appear tiny (your good and desirable qualities or someone else's limitations).

7. **Emotional Reasoning.** You assume that your negative emotions necessarily reflect the way things really are, "I feel it, so it must be true."

8. **"Should" Statements.** You try to motivate yourself with "shoulds" and "shouldn'ts", as if you had to be whipped and punished before you could accomplish anything. "Musts" and "oughts" also fall into this faulty-thinking category. The emotional consequence is guilt. When you direct "should" statements toward others, you feel anger, frustration, and resentment.

9. **Labeling and Mislabeling.** This is an extreme form of overgeneralization. Instead of describing your error, you attach a negative label to yourself, "I'm a loser." When someone else's behavior rubs you up the wrong way you attach a negative label to the other person, "He's a jerk." Mislabeling involves describing an event with language that is highly colored and emotionally loaded.

10. **Personalization.** You see yourself as the cause of some problem, or take on someone's opinion as having more value than it does.

Therapist's Guide to Clinical Intervention, Second Edition by Sharon L. Johnson (© 2003 Elsevier Inc.)

Behavioral Monitoring Logs

Chapter Contents

Logging a patient's progress during therapy as well as in daily life situations is an important task of a therapist. Logs help the therapist educate and instruct patients. Logs help the therapist inform patients of their progress and the significance of their problem behavior. Logs become one of the most useful tools of a therapist in bringing about the desired changes in behavior for each patient coming to therapy.

The logs in this chapter will be helpful to a therapist in many ways. Guidelines, templates, and questionnaires are provided to help the therapist be even more effective in therapy and to chart progress so that patients can observe it objectively.

BEHAVIOR MONITORING GRAPH

Key or target behavior patterns need to be monitored and systematically charted to demonstrate the patient's progress in therapy. The target behaviors need to be counted daily as they occur and recorded on a graph such as the one below. Be sure a sufficient sampling of the target behavior over time has been taken into account. Record the number of occurrences of the target behavior over time, e.g., per week or per month. The graph can be reviewed with the patient for constructive feedback and encouragement.

Behavior #1:_____

Number of occurrences		JAN	FEB	MAR	APR	MAY	JUN	JUL	AUG	SEP	OCT	NOV	DEC
	100												
	90												
	80												
	70												
	60												
	50												
	40												
	30												
	20												
	10												
	0												

Behavior #2:_____

Number of occurrences		JAN	FEB	MAR	APR	MAY	JUN	JUL	AUG	SEP	OCT	NOV	DEC
	100												
	90												
	80												
	70												
	60												
	50												
	40												
	30												
	20												
	10												
	0												

PATIENT NAME: _____

TIME DURATION FOR MAKING OBSERVATIONS: _____

COMMENTS:

MONITORING OF ANTECEDENT DIAGNOSTIC EVENTS TO SELF-DEFEATING BEHAVIOR

There are times when self-defeating behavior is engaged in and needs to be addressed. Examples might include: panic attacks, delusional thinking, cutting, hallucinations, excessive sleeping, ditching school or work, and mood changes, to name a few. Keep track of these events as best as possible so that any pattern can be identified and addressed. Do this exercise for a few weeks to get a clear perspective.

Date	Time	Where were you at the time?	What seemed to cause the behavior?	Describe the specific behavior	What action did you take?

COMMENTS:

A LOOK AT MY SELF-DEFEATING BEHAVIOR PATTERN

We engage in a variety of self-defeating behavior patterns most days. These only get worse over time. We learn bad habits. We find it difficult to change them and learn new and better patterns of behavior instead. Here is where we need help. This assignment may help you become less self-defeating and more effective in your daily life.

What are my self-defeating behavior patterns and what is their effect on me?

Self-defeating behavior in which I engage	Negative outcomes I experience	Positive outcomes I miss if I am self-defeating
1.		
2.		
3.		
4.		
5.		

MY PLAN TO CHANGE FOR MY BETTERMENT AND THAT OF OTHERS:

1.

2.

3.

4.

5.

OTHER COMMENTS AND IDEAS:

BEHAVIORAL MANAGEMENT PROGRAM IN THE HOME

Any behavioral program must have three basic components. These are: (1) the expectations clearly articulated, (2) the consequences associated with keeping and not keeping the expectations, and (3) some type of charting procedure to visually show progress or lack of progress. Spell out clearly on paper the expectations and follow them daily.

EXPECTATIONS:

1.

2.

3.

4.

5.

CONSEQUENCES IF EXPECTATIONS ARE NOT MET:

1.

2.

3.

4.

5.

CONSEQUENCES IF EXPECTATIONS ARE MET:

1.

2.

3.

4.

5.

CHARTING OF THE DAILY PROGRESS AT HOME AND WORK

On a daily calendar or a sheet of paper, chart the progress made each day for each expectation. Use a point scale or a letter to show different degrees of success. Be consistent from day to day.

BEHAVIORAL OBSERVATIONS CHART FOR DAYCARE AND HOSPITAL PATIENTS

Name of resident: _____

Directions: All staff should observe the resident carefully for problem behavior. Identify each apparent behavior or indication of hostility/anxiety, delusional thoughts, hallucinations, confusion, or disorientation. Note the apparent cause(s) in such a way and with sufficient detail that the problems are clear to anyone reading this report.

Date	Time	Where was the resident?	Describe behavior: What did resident say/do? Intensity?	What seemed to cause the behavior, if anything?	What did staff do to intervene?	What was the response to intervention?

SUMMARY OF BEHAVIORS OF CONCERN: 1. _____   2. _____   3. _____

4. _____   5. _____   6. _____

ACTION PLAN:

Dealing with Crisis

Chapter Contents

When most patients present themselves for therapy, they are in a crisis. Rarely are crises anticipated. Therapists are rarely consulted beforehand to prepare a patient for the unexpected or unanticipated crisis. Therapists need to be prepared to effectively intervene in a crisis that is beginning to unfold or one that has already escalated. The progression of a crisis usually needs to be slowed or brought to termination. New life needs to come out of the crisis situation for those involved.

Therapists themselves can experience a revived memory of a prior crisis in their life when working with patients going through similar experiences. Therapists need to manage their own emotional states so patients are not adversely affected.

This chapter contains forms and guidelines on how to effectively deal with a patient's crisis experience as well as the vicarious crisis that a therapist may sometimes experience.

HOW BEST TO RESPOND TO A CRISIS

Here are some basic helping skills that can enhance your ability to provide effective services in a crisis using generally accepted actions and principles for crisis management.

- **Just being there helps.** Being present and offering companionship to a hurting person provides a sense of community that calms.
- **Be a listening ear.** Focused listening rather than focusing on quick and easy solutions is preferred.
- **Mirror the experience.** People are apt to listen better when they know they will be asked to recall what they have just seen or heard. Mirroring also helps to clarify your own thoughts and feelings.
- **Confidentiality is essential.** Fear of becoming the topic of gossip inhibits people from confiding in others. Embrace the importance of maintaining confidentiality as well as the rare occasions (e.g., suicidal, homicidal ideation) where confidentiality may/must be broken.
- **Share basic and relevant information.** Be equipped with basic information about grief and related topics. For example, be prepared to help those who grieve to understand that mourning is important to the recovery process, and prepare them for intense times (e.g., birthdays, anniversaries, and special days) where the grief experience may be relived.
- **Find the help needed in taking the next step.** Draw upon the model of the Good Samaritan who took the injured traveler to an inn where more extensive needs were able to be met.
- **Support for the basic needs of the moment is vital.** Learn how to assess and provide the needed support for the moment. Basic needs like food and shelter usually take precedence over the higher level needs and assistance.

WHAT I NEED TO LEARN TO IMPROVE MY EFFECTIVENESS:

Modified from an article by Edward E. Moody, PhD.

CRISIS INTERVENTION

When a person experiences an unexpected traumatic experience, an intervention is most beneficial when it comes as soon after the event as possible. A discussion about what happened and the associated response facilitates working through and resolving the crisis experience. The personal response to a traumatic crisis includes emotional, psychological, physical, and behavioral factors, and the response pattern varies among individuals.

The individual response pattern is a function of the following:

1. Past experiences and how the person has coped
2. Access and utilization of a support system
3. Emotional health at the time of the crisis
4. Physical health at the time of the crisis
5. Beliefs
6. Attitudes
7. Values
8. How others/society respond to the individual and the event that the person experienced.

Here are some of the more common responses:

Emotional	Mental	Physical	Behavioral
anxiety	confusion	fatigue	angry outbursts
fear	forgetfulness	exhaustion	increased substance use
agitation	difficulty concentrating	gastrointestinal problems	isolation
irritability	distractibility	respiratory problems	withdrawal
anger	intrusive thoughts	headaches	restless
guilt	flashbacks	twitching	interpersonal problems
grief/loss	nightmares	sweating	appetite disturbance
vulnerability	obsessing	dizziness	sleep disturbance
fragility	hypervigilance		change in libido
disbelief			easily agitated

In an effort to decrease the intensity of the emotional and psychological response, decrease physiological arousal, and facilitate resolution of the crisis with a return to previous level of functioning, discussion of the traumatic experience should be initiated as soon as possible following the crisis. Early intervention will prevent the development of post-traumatic stress disorder (PTSD) for some individuals. Be careful not to overstimulate the individual and add to the experience of trauma.

1. Listen carefully and pay close attention to the responses of these individuals (detachment, agitation, emotional reactiveness, flashbacks, etc.).
2. Decrease physiological arousal.
3. Facilitate appropriate support(s).
4. Normalize their responses to crises.
5. Educate them about the range of responses to crises, with care to avoid the following:

    A. Compounding social stigmatization of those with more symptoms.
    B. Creating feelings of guilt for experiencing fewer symptoms than others.
    C. Using confusing jargon/language not used by the general public.
    D. Overpathologizing and focusing on disability.

Therapist's Guide to Clinical Intervention, Second Edition by Sharon L. Johnson (© 2003 Elsevier Inc.)

6. Assure them that their response is temporary.
7. Let them know that there is not a specific time frame in which to recover from a crisis. However, if they engage in self-care behaviors, healing is likely to be expedited.
8. Foster resilience and recovery.
9. Assess for substance abuse.
10. Follow up.

When providing psychological interventions to those recently traumatized and experiencing acute stress, or individuals with PTSD, validated treatment elements include direct therapeutic exposure and cognitive restructuring. Early cognitive-behavioral interventions include the following techniques:

1. Deep breathing
2. Progressive muscle relaxation
3. Imaginal and *in vivo* exposure therapy
4. Regular physical activity
5. Positive daily structure with reinforcers
6. Utilization of resources
7. Journaling
8. Self-monitoring

FACING AND OVERCOMING A CRISIS

COMMON SIGNS OF A CRISIS REACTION

Physical

Fatigue
Rapid heartbeat
Headaches
Nausea
Hunger
Chills

Insomnia
Chest pain
Hypertension
Visual distortion
Dizziness
Sweating

Cognitive

Blame others
Disturbed thoughts
Poor concentration
Poor problem solving
Inescapable images
Suicidal ideas
Search for meaning
Hypervigilant

Inattentive
Nightmares
Flashbacks
Disbelief
Indecisive
Confusion
Forgetfulness

Emotional

Anxiety
Denial
Uncertainty
Apprehension
Panic feelings
Agitation
Mistrust
Worthless feelings

Grief
Depression
Lack of enjoyment
Anger
Irritability
Helplessness
Apathy/Boredom

Behavioral

Withdrawal
Emotional outburst
Tiredness
Erratic movements
Loss of sex drive
Appetite disturbance

Suspiciousness
Substance abuse
Antisocial acts
Pacing
Silences
Accident proneness

EXPERIENCING A CRISIS

What is a crisis?

- A crisis is an unstable time or state of affairs with risk and uncertainty.
- It may be a sudden, unexpected, unanticipated event.
- It causes us to feel upset and off-balance.

Along the path of a crisis

- We trust that our reactions are normal.
- We talk about the experience.

Cont.

Facing and Overcoming a Crisis (*Continued*)

- We express feelings, emotions.
- We support each other.
- We use humor as appropriate.

During a crisis

- We feel numb from initial shock and disbelief.
- We discover that time may seem to stop or events run together.
- We experience shortness of breath and a tightness in the chest.
- We do what has to be done.
- We choose not to think about it.

Recovering from a crisis

- Find someone you trust.
- "Tell your story to others."
- Give yourself permission to feel what you are feeling.
- Take care of yourself. Get enough rest and eat regularly.
- Practice relaxation.
- Create a quiet scene.
- Take one thing at a time.
- It causes us to feel upset and off-balance.
- Allow time for task.
- Spruce up your surroundings.
- Escape for a while.
- Seek professional counseling.
- Healing is a process.
- Time is needed to heal, often 4–20 weeks.

Outcome of a crisis

- We become more alert and vigilant.
- We develop a positive perspective.
- We create preparedness plans.
- We integrate the experience in our life.
- We reach our conclusion or resolution point

Quotable quotes on crisis

- "The same sun melts ice and hardens clay."
- "Don't be afraid of opposition. A kite rises against the wind."
- "Great trials often precede great triumphs."

Post-trauma Do's

(Suggestions to reduce likelihood of long-term stress reactions)

- Do get enough rest.
- Do maintain a good diet and exercise program.
- Do follow a familiar routine.
- Do find and talk to supportive peers and family about the incident.
- Do take time for leisure activities.

Facing and Overcoming a Crisis (*Continued*)

- Do take one thing at a time.
- Do attend any meetings regarding this traumatic event.
- Do spend time with family and friends.
- Do create a serene scene to briefly escape to either visually or in reality.
- Do expect the experience to bother you.
- Do seek professional help if your symptoms persist.

Post-trauma Don'ts

(Suggestions to reduce likelihood of long-term stress reactions)

- Don't drink alcohol excessively.
- Don't use drugs or alcohol to numb feelings.
- Don't withdraw from significant others.
- Don't reduce leisure activities.
- Don't stay away from work.
- Don't increase caffeine intake.
- Don't have unrealistic expectations from recovery.
- Don't look for easy answers.
- Don't take on new major projects.
- Don't pretend everything is OK.
- Don't make major changes if you don't need to.

The therapist could reformat these lists to produce a handout or brochure.

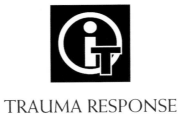

TRAUMA RESPONSE

The sequential responses to trauma include the following stages: stressful event, outcry, denial, intrusion, working through, and resolution. Sometimes an individual will bypass the outcry stage and proceed from the traumatic event to denial. Corresponding to the stages of sequential responding are normal reactions or intensification/pathological reactions. Intensifications result when the normal reaction is unusually intense or prolonged.

1. **Traumatic/stressful event**

   A. Normal emotional response: anxiety, fear, sadness, distress

   If normal response is unusually intense or prolonged, the result is a pathological response.

   B. Pathological response: overwhelmed, confused, dazed

2. **Outcry**

   A. Normal emotional response: anxiety, guilt, anger, rage, shame, protest

   If normal response is unusually intense or prolonged, the result is a pathological response.

   B. Pathological response: panic, exhaustion, dissociative symptoms, psychotic symptoms

3. **Denial**

   A. Normal emotional response: minimizing, hypersomnia, anhedonia, depression, suppression, repression, obsession, fatigue/lethargy, denial

   If normal response is unusually intense or prolonged, the result is a pathological response.

   B. Pathological response: maladaptive avoidance, withdrawal, substance abuse, suicidality, fugue state, amnesia, rigid thinking, psychic numbing, sleep dysfunction, massive denial of initial trauma or current problems, somatization (headaches, fatigue, bowel problems/cramps, exacerbation of asthma, etc.)

4. **Intrusion**

   A. Normal emotional response: anxiety, somatosizing, decreased concentration and attention, insomnia, dysphoria

   If normal response is unusually intense or prolonged, the result is a pathological response.

   B. Pathological response: flooded states, hypervigilance, exaggerated startle response, psuedohallucination, illusions, obsession, impaired concentration and attention, sleep/dream disturbance, emotional lability, preoccupation with the event, confusion, fight or flight activation (diarrhea, nausea, sweating, tremors, feelings of being on edge), compulsive re-enactments of trauma, impaired functioning

5. **Working through**

   A. Normal emotional response: find meaning in experience, grieve, personal growth

   If working through is blocked, the result is a pathological response.

   B. Pathological response: frozen states or psychosomatic reaction, anxiety/depression syndromes

6. **Resolution**

   A. Normal response: return to pre-event level of functioning, psychological/personal growth/integration

   If not achieved the result is a pathological response.

   B. Pathological response: Inability to work/act/feel, personality change, generalized anxiety, dysthymia.

Adapted from J.S. Maxmen and N.G. Ward (1995) *Essential Psychopathology and Its Treatment* (New York, WW Norton); modified from M.J. Horowitz.

THE THERAPIST'S EXPOSURE TO AND THE MANAGEMENT OF TRAUMA

Every therapist works with patients that have been deeply traumatized. Daily exposure to the trauma experiences of others can have a significant personal impact on the therapist. This experience might be called, "second hand trauma." It can cause the therapist to become distressed and impair the progress of therapy. It can resurrect an old trauma experience in the therapist that may not have been resolved. The guidelines below can help a therapist work with such patients productively and effectively.

TYPES OF TRAUMA

Covert trauma is harm caused by the absence of an expected or much-needed experience which, by its absence, has a damaging effect on one's emotions. For example, the absence of compassion by a parent when a child experiences a defeat, severe injury or crisis, can result in a traumatic experience for the child. It is what should have been present or occurred, but did not. Unfortunately, we all can recall at least one covert trauma wound on our past that needs healing attention.

Overt trauma is harm caused by the direct occurrence or presence of some overwhelming adverse experience. Being on the receiving end of a severe public criticism or being falsely accused of some wrongdoing can create an overt trauma experience that will require therapeutic assistance.

Secondary trauma. Secondary trauma is considered an inevitable response to spending significant time working with, or studying, trauma survivors. If can have several effects:
  Working with a population of trauma patients can be very tiring.
  The transmission of traumatic stress can come about through witnessing the effects of trauma.
  A therapist may have experienced a similar or different type of trauma and may have intrusive thoughts and feelings about it during a therapy session.
  A therapist may not have experienced trauma but can be overwhelmed by the stories told by their patients.

A THERAPIST'S SELF-HELP STRATEGY

- Trauma work is best conducted in a team approach by trusted colleagues.
- A therapist must be educated regarding trauma syndromes and their treatment.
- The goal is to normalize one's responses to trauma of any kind.
- Recognition of the trauma impact cannot be neglected.
- Ventilation in a supportive environment can be helpful to a therapist.
- Setting boundaries between personal and professional activities is vital.
- A therapist must carefully manage their caseload in terms of trauma cases.
- A therapist must engage in other activities to defuse the impact of trauma.

GETTING UNSTUCK IN RECOVERY FROM TRAUMA

It is important to get unstuck from any unresolved trauma experience the therapist may have in their own life that may impair their work with traumatized patients.

- Identify any covert and overt traumas in your own life, in order to clarify what resources you will need for healing.
- Identify specific emotions that you get stuck in, or those that you work extra hard to avoid. Intentionally allow yourself to experience these, and then look for ways to get back to joy, primarily by receiving love and support from those close to you.
- Identify the lies that were/are imbedded within the wounds that may be yet be unhealed in your life.

Part V

Dealing with Specific Types of Patient Problems and Issues

It is generally accepted that a strong support system mitigates stress, prolongs life, and significantly contributes to one's quality of life. Without a strong and multi-level support system, individuals tend to be isolated and experience significant styles of dysfunctional living, have poor communication patterns, over-eat, engage in drug use, take high-risk chances, and generally live a self-defeating lifestyle. A strong therapeutic system, on the other hand, provides a reality check, encouragement, and provides for a lifestyle of healthy living and positive relationships.

Therapists are generally turned to at times of great stress and relationship breakdown. Also, therapists are sought out at times of major decision making and life changes, as well as times of trauma, hurt, and anguish. While a therapist cannot be the sole support system for a patient, therapists play a significant role in the healing process. It is essential that therapists work towards the goal of helping patients reach out and establish a much more healthy lifestyle that will carry them for years to come. Besides individuals and one's family, a supportive social network needs to be established. With a support network in place, specific problems and issues can be independently and constructively addressed in a timely manner by the patient, with less reliance on professional assistance.

The forms in Part V of the book are designed to give the therapist tools by which to help patients to generate a behavior change system, learn better communication skills, and help others rebuild their relationships in the home and elsewhere. The forms, checklists, exercises, and guidelines included in this section will be useful tools for the therapist to help their patients establish a strong belief that change is possible and that isolation and loneliness are states that can be dramatically altered for the good of all.

Chapter 33

Serving Children and Their Families

Chapter Contents

Children who are reared in a healthy family life flourish. Support and guidance for personal growth and the freedom to explore and understand the universe is the gift healthy parents give to their children. While most children are fortunate to live within the secure structures of a healthy family, there are those who must endure the stress and disorganization of dysfunctional home life. The results of these two types of homes are soon noticed as the children come together in school and begin to associate and compete in the open marketplace of academia and the general community.

This chapter provides the guidelines, templates, and informational forms that can help the therapist serve the families that come to the office for help and guidance. The forms, arranged in 12 topic groupings, assist the therapist in teaching and redirecting parents and their children towards the lifestyle of a healthy home.

The Family Needs Help to Change

Section Contents

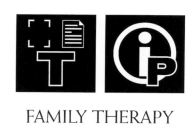

FAMILY THERAPY

WHAT WILL HAPPEN IN THE FIRST MEETING?

The first session can take many forms. On rare occasions, I have had a client who came with a very specific issue that we resolved in a single session. Usually, though, the first meeting serves several purposes:

- I obtain a personal and family history so that I can better place the current problems in context. In the case of a child or teen, this helps me get a sense of whether it will be more effective to work primarily with the entire family, the parents and the child/teen, or predominantly with just the child/teen in individual therapy.

- It serves as a time to further define just what you want from therapy. A common question I ask takes the form of, "When you have accomplished what you came here to do, how will things be different? What will have changed in your life?"

- The session gives both of us a chance to begin to confirm that we are a "good fit." In those rare situations where one or both of us decides it won't be a good fit, I can often suggest names of some other therapists that may be a better match based on what I learned about you in this session.

WHAT KINDS OF THERAPY DO I USE?

I once browsed through a textbook that described more than 500 different kinds of psychotherapy! I find it hard to condense my approaches to a few terms, though there are some common themes that seem to characterize how I work. Here are a few, in no particular order.

- I'm a pragmatist: If it works, do it; don't form a committee.
- I often look at things from a "family/systems" model. Like two kids on a see-saw, relationships involve balance. Sometimes life may feel as if you're in the one down position, sometimes the other way around. Being stuck is often an illusion.
- I find it much more useful to look at who can help resolve a problem rather than look at who is to blame for it.
- I love using stories and metaphors to teach.
- I pay careful attention to the impact of particular words. Many times, disagreements get started from the same few words.
- I value the use of humor as an antidote to many things such as power struggles and tunnel vision.
- I believe that coincidences usually aren't.
- I encourage clients to pay very careful attention to intuitive hunches. Intuition is more reliable than the other senses. Fear is never part of an intuition.
- Lastly, I like to work myself out of a job quickly. In the process, I hope to give you more problem solving tools.

HOW OFTEN ARE SESSIONS SCHEDULED?

Most of my clients choose to meet once a week. When financial or scheduling constraints dictate, sessions are scheduled less often. A few meet twice a week when getting started or during a tough period. Many clients reduce the frequency of their sessions to once every other week for a few sessions before their final appointment. I sometimes joke that if I am staying on top of things well, I'll sense that you're about ready to stop therapy about 5 minutes before you tell me.

HOW LONG WILL THERAPY TAKE?

Some presenting concerns lend themselves to brief therapy, defined as 6 to 12 sessions. Acute situations often respond fairly quickly; long-standing problems (e.g., poor self-worth, chronic depression) understandably take longer.

WHAT ARE THE LIMITS OF CONFIDENTIALITY?

In the state of _____ , information given to a psychologist is termed "confidential", a term providing even more protection than "privileged" information. In essence, I am not allowed to share any information with anyone else without your written consent, with a few important exceptions:

- Suicidal risk. If I believe that a client is at imminent risk of harming himself or herself, I am required to intervene. In the unlikely event that I thought this applied to you, I would tell you before I contacted anyone else.

- Homicidal risk. If I believe that a client is at imminent risk of harming someone else, I am required to intervene. Stemming from "duty to warn" legislation, I would have to notify the person whose life I believed was at risk. Again, in the unlikely event that I thought this applied to you, I would tell you before I contacted anyone else.

- Abuse of a minor child or an elderly person. Psychologists are required to report suspected abuse to DFCS. Again, in the unlikely event that I thought this applied to you, I would tell you before I contacted DFCS.

- In very rare cases, a judge can order a psychologist to release records. In my _____ years of practice, I have never had this happen.

- If parents are involved in child custody litigation, the situation can arise where one parent waives confidentiality for the child's psychological records. In such cases, it is important to talk things over with your attorney.

- For children and teens under age 18, there are two additional exceptions. If I believe a child/teen is either engaged in criminal activity (e.g., breaking into homes, stealing cars) or is involved in drug/alcohol use, it is my policy to tell parents – after discussing it with the child/teen first. Technically, this is not a violation of confidentiality, because with few exceptions, parents have the legal right to access to their minor children's medical/psychiatric records.

So what about confidentiality for children and teens? The HIPAA regulations have made some changes that therapists are still sorting out. Historically, I have worked under the assumption that parents have the legal right to access everything in my notes. However, the reality is that teens (and children) are more likely to open up to me if they trust that I will honor their confidence. So I ask that parents trust that I will alert them if any of the above exceptions come into play.

WHAT ABOUT PSYCHOLOGICAL TESTING?

For adults, there are several pencil-and-paper questionnaires I frequently use. Most of the forms can be completed at home. The information helps me insure I'm not overlooking something important. I'll discuss the results with you.

For children/teens, I like to have parents complete a couple of questionnaires. If there are concerns about behavior at school or academic performance I like to have the teacher(s) complete a similar questionnaire. I'll discuss the results with you. With some older teens I will administer additional pencil-and-paper tests.

FOR FAMILY THERAPY, WHO WILL ACTUALLY COME TO THE SESSIONS?

Years ago I used to push to have everyone in the family come if a child/teen was the focus of concern. I still like to meet everyone, but I often work with subsets of the family. Typically, I mix individual sessions with the child, sessions with the parent(s), and sessions with the child and parent(s). Often I do this within a single session to facilitate getting critical updates from a parent.

TEACHING CHILDREN HOW TO MAKE WISE CHOICES

Being an effective teacher or parent in today's world is not easy. Many parents simply "cop out" and allow their children to determine their own course of action, behavior patterns, and future destiny. Teachers do likewise. Fortunately, the vast majority of teachers and parents approach their responsibility seriously, diligently, and courageously. They do not allow their children to be blind followers or merely passive participants in life events. Responsible teachers and parents assume the role of an active influencer in the lives of their children.

Among the critical areas of influence is teaching wise decision making. To be good decision makers children must have formal instruction and lifestyle models in the clarification of values, moral development, assertive communication skills, relationship skills, and conflict and stress management skills.

Effective decision making also depends on the skills of formulating questions, accepting unpopular decisions, and understanding why a particular decision has greater future value than immediate gratification. Here are a few guidelines to help you teach your children to make wise choices:

1. **Talk with your children daily.** Set aside a time each day to talk with your children. Learn what is on their mind and what they are feeling. Be careful not to criticize or put them down, or to cast aside or minimize their feelings and opinions as being unimportant. The issues children face are just as important to them as are the issues we adults face. Wise decision making requires the ability to talk with others and share thoughts and feelings and concerns. This basic skill begins at home and in the classroom.

2. **Teach values and morals.** Teachers and parents cannot sit back and let others teach basic values and morals. Training in these basic areas is a critical responsibility of each teacher and parent. Use stories, illustrations, personal examples, and daily life events as teaching tools. Be practical and help the children identify decision making points within each story discussed. Always pinpoint options, associated consequences, and the advantage of one course of action over another.

3. **Use the if–then technique in teaching decision making.** Every choice is associated with a particular consequence that has a likelihood of occurrence. Hence, it is important to help children think through the effects of one choice over another. This is done by helping them think through "if–then" statements. For example, if option A is selected, then such-and-such consequence is likely to result. Help children think through the natural consequences of their actions or decision.

4. **Praise wise decisions and choices.** Children do make decisions and judgments. Many of these decisions may be very wise and deserving of compliments and praise. When this occurs, be liberal and direct in recognizing and liberal in praising a wise decision when it occurs. Point out not only that it was a wise decision, but why it was a decision worthy of commendation. Avoid the temptation to preach, moralize, or show how the decision could have been even better. There will be opportunity to recognize and encourage children in their good decision making in the future.

5. **Teach decision making.** Have children break down their problem into smaller components. Help them solve the simpler component before moving on to the more complex aspects of the problem. Encourage children to do what can be done under the circumstances even though it would be best if the problem could be approached in a different manner. Be practical. Be available as a decision making partner and a strong support person for your children.

6. **Encourage friendships with other wise decision makers.** We learned to make wise decisions and choices by following the example set by others. Hence, social relationships should not only *include* others who model and demonstrate wise decision making, but also *exclude* those who live to the contrary. Teachers and parents need to be particularly careful with whom they associate as children watch very closely the lives of their teachers, parents, and their own peers. Teachers and parents, indeed all adults, also need to be very careful in helping children select and develop friendships with those that live a lifestyle based upon wise choices and decision making, and this requires giving their children guidance in friendship selection.

In summary, as teachers and parents we commit ourselves to the teaching of our children so that they will choose right over wrong and become wise decision making adults. Dipping back into the history of Hebrew instruction we see the basic thought that still applies today: "Teach children how they should live, and they will remember it all their lives" (Prov. 22:6).

The crux of this theme of effective instruction of children by adults was nailed by the Rev. Jesse Jackson, who said: "You can't teach what you don't know and you can't lead where you don't go."

Functional and Dysfunctional Families

Section Contents

THE EIGHT VITAL CHARACTERISTICS OF A FUNCTIONAL FAMILY

The family best functions together as a unit rather than as separate and independent members. All members uniquely contribute to the life of the family. One member has need of all the other members. There is a sense of honor among all the members in the well-functioning family. Even the smallest member is vital and worthy of honor. All members are connected and function as a whole. If one member suffers, all suffer. This suggests the unity and integration of the well-functioning family into a working and inseparable whole.

The Functional Family	The Dysfunctional Family
One suffers, all suffer	No one cares who is suffering
All belong to each other	No connection, bond or commitment
Unique contributions by each member	No intent to contribute to each other
One honors and values another	No honor or respect for each other
Honor even for an absent member	No value for those absent
Others are first and before self	No honor for others, only self
Respect for each other's role	No regard for a role order or system
Work together to reduce family stress	No concern for overall stress levels

CHILD MANAGEMENT PERSPECTIVE

The management of children from the very beginning of life through the young adult years can be thought of by using the model of a megaphone. Picture a megaphone in your mind, with the small or narrow end representing infancy and the broad open end representing young adulthood and maturity.

THE HEALTHY PROCESS OF RAISING CHILDREN

1. The small end of the megaphone represents infancy, where the parent is in total control and manages the life and affairs of the child.
2. Moving from the narrow end to the broad open end of the megaphone represents the growth and development and maturity process of a child, with increased levels of trust and independence.
3. The acquisition of independence is a slow and gradual process, taking place in stages. The stages generally parallel school grade levels and landmark ages as a child in our society.
4. The steps of increase in independence generally take place at grade 3 or 4, grade 6 or 7, grade 9 or 10, grade 12 and the college years, age 16, 18, and 21, graduation from college, and career and marriage.
5. While a parent never ceases to be a parent to their children, the level of control and dependency becomes less as the years increase and as the child presents evidence of increased maturity, wisdom, decision making, and good judgment.

THE UNHEALTHY PROCESS OF RAISING CHILDREN

There are parents that start out a child's life with the megaphone the other way round. They allow their children at very young ages to have far more independence, freedom, and leniency than is proper or they can handle. Things tend to go badly. Children lose interest in school, obtain failing grades, become involved in social problems, are disrespectful to parents, and engage in various forms of illegal and antisocial behavior patterns. In such cases, a parent then has a choice of either letting the child continue throughout life without boundaries and restrictions and respect for authority or to reverse the process by turning the megaphone around and starting life over with a great deal of restriction and then gradually increasing the levels of freedom as the child is able to accept and work within the framework of the boundaries imposed. This is a very difficult process and may be as many as five years in the making to reverse the undesirable behavior patterns previously established. In such cases, professional guidance and assistance would be an essential component and aid to the parents and child.

CHECK YOUR FAMILY'S VITAL SIGNS

It takes hard work to build a strong family life. Even the most successful families need to pause, now and then, to check their "health indicators." Take a moment to see how your family is doing.

1. **Adults feel close to each other and share authority.** They support each other, feel proud of each other. They are able to confide in each other and share leadership and responsibilities. The single parent is confident and in charge. In your family, you can:

   a. Take time daily to discuss each other's activities, share your feelings, and make family plans. As a single parent, spend time taking care of yourself, doing things you enjoy.

   b. Talk about your differences. Try to settle them by compromising or taking turns in making family decisions.

   c. Admit your mistakes. Apologize when you behave thoughtlessly.

2. **Family members discuss their thoughts and feelings freely.** They speak honestly but affectionately. They encourage each other to open up even when they feel angry or sad. They listen. Conflicts are discussed in an atmosphere of love and sometimes gentle humor. In your family, you can:

   a. Tell others when you appreciate something they have done or said. Sincere compliments build trust and loyalty.

   b. Behave in the way you want other family members to act toward you. If you want them to pay attention when you have problems, listen when they talk to you. If you sometimes need help, look for ways to be helpful to them.

3. **Family members are allowed to be different and to feel different.** These families don't insist that all have the same beliefs or feelings or enjoy identical activities. One might like sports and rock music; another may prefer books or stamp collecting. Everyone is unique and loved. In your family, you can:

   a. Spend time alone with each family member doing what he or she enjoys.

   b. Recognize that people disagree. If you don't like what others say or do at times, give your opinions calmly and explain why you feel that way.

4. **The parent or parents set high standards and clear guidelines for children.** They explain the reasons for rules and, while they enforce rules consistently, they are flexible in special situations. Children know what to expect and feel they are treated fairly and with respect. In your family, you can:

   a. As a parent, set a few important rules, explain them and the values you hold to your children. Reward good behavior with praise, hugs, smiles, and special privileges.

   b. As a child, discuss rather than disobey rules that you think are unfair. Try to find a compromise that both you and your parents can live with.

5. **Family members spend time together and in the community.** They make time to do things together as a family, just for fun. Often they are active in school, church, community, or recreational organizations. A shared religious life provides these families with common values and a sense of purpose. In your family, you can:

   a. Plan an activity that all family members will enjoy, and do it together soon. Or, set aside a regular time reserved for the family, and take turns choosing the activity.

   b. Talk to others about their families. Share ideas on rules, solving problems, or planning activities.

6. **The family faces problems and works together to solve them.** Parents and children try to figure out what is wrong. They talk about possible solutions. Finally, one or both parents make a decision. Everyone cooperates to try to make the solution work. In your family, you can:

   a. Set aside time this weekend to sit down together and talk about what each of you likes and doesn't like about home life. Ask how each thinks problems could be solved.

   b. Hold such family discussions regularly.

   c. If you think your family problems are serious, seek help from a church leader, crisis intervention service, mental health center, family counselor, or psychologist.

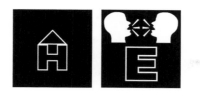

THE DYSFUNCTIONAL FAMILY

We often hear references to the fact that the "Jones" family is dysfunctional. We tend to use that same descriptive phrase in reference to a marriage, business, club, or any organization where we perceive people are having difficulty in coexisting. Much psychological research has been devoted to the definition and characterization of a dysfunctional unit of people, however they coexist. While there is fairly good agreement of what constitutes a dysfunctional relationship or unit, there is still much variation in our understanding of how dysfunctional relationships actually operate. The degree to which a dysfunctional relationship is hurtful, and in what way, to the parties involved is different in each situation. To be sure, and to some degree, all dysfunctional relationships are destructive, self-defeating, and unproductive. They are inefficient in all areas of family life.

Below are the components of most dysfunctional relationships. Rate your family on a 5-point scale, with 1 being "not true of us" and 5 being "very true of us." The number 3 would be "sometimes yes and sometimes no."

- **Role reversal prevails**. The children are in charge and tell parents what to do. Parents tend to obey the most demanding child out of fear and intimidation. Further, the parents take their direction from the prevailing popular opinion among the children. (_____)

- **Illness prevails**. The family members are often ill or have times of non-productivity due to poor health or depressed mood. Chronic illness or fatigue is commonly present. The family may not be fully sick, but they are not fully well either. (_____)

- **Traditions are absent**. The family unit has been subject to or creates constant change and fails to establish and maintain long-term traditions and customs. (Traditions give depth and stability to a family.) (_____)

- **Communication is distorted or non-existent**. Communication is the backbone to any informed group of people. It is only through regular communication that the family members come to know each other, bond together, and strengthen each other. Without communication family members create assumptions of what is reality and act accordingly. They begin to act independently with little care for how well the whole family functions. (_____)

- **Argument and conflict is rampant.** Instead of positive support and mutual encouragement, the dysfunctional family operates on criticism, negative feedback, distrust and demeaning talk towards each other. Differences of opinion are ignored, denied or suppressed, and not resolved. Conflict resolution is avoided and interpersonal schisms are allowed to become embedded in the fabric of the family. (_____)

- **Unending crisis results in feelings of helplessness.** Dysfunctional family relationships create a series of never-ending crises. The family allows a crisis to continue by avoiding or denying its powerful and destructive influence. The lack of skill or courage to resolve a crisis contributes to a sense of helplessness on the part of all family members. Helplessness is one of the foundational components of depression. (_____)

- **Identified leaders present as "apparently" competent.** Oftentimes the head of the family may appear to be competent in fulfilling his/her responsibilities that have been assumed. However, this false presentation of competency may only reflect the parents' attempt to appear in control and not their true ability to function effectively. Expectations that prove to be false result in a sense of betrayal, failure, and defeat when the actual truth is ultimately revealed. (_____)

There are other considerations of a dysfunctional family system that could be mentioned. The list could go on. Every situation is different. Every family plays out the dysfunctional dynamic in a different manner. However, the pattern is similar. The commonalties of most dysfunctional family relationships are outlined above.

The basic question that each family must ask is, are we dysfunctional? If so, in what areas of our relationships are we dysfunctional? First, look over the scores and select the areas of family life in which change is needed and where a strategy of change must be developed. Then spend time developing a strategy to bring about change to a well-functioning family life in the home. The goal is to face problem areas and make all family relationships functionally productive, achievement-oriented, and person-driven.

MUNCHAUSEN SYNDROME BY PROXY

SIGNS OF TROUBLE: A CHECKLIST

Since January, the Federal Bureau of Investigation has begun to advise law enforcement officers and medical workers on how to identify the child abuser whose motive is to draw sympathy and attention as the parent of a sick child. Researchers have found 200 cases since 1977 of abuse by people suffering from the psychological disorder called Munchausen Syndrome by Proxy. Below are some of the key signs of this disorder.

THE CHILD

- Has unexplained, prolonged illness that is so extraordinary that it prompts medical professionals to remark that they've never seen anything like it before.
- Has repeat hospitalizations and medical evaluations without definitive diagnosis.
- Has inappropriate or incongruous symptoms that don't make medical sense.
- Shows persistent failure to tolerate or respond to medical therapy without clear cause.
- Has signs and symptoms that disappear when the child is away from the parent.

THE PARENT

- Shows less concern than the medical staff over the child's illnesses, seems at ease on the children's ward, and forms unusually close relationships with the staff.
- Has medical experience similar to the child's.
- Welcomes medical tests for the child, even if they are painful.
- Shows increased uneasiness as the child recovers or approaches discharge.
- Attempts to convince the staff that the child is more ill than is apparent.

THE PLAN OF CARE

- Individual, group, family, and marital therapy are the primary options.
- Mother and child may need to be separated for a time until therapy begins to be effective. Look for an immediate resolution of the symptoms in the child.
- Parents may need to be required to attend therapy by Department of Social Service or the Court.
- A team approach is most helpful but the team must work together, not separately. Watch out for triangulation strategies. The tenets of feminist therapy may be relevant.
- Treat the mother for her own history of victimization, rage patterns, and unfinished business from childhood and adolescence.

Family Based Assessment

Section Contents

PSYCHOLOGICAL TESTING FOR CHILDREN AND TEENS

AN IMPORTANT WORD ABOUT "PSYCHOLOGICAL TESTING"

For many years now, most insurance companies have NOT covered "psychological testing" when it includes the kinds of instruments that are used to assess for problems with learning. For example, the HMO and POS plans from Blue Cross Blue Shield say that psychological testing "should not be for the primary purpose of assessing learning disorders, vocational testing or educational planning, unless allowed by local plan clinical guidelines."

When I am evaluating a student for suspected learning problems, I make regular use of the following instruments (among others) that insurance companies usually will NOT cover:

- Weschler Intelligence Scales for Children – 4th Revision (WISC-IV)
- Woodcock–Johnson Tests of Cognitive Ability (WJ–III Cognitive)
- Woodcock–Johnson Tests of Achievement (WJ–III Achievement)
- Beery–Buktenica Developmental Test of Visual-Motor Integration
- Gray Oral Reading Test 4th Revisions (GORT–4)
- Gray Silent Reading Test (GSRT)
- Nelson–Denny Reading Test (for older teens)
- Comprehensive Test of Phonological Processing (CTOPP) (early elementary)

My perception of the rationale for the refusal to cover these tests is that, because local school systems employ school psychologists to do such testing when indicated, there is no reason for the insurance company to pay for such testing.

Insurance companies usually WILL cover psychological testing when it involves tests used to help diagnose emotional problems. The most common one that I use with teenagers is the Minnesota Multiphasic Personality Inventory – Adolescent. I do not bill for most of the other self-report questionnaires that I use.

When a child/teen is referred to me for evaluation of suspected ADHD, most of the time I include an evaluation for learning problems. At least one in three students diagnosed with ADHD also has some kind of learning problem. Complicating the picture is that some learning problems can present in ways that look like ADHD.

Identifying a learning problem early means more opportunity to address it successfully. Further, when it is time for your son or daughter to take the SAT, it is difficult to get "accommodations" (such as extended time) if the school has not already been providing these accommodations. The longer these accommodations have been in place, the easier it may be to get similar ones when taking the SAT.

Therefore, PLEASE use the Insurance Benefits Worksheet when you talk with your insurance carrier if you are hoping to get coverage for psychological testing. Take careful notes and be specific.

FAMILY LIFE IN THE HOME

DESCRIBE YOUR FAMILY LIFE IN THE HOME:

1 = ALMOST NEVER   2 = ONCE IN A WHILE   3 = SOMETIMES
4 = FREQUENTLY   5 = ALMOST ALWAYS

FAMILY

1. Family members ask each other for help. _____
2. We approve of each other's friends. _____
3. We like to do things with just our immediate family. _____
4. Different persons act as leaders in our family. _____
5. Family members feel closer to other family members than to people outside the family. _____
6. Our family changes its way of handling tasks. _____
7. Family members like to spend free time with each other. _____
8. Family members feel very close to each other. _____
9. When our family gets together for activities, everybody is present. _____
10. We can easily think of things to do together as a family. _____
11. Family members consult other family members on their decisions. _____
12. It is hard to identify the leader(s) in our family. _____
13. Family togetherness is very important. _____

CHILDREN

1. In solving problems, the children's suggestions are followed. _____
2. Children have a say in their discipline. _____
3. Parent(s) and children discuss punishment together. _____
4. The children make the decisions in our family. _____

RULES AND RESPONSIBILITIES

1. Rules change in our family. _____
2. We shift household responsibilities from person to person. _____
3. It is hard to tell who does which household chores. _____

TOTAL _____

ANALYSIS: The therapist is advised to review each item and give attention to those items that were scored at either extreme, as a 1 or 2 or as a 4 or 5. Extreme scores would provoke a therapist to initiate and address in therapy the problem associated with that item.

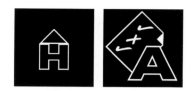

CHILD/TEEN BRAIN SYSTEM CHECKLIST

Name of child/teen: _____ Date: _____

Please rate your child/teen on each of the symptoms listed below using the following scale [Other]. Ask the child, if a teenager, to rate himself/herself also [Self]. Try to give the most complete picture as possible. State who filled out this form: _____

Never (0)   Rarely (1)   Occasionally (2)   Frequently (3)   Very Frequently (4)   Not Applicable/Not Known (N)

Other	Self		
_____	_____	1.	Fails to give close attention to details or makes careless mistakes
_____	_____	2.	Trouble sustaining attention in routine situations (i.e., homework, chores, paperwork)
_____	_____	3.	Trouble listening
_____	_____	4.	Fails to finish things
_____	_____	5.	Poor organization for time or space (such as backpack, room, desk, paperwork)
_____	_____	6.	Avoids, dislikes, or is reluctant to engage in tasks that require sustained mental effort
_____	_____	7.	Loses things
_____	_____	8.	Easily distracted
_____	_____	9.	Forgetful
_____	_____	10.	Poor planning skills
_____	_____	11.	Lacks clear goals or forward thinking
_____	_____	12.	Difficulty expressing feelings
_____	_____	13.	Difficulty expressing empathy for others
_____	_____	14.	Excessive daydreaming
_____	_____	15.	Feeling bored
_____	_____	16.	Feeling apathetic or unmotivated
_____	_____	17.	Feeling tired, sluggish or slow-moving
_____	_____	18.	Feeling spacey or "in a fog"

SUBTOTAL _____

_____	_____	19.	Fidgety, restless or trouble sitting still
_____	_____	20.	Difficulty remaining seated in situations where remaining seated is expected
_____	_____	21.	Runs about or climbs excessively in situations in which it is inappropriate
_____	_____	22.	Difficulty playing quietly
_____	_____	23.	"On the go" or acts as if "driven by a motor"
_____	_____	24.	Talks excessively
_____	_____	25.	Blurts out answers before questions have been completed
_____	_____	26.	Difficulty awaiting turn
_____	_____	27.	Interrupts or intrudes on others (e.g., butts into conversations or games)
_____	_____	28.	Impulsive (saying or doing things without thinking first)

SUBTOTAL _____

_____	_____	29.	Excessive or senseless worrying
_____	_____	30.	Upset when things do not go your way
_____	_____	31.	Upset when things are out of place
_____	_____	32.	Tendency to be oppositional or argumentative
_____	_____	33.	Tendency to have repetitive negative thoughts
_____	_____	34.	Tendency toward compulsive behaviors
_____	_____	35.	Intense dislike for change
_____	_____	36.	Tendency to hold grudges
_____	_____	37.	Trouble shifting attention from subject to subject
_____	_____	38.	Trouble shifting behavior from task to task
_____	_____	39.	Difficulties seeing options in situations
_____	_____	40.	Tendency to hold on to own opinion and not listen to others
_____	_____	41.	Tendency to get locked into a course of action, whether or not it is good

_____	_____	42. Needing to have things done a certain way or you become very upset
_____	_____	43. Others complain that you worry too much
_____	_____	44. Tend to say no without first thinking about question
_____	_____	45. Tendency to predict fear

SUBTOTAL _____

_____	_____	46. Frequent feelings of sadness
_____	_____	47. Moodiness
_____	_____	48. Negativity
_____	_____	49. Low energy
_____	_____	50. Irritability
_____	_____	51. Decreased interest in others
_____	_____	52. Decreased interest in things that are usually fun or pleasurable
_____	_____	53. Feelings of hopelessness about the future
_____	_____	54. Feelings of helplessness or powerlessness
_____	_____	55. Feeling dissatisfied or bored
_____	_____	56. Excessive guilt
_____	_____	57. Suicidal feelings
_____	_____	58. Crying spells
_____	_____	59. Sleep changes (too much or too little)
_____	_____	60. Appetite changes (too much or too little)
_____	_____	61. Chronic low self-esteem

SUBTOTAL _____

_____	_____	62. Negative sensitivity to smells/odors
_____	_____	63. Frequent feelings of nervousness or anxiety
_____	_____	64. Panic attacks
_____	_____	65. Symptoms of heightened muscle tension (headaches, sore muscles, hand tremor)
_____	_____	66. Periods of heart pounding, rapid heart rate or chest pain
_____	_____	67. Periods of trouble breathing or feeling smothered
_____	_____	68. Periods of feeling dizzy, faint or unsteady on your feet
_____	_____	69. Periods of nausea or abdominal upset
_____	_____	70. Periods of sweating, hot or cold flashes
_____	_____	71. Tendency to predict the worst
_____	_____	72. Fear of dying or doing something crazy
_____	_____	73. Avoid places for fear of having an anxiety attack
_____	_____	74. Conflict avoidance
_____	_____	75. Excessive fear of being judged or scrutinized by others
_____	_____	76. Persistent phobias
_____	_____	77. Low motivation
_____	_____	78. Excessive motivation
_____	_____	79. Tics (motor or vocal)
_____	_____	80. Poor handwriting
_____	_____	81. Quick startle
_____	_____	82. Tendency to freeze in anxiety-provoking situations
_____	_____	83. Lacks confidence in their abilities
_____	_____	84. Seems shy or timid
_____	_____	85. Easily embarrassed
_____	_____	86. Sensitive to criticism

SUBTOTAL _____

_____	_____	87. Bites fingernails or picks skin
_____	_____	88. Short fuse or periods of extreme irritability
_____	_____	89. Periods of rage with little provocation
_____	_____	90. Often misinterprets comments as negative when they are not
_____	_____	91. Irritability tends to build, then explodes, then recedes, often tired after a rage
_____	_____	92. Periods of spaciness or confusion
_____	_____	93. Periods of panic and/or fear for no specific reason
_____	_____	94. Visual or auditory changes, such as seeing shadows or hearing muffled sounds
_____	_____	95. Frequent periods of déjà vu (feelings of being somewhere you have never been)
_____	_____	96. Sensitivity or mild paranoia
_____	_____	97. Headaches or abdominal pain of uncertain origin

Cont.

_____ _____ 98. History of a head injury or family history of violence or explosiveness
_____ _____ 99. Dark thoughts, may involve suicidal or homicidal thoughts
_____ _____ 100. Periods of forgetfulness or memory problems
SUBTOTAL _____

SCORING KEY: Attention problems: Items 1–18
Hyperactivity and impulsivity: Items 19–28
Obsessive compulsive behaviors: Items 29–45 (Anterior Cingulate Gyrus)
Depressive behaviors and disorders: Items 46–61 (Deep Limbic System)
Generalized anxiety behaviors and disorders: Items 62–86 (Basal Ganglia)
Explosive behaviors and disorders: Items 87–100 (Temporal Lobe)

INTERPRETATION: To obtain a meaningful score, add up the 3 and 4 ratings (all items scored as Frequently and Very Frequently). While there are no specific cutoff points, the higher the Score in each subcategory, the greater the probability the child is having a significant problem needing therapeutic intervention. The Checklist can also be used to assess change or improvement over time, such as after a therapeutic intervention has been attempted.

Adapted with permission from Dr Daniel Amen and Dr Bradley Schuyler, 2009.

A DIAGNOSTIC ANALYSIS OF TEENAGE MENTAL HEALTH PROBLEMS

The Warning Signs

The teen years can be tough for both parent and child. Adolescents are under stress to be liked, do well in school, get along with their family and make important life decisions. Most of these pressures are unavoidable and worrying about them is natural. But if your teen is feeling very sad, hopeless, worthless or acting out, these could be warning signs of a mental health problem.

Mental health problems are real, painful, and can be severe. They can lead to school failure, loss of friends, or family conflict. Some of the signs that may point to a possible problem are listed below. If you are a parent or another caregiver of a teenager, pay attention if your teen:

Is troubled by negative "stinkin' thinkin'":

- sad and hopeless thoughts without good reason
- angry thoughts most of the time, overreacts to things
- worthless or guilty thinking
- anxious or worried thoughts
- suicide thoughts and threats
- extremely fearful – has unexplained fear thoughts or more fears than most kids
- constantly thinks about physical problems or appearance
- frightened that his/her mind is controlled by some force or is out of control

Is limited by:

- inability to make decisions
- poor concentration
- inability to sit still and focus attention
- speech impairment
- thoughts that race almost too fast to follow
- persistent nightmares
- poor social skills
- poor assertive communication skills
- poor reading/math skills
- lack of computer skills
- poor writing skills
- lack of impulse control

Experiences changes in lifestyle:

- suddenly does much worse in school
- loses interest in things usually enjoyed
- has unexplained changes in sleeping or eating habits
- notable change in dress and appearance, especially if all black
- avoids friends or family and wants to be alone much of the time
- daydreams too much and does not get things done

- feels life is too hard to handle or talks about a desire to die
- hears voices that cannot be explained

Undergoes disruption in his/her support system:

- divorce of parents
- parents working long hours
- death of family members, friend, grandparents or pet
- loss of friends and family that move away or abandon him/her

Behaves in ways that cause problems:

- uses alcohol or other drugs
- often hurts other people, destroys property
- does things that can be life-threatening
- runs away from home
- cuts on his/her skin (arms, legs, feet, hands)

Is in need of help:

- needs friends desperately
- needs much attention, affirmation and compassion
- needs religious instruction and connections
- needs friends that are strong, active, competent and have good values

PARENTAL ACTIONS TO TAKE:

1. Talk to your teen and demonstrate interest in their world.
2. Spend extra time with your teen.
3. Go to his/her activities and be a support person to them.
4. Go to counseling together.
5. Monitor their comings and goings closely.
6. Check their room for contraband.
7. Be loving and affirming; build self-esteem.
8. Talk of expectations and praise even small steps of progress.
9. Be a caring parent, not a friend; keep roles clear.
10. Be a positive role model, thereby encouraging your teen to do as you do.
11. Be a teaching parent and seek out teaching opportunities in everyday life.
12. Be quick to reward and slow to criticize.

Adapted from a seminar on drinking and teenagers.

Learning Disabilities

Section Contents

CHILDREN WITH SPECIAL NEEDS: EARLY WARNING SIGNS

Some children are born with physical, mental and/or cognitive impairments, while others acquire such disorders that adversely influence ongoing normal growth and development. If parents recognize the problems of children early and seek appropriate professional treatment, most impairments can be corrected or improved. Failure to deal with a child's problem early in the life course when the warning signs are present may lead to unnecessary life-long and chronic handicaps. Parents, grandparents, friends, and professionals facilitate normal development by taking supportive and encouraging action.

Below are some early warning signals which indicate that a problem may exist and corrective action is needed. Don't wait. Bring your concerns to a professional who specializes in the diagnosis and treatment of child-related disabilities and problems, such as a child psychologist, educator, marriage and family counselor, or pediatrician. They will help you determine if further study, treatment or referral is indicated.

The areas noted below can guide you in your informal assessment of your child's developmental status.

VISUAL
- Is often unable to locate and pick up small objects which have been dropped
- Frequently rubs eyes or complains that eyes hurt
- Has reddened, watering or encrusted eyelids
- Holds head in a strained or awkward position (tilts head to either side – thrusts head forward or backward) when trying to look at a particular person or object
- Sometimes or always crosses one or both eyes

SPEECH
- Is unable to say "Ma-ma" and "Da-da" by age 1
- Is unable to say the names of a few toys and people by age 2
- Is unable to say repeat common rhymes or TV songs by age 3
- Not talking in short sentences by age 4
- Is not understood by people outside the immediate family by age 5

AUDITORY
- Does not turn to face the source of sounds or voices by 6 months of age
- Has frequent ear aches or running ears
- Talks in a very loud or very soft voice
- Does not respond when called from another room
- Turns the same ear toward a sound he/she wishes to hear

SOCIAL
- Does not play games such as peek-a-boo, pat-a-cake, waving bye-bye by age 1
- Does not imitate parents doing routine household chores by age 2
- Does not enjoy playing alone with toys, pots and pans, sand, etc. by age 3
- Does not play group games such as hide-and-seek, tag-ball, etc. with other children by age 4
- Does not share and take turns by age 5

COGNITIVE
- Does not react to his/her own name when called by age 1
- Is unable to identify hair, eyes, ears, nose and mouth by pointing to them by age 2
- Does not understand simple stories told or read by age 3
- Does not give reasonable answers to such questions as "What do you do when you are sleepy?" or "What do you do when you are hungry?" by age 4
- Does not seem to understand the meanings of the words "today," "tomorrow," "yesterday" by age 5

PHYSICAL
- Unable to sit up without support by age 1
- Cannot walk without help by age 2
- Does not walk up and down steps by age 3
- Is unable to balance on one foot by age 4
- Cannot throw a ball overhand and catch a large ball bounced to him/her by age 5

ATTENTION DEFICIT HYPERACTIVITY DISORDER

- Onset before age 9.
- Must not have pervasive developmental disorder.
- Symptoms must be more frequent and severe than in children of similar mental age.
- Eight of the following 14 criteria must be present for more than 6 months:
    1. Often fidgets with hands or feet or squirms in seat (in adolescents, may be limited to subjective feelings of restlessness).
    2. Difficulty remaining seated when required.
    3. Easily distracted by extraneous stimuli.
    4. Difficulty waiting turn in games or group situations.
    5. Often blurts out answers to questions before they have been completed.
    6. Difficulty following through on instructions from others (not due to oppositional behavior or failure to comprehend).
    7. Difficulty sustaining attention in tasks or play activities.
    8. Often shifts from one uncompleted activity to another.
    9. Difficulty playing quietly.
    10. Often talks excessively.
    11. Often interrupts or intrudes on others (other children's games or activities).
    12. Often does not seem to listen to what is being said to him/her.
    13. Often loses things necessary for tasks or activities at school or at home (assignments, books, pencils, toys).
    14. Often engages in physically dangerous activities without considering possible consequences (not thrill seeking).

Adapted from Easter Seals.

THE EVALUATION OF LEARNING DISABILITIES

When considering having me perform a psychological/educational evaluation for your son or daughter, please remember that the public school system provides psychological services that include testing for learning problems. Your tax dollars have already paid for the staff who provide these services in your county. Most insurance companies do not cover testing of this kind for just this reason. If you hope to use your insurance coverage please check with me before we begin the evaluation so that we may ascertain whether your carrier will cover any part of the evaluation. It is critical that this is done in advance as very few insurance companies will backdate an authorization for services (when authorization is required).

What Else Might Explain My Child's Academic Problems?

Academic problems sometimes have their roots in other areas. These include a wide variety of personal or family factors such as the following:

- visual or hearing problems
- allergies or food intolerances
- health problems (including side effects of medications)
- other medical/neurological conditions such as ADHD/ADD
- worry, anxiety or depression stemming from:
  - peer problems
  - parental job stresses
  - financial difficulties
  - illness or death of a family member, relative or pet

What Are the Components of an LD Evaluation?

Part of the evaluation involves ruling out other possible factors by taking a careful family and medical history. In addition to having parents complete a detailed history form, I like to meet with them for an hour to gather additional background information prior to meeting with the child to do the formal testing. This is followed by a series of testing sessions with the child. Following this I prepare a draft of the report and meet with the parents (and older teens) to discuss the results of the evaluation and my recommendations. After the parents have had an opportunity to review the draft, I give the parents a final copy with additional copies as needed for the school, pediatrician, etc.

Information I Need from You

Please bring me photocopies of as much of the following as you can locate:

- Report cards from as far back as you have them
- Standardized Achievement Test (SAT) scores such as the ITBS, Stanford, and CAT
- Prior psychological evaluations
- Samples of homework – the more varied the better, including math homework and handwritten compositions such as book reports. You do *not* need to copy homework. I will return all originals. Please do *not* bring any personal writings (journals/diaries) without first getting permission from your son or daughter

In general, the more you would like to bring to have me look at, the better. Sometimes I find a critical clue buried in a stack of papers.

IQ and Achievement Testing

IQ and achievement testing typically requires about 6 hours spread out over several sessions (usually 45 to 90 minutes each). My typical evaluation includes the following test instruments as a core battery:

- Weschler Intelligence Scales for Children – 4th Revision (WISC-IV)
- Woodcock–Johnson Tests of Cognitive Ability (WJ-III Cognitive)
- Woodcock–Johnson Tests of Achievement (WJ-III Achievement)
- Gray Oral Rating Tests – 4th Revision (GORT-4)
- Gray Silent Reading Tests (GSRT)
- Nelson–Denny Reading Test (for senior high and college students)
- Comprehensive Test of Phonological Processing (CTOPP) (early elementary)
- Beery–Buktenica Developmental Test of Visual Motor Integration (Beery)
- Several Pencil-and-Paper Symptom Checklists

If weaknesses emerge in a specific area such as spelling, math or reading, I administer additional subtests from other instruments to explore the area in greater depth. For example, I may use subtests from the K-TEA or WIAT to get additional measures about spelling or arithmetic if problems emerge on the WISC-IV or WJ-III.

What Will It Cost?

The evaluation has five components:

- Diagnostic Interview with the parents (1 session)
- The actual testing with the student (typically 7 sessions 50 minutes each)
- 3 hours to score and interpret the results and prepare a 15–20 page report
- A 90-minute feedback session with the parents (optionally, including the student)

This translates to a typical cost of about $ _____. Insurance may cover part of the diagnostic interview and the feedback session, but it rarely covers the testing or report preparation.

Multiple Intelligence

It is important to understand that "intelligence" is not a single construct. Researchers such as Gardner, Armstrong, and Phipps have identified seven distinct kinds of intelligence. (My personal opinion is that more will be defined as time goes on.) The testing that I do looks at several of these, but for a variety of reasons is not meant to be an exhaustive assessment of all seven types. Here are the seven that have been defined thus far:

- Verbal (writing, poetry, etc.)
- Logical mathematical (analytical, math)
- Musical
- Bodily kinesthetic (movement, dance, athletics, craftsmen, etc.)
- Visual spatial (designers, painters, artists, etc.)
- Intrapersonal
- Naturalist intelligence

Our school system is heavily skewed to the first two. In the early grades (K to 3) there is more emphasis on visual spatial. After that point there is a progressive shift to more auditory-based teaching with an emphasis on verbal and logical/mathematical skills.

For some additional reading on a related issue of learning styles, see the article "What *Sounds* Right to You May *Look* Better to Your Child" (Paul Scherk, 1999).

Attention Deficit-Hyperactivity Disorder (ADD/ADHD)

Section Contents

ADHD: AN OVERVIEW

POSSIBLE CAUSES OF ADHD

- Genetic factors, a family line usually on the side of the males
- Brain trauma, left frontal lobe, and usually in early childhood
- Toxic exposure pre-natally or in very early childhood
- Oxygen deprivation, usually accident- or birth-related
- Brain infection
- Slower than normal brain development

ESSENTIAL COMPONENTS OF A TREAMENT PROGRAM

- Parent education, lectures, books, articles, workshops, counseling sessions
- Support group for parents and/or child
- Parent training in child management techniques to help teach focusing
- Use of medication and supplements
- Home lifestyle changes in diet, exercise, routine living, and reduced stimulation
- School and home coordination and communication
- Contract with an ADHD expert psychologist for therapy and self-control training
- Start treatment as early as 3–4 years of age
- Teach internal monitoring and supervision of thought, feelings, and movements
- Teach stress management techniques

PROBLEMS FOR WHICH TO BE ALERT AND AVOID

- Abusive behavior of a physical, sexual, and/or emotional nature
- Suicide potential
- Social inadequacy and interpersonal conflict
- Alcohol and substance abuse
- Weight loss and sleeping difficulty; insomnia
- School work unfinished, underachievement, and poor grades
- Excitement seeking
- Multiple relationships and multiple marriages
- Job failure and frequent changes
- Impulsive decision making
- Driving-related problems
- Poor handwriting and poor organizational skills
- Many interests and poor follow-through; many unfinished tasks

POTENTIAL DIAGNOSTIC CONFUSION

- ADHD vs. Bipolar disorder
- ADHD vs. Learning disorder
- ADHD vs. Anxiety/Depression
- ADHD vs. Pervasive developmental disorder
- ADHD vs. Autism
- ADHD vs. Asperger's
- ADHD vs. Obsessive-compulsiveness (over-focus)

ADHD EVALUATION

Both healthcare professionals and lay people have become increasingly aware of the prevalence of ADHD in children and adults. However, the assessment tools that have been available have had certain limitations. Symptom checklists (e.g., The Connors Test) are very helpful as screening instruments but one should not arrive at a diagnosis based on this type of information alone. The best of these symptom checklists is only 70% accurate in diagnosing ADHD because so many other disorders can produce many of the symptoms of ADHD (i.e., depression, anxiety, oppositional defiant disorder, learning disabilities, and some medical disorders). Further, 80% of individuals with ADHD have at least one other co-existing disorder. Consequently, a thorough diagnostic evaluation is essential.

Psychometric testing has been a common method of assessment for ADHD. However, most of the tests that have been available, until recently, are time-consuming to administer and therefore costly. In addition, almost all of these tests were designed to measure other mental functions such as immediate memory, fine motor speed, visual perception, and mental calculation skills. While these tests can be affected by concentration problems, they are not directly assessing attention and concentration. Therefore, these tests are not very accurate.

In the past several years, much more sophisticated tests have been developed which are very sensitive and specifically measure concentration and impulse control without requiring other cognitive processing. The two with the highest diagnostic accuracy are the **Test of Variables of Attention (TOVA)** and the **IVA Continuous Performance Test.** These instruments have a **92% accuracy rate** in identifying adults and children with ADHD.

Further, the TOVA and the IVA are designed for serial administrations in order to assess response to medication. Research with these instruments has shown that either too little or too much medication will result in less than optimal symptom control. By performing drug challenge administrations, it is possible to objectively assess the patient's response to medication and make adjustments accordingly. Because these tests take less than an hour to administer, they are very cost-effective.

Generally, the initial interview with the doctor or therapist can identify whether there are any other possible disorders that might account for the patient's presenting problems and an additional evaluation is performed if necessary. Otherwise, either the IVA or the TOVA are quite accurate in identifying children and adults with ADHD.

KEY BENEFITS

- Accurate diagnosis
- Accurate adjustment of medication
- Identification of possible co-existing disorders
- Cost-effective

POSSIBLE CAUSES OF IMPULSIVITY AND HYPERACTIVITY

Impulsiveness and hyperactivity are behavioral problems with many possible causes, as well as courses of action to bring about control. One is not helpless over such conditions and behavioral patterns. However, it calls for serious and forthright professional action, often involving several different types of providers. Consultation among providers is necessary for good and effective treatment. The most likely cause of the disorder may give some direction for treatment, but not necessarily. A multi-dimensional approach may be indicated.

Possible Causes of Impulsivity and Hyperactivity

- Chaotic/aggressive family style and organization
- Permissive/discipline-free parenting
- Egocentricity/narcissism
- Immaturity
- Anti-social personality
- Psychopathic personality
- Drugs/alcohol intoxication or withdrawal
- Sensory integration/Lateralization deficits
- Neurological impairments (brain damage, mild fetal alcohol syndrome)
- Environmental stress, and inappropriate demands
- Psychiatric conditions (psychosis, anxiety, manic phase)
- Brainwave disorder
- Attention-deficit hyperactivity disorder (ADHD)

What Is the Most Likely Cause of My Child's Condition?

What Can I Do to Improve the Impulsivity or Hyperactivity of My Child?

1.

2.

3.

4.

5.

6.

Comments:

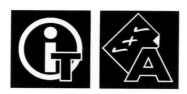

ADHD BEHAVIORAL REVIEW

Below is a list of behaviors one can review in establishing difficulties experienced by a child with a potential diagnosis of ADHD. When a therapist is consulting with teachers or parents, this information can be used to indicate the importance of an ADHD evaluation and referral for medical treatment.

Child's name: _____

Gender: M   F

Age: _____   **Grade:** _____

1. Does not give close attention to details.
2. Makes careless mistakes in schoolwork.
3. Squirms in seat and fidgets hands/feet.
4. Demonstrates difficulty maintaining attention on tasks/play activities.
5. Does not stay in seat or room as directed.
6. Does not appear to listen when being directly spoken to.
7. Exhibits behavior that is inappropriate to situations (climbing on things/getting into things when it is appropriate to be relatively quiet).
8. Does not follow instructions.
9. Fails to complete work.
10. Demonstrates difficulty playing quietly.
11. Demonstrates difficulty organizing tasks/activities.
12. Seems to be constantly on the go.
13. Avoids tasks that require consistent/sustained mental effort.
14. Talks constantly.
15. Constantly losing things that are needed for tasks/activities.
16. Is not able to wait his/her turn to talk or blurts out answers.
17. Is not able to wait for questions to be fully stated before answering.
18. Demonstrates difficulty waiting his/her turn.
19. Is easily distracted.
20. Demonstrates forgetfulness in daily tasks/activities.
21. Interrupts others.
22. Is intrusive in behavior/talking.

Adapted from G. J. Di Paul et al. (1998) ADHD Rating Scale-IV, School Version.

School Performance and Teacher Feedback

Section Contents

DAILY/WEEKLY SCHOOL REPORT

Daily School Report

Use this form when a child has only one teacher. The teacher should fill out the form and sign it and then give it to the child to take home to review with the parents.

Pupil name: _____

    School work was done on time   Yes ☐   No ☐

    School work was done properly   Yes ☐   No ☐

    Classroom behavior was acceptable   Yes ☐   No ☐

    Comments:

Teacher's signature: _____ Date: _____

Weekly School Report

Use this form when the child has several teachers in a day or week. The chart should be filled out by each teacher based on the child's performance for an entire week.

Pupil name: _____

Please answer "Yes" or "No" based on the following questions:

A. School work was done on time.

B. School work was done properly.

C. Classroom behavior was acceptable.

Sign the form and date it for future reference.

Subject	Teacher name	Yes/No	Teacher signature	Date
		A. B. C.		
		A. B. C.		
		A. B. C.		
		A. B. C.		
		A. B. C.		
		A. B. C.		
		A. B. C.		
		A. B. C.		

WEEKLY SCHOOLWORK REVIEW

Evaluate your child's homework for a week. When the form has been completed, ask your child to take it to their teacher for review and comment. Repeat the process weekly until stable improvement has been noted.

Pupil name: _____

Date	I am pleased with this week's work	I am pleased with most of this week's work	I am concerned about this week's work	I would like a conference to discuss this week's work	Parent signature	Teacher signature

TEACHER FEEDBACK FORM ON STUDENT PERFORMANCE

Teacher's name: _____   Today's date: _____

Child's name: _____   Grade level: _____

DIRECTIONS: Each rating should be considered in the context of what is appropriate for the age of the child you are rating and should reflect that child's behavior over the past two (2) weeks. Please check your answers with a X.

This evaluation is based on a time period when the child:

☐ was on medication   ☐ was not on medication   ☐ not sure?

Classroom behaviors	**Never**	**Occasionally**	**Often**	**Very Often**
1. Does not seem to listen when spoken to directly	☐	☐	☐	☐
2. Has difficulty organizing tasks and activities	☐	☐	☐	☐
3. Loses things necessary for tasks or activities (school assignments, pencils, or books)	☐	☐	☐	☐
4. Is easily distracted by external stimuli	☐	☐	☐	☐
1. Fidgets with hands, feet, and/or squirms in seat	☐	☐	☐	☐
2. Has difficulty engaging in leisure activities quietly	☐	☐	☐	☐
3. Is "on the go" or often acts as if "driven by a motor"	☐	☐	☐	☐
4. Talks excessively	☐	☐	☐	☐
1. Actively defies or refuses to comply with adult's requests or rules	☐	☐	☐	☐
2. Bullies, threatens, or intimidates other kids	☐	☐	☐	☐
3. Lies to obtain favors or to avoid obligations (e.g., "cons" others)	☐	☐	☐	☐
4. Deliberately destroys the property of others	☐	☐	☐	☐
1. Is self-conscious or easily embarrassed	☐	☐	☐	☐
2. Is afraid to try new things for fear of making mistakes	☐	☐	☐	☐
3. Presents as lonely, unwanted, or unloved; complains that "no one loves him/her"	☐	☐	☐	☐
4. Appears sad, unhappy, or depressed	☐	☐	☐	☐

COMMENTS:

STUDENT RATING SCALE FOR EDUCATIONAL PLANNING

Please complete the rating scale below on a 5-point scale based on how the student has been performing and behaving over the past _____ weeks. Consider a 1 to be poor and needs much improvement. Consider 5 being excellent and keep it up, while 3 is an average score and some improvement is needed. When completed, provide a copy to the parents so they can help the child improve in any of the areas noted below as a problem area of learning or classroom behavior.

Student's name: _____ Grade: _____ Date: _____

School: _____ Teacher: _____

Personal and Interpersonal Behavior:
Compliance/cooperation   _____

Sustained attention   _____

Organizational skills   _____

Copes with new situations   _____

Social acceptance by peers   _____

Responsibility for self/others   _____

Completes assignments   _____

Politeness/kindness   _____

SUBTOTAL _____

Speech and Language Skills:
Use of vocabulary   _____

Use of grammar   _____

Relates personal experience in a meaningful manner   _____

Formulates ideas and shares them with the class   _____

SUBTOTAL _____

Auditory Attention and Comprehension:
Follows instruction of teacher   _____

Comprehends class discussion and participates   _____

Retains new information presented in class by teacher _____

SUBTOTAL _____

Teacher comments, observations, homework, instructions, and suggestions for improvement:

Communication with Children

Section Contents

10 STEPS IN TALKING WITH CHILDREN

1. Listen more than you talk.

2. Convey you understand the child's point or issue.

3. Paraphrase what they say to minimize miscommunication.

4. Clarify what you think you heard by asking for more information.

5. Empathize with the child and his message.

6. Express your need for the child to act in some particular manner.

7. Give expectations clearly and in simple terms.

8. Encourage mutual problem solving when a problem develops.

9. Provide limited choices and options.

10. Express appreciation and affirmation.

TALKING TO KIDS SO THEY WILL FEEL VALUED

Talking with kids involves the exchange of words, ideas, feelings, and thoughts. It includes both what we say and how we say it, the latter often being the more important. We express ourselves with kids through looks, words, gestures, silence, and actions. Children place much attention on the feeling tone of our expressions with them, while adults often place the focus on the directions given children in a given situation. This difference can be a basis for relationship difficulties with children.

Below are 15 ways to talk with children and win mutual attention, respect, and affection in the process.

WIN–WIN WAYS OF TALKING WITH CHILDREN

1. Clearly communicate acceptance of the child and what they are trying to say.
2. Use inviting questions, remarks, and comments to open the door of communication.
3. Listen attentively and actively with an open mind and without distractions.
4. The empathic use of "You-Messages" can help a child express feelings and ideas more freely.
5. The empathic use of "I-Messages" can help a child better understand your thoughts and feelings on a topic or situation that developed.
6. Use abundantly more Do's than Don'ts as children want to know what to do rather than just what not to do.
7. Be sure to get the child's attention before speaking to him/her, especially if the issue is important to both of you.
8. Talk *with* children, as in a two-way conversation, rather than *at* them as in giving a lecture.
9. Requests are best made in a simple, positive, and one- or two-step process.
10. Make requests that are important in a firm manner so the child knows you mean it.
11. Be very quick to say, "please," "thank you," and you're welcome" to children.
12. When children are talking and telling a story or explaining an event, do not interrupt them or scold them at the time.
13. Be very careful not to use unkind, deprecating, or put down comments which tear down a child and counteract their self-esteem
14. Use kind and encouraging words to build up the child and establish self-esteem.
15. Communicate with children at eye-level.

A SELF-TEST ON YOUR COMMUNICATION WITH CHILDREN TODAY

1. Did I build up or tear down the child today by how I talked with him/her?
2. Did I give the child a feeling of acceptance and value today in how I interacted with him/her?
3. Did I look for opportunities to connect with my child today and opened doors of communication?

Adapted from Virginia State University, Extension Division.

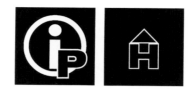

THE GOODNIGHT FORMULA FOR CHILDREN AND PARENTS

The Goodnight Formula consists of four steps:

1. Parent and child take turns saying something that they like about the other person. The parent might say, "I like the way you always help out the baby when he's in trouble."
2. Both parent and child share something positive that they did that day. Your child might say, "I feel good that I told Sarah I was sorry that I embarrassed her."
3. Both parent and child share what they are looking forward to doing tomorrow. Your daughter, talking about her basketball game, might say, "I'm looking forward to your coming to watch me play tomorrow."
4. Following the verbal sharing, parent and child exchange hugs, kisses, and "I love you" statements.

It may take several nights for you and your child to become comfortable with this exercise, but if you persist, eventually both of you will anticipate this special time together. Experience has shown that the Goodnight Formula provides a good opportunity for parents to show children how to care for themselves and others – important factors in helping children handle stress.

WEEKLY FAMILY MEETINGS

Family life is ever changing and ever improving. It is generally considered to be a good exercise to have a weekly family meeting so that issues can be dealt with in a timely manner, cleared up and improvements made where needed within family life. It is recommended that the family set aside 15–20 minutes at least one night a week, after dinner, for a family meeting with notes taken below so that there is a trail of what was agreed upon and what was planned. Not only does such a meeting minimize conflict within the family, it also increases the chance that the family unit will function in a more communicative and thoughtful manner. Communication skills, problem solving skills, decision making skills, and cooperation skills are taught in this process of a weekly family meeting.

AGENDA

1. Have there been any problems at school in the past week that need to be discussed?
2. Have there been any problems at home in the past week that need to be discussed?
3. Are there any activities during the next week that all family members must know about and participate in?
4. Are there any activities or events that any family member would like to do during the coming week or month?
5. What are the areas of praise and accommodation that need to be identified and discussed?
6. Are there any areas of our family relationships that need to improve during this next week?

   ... and have a good week!

FAMILY LOCATOR AND CONNECTION WORKSHEET

Please answer these questions in terms of your perception of how a typical week proceeds. Place an asterisk (*) next to any entry which is a problem area for you. State what the problem is for you.

HUSBAND	WIFE
Breakfast with family	Breakfast with family
Time leaves morning	Time leaves morning
Connect with family #1	Connect with family #1
Connect with family #2	Connect with family #2
Time returns	Time returns
Dinner with family	Dinner with family
How time spent in evening with family	How time spent in evening with family
Time leaves evening	Time leaves evening
Time returns	Time returns
Connect with family upon return	Connect with family upon return
Weekend times with family	Weekend times with family

Hours worked per week: _____
Hours with family per week: _____

Hours worked per week: _____
Hours with family per week: _____

HUSBAND:
My plan for making family life a higher priority in my life and daily schedule:

WIFE:
My plan for making family life a higher priority in my life and daily schedule:

54 WAYS TO SAY "GOOD FOR YOU"

A little praise goes a long way in any situation. But "a little praise" really needs to be something more than the same few phrases repeated over and over again. Your child needs more than the traditional "good," "very good," and "fine" for encouragement. Here are some additional possibilities:

That's really nice.

Thank you very much.

That's great.

That's clever.

I'm proud of you.

Keep it up.

Good job.

Very creative.

Much better.

Wow!

Terrific!

Fantastic!

Beautiful!

Excellent work!

Marvelous!

You make it look easy.

I like the way you're working.

That's right! Good for you!

Now you've figured it out.

You are waiting so quietly.

It is really hard to wait.

You are really listening.

That's a good point.

You are doing a good job.

That's coming along nicely.

Keep up the good work.

I appreciate your help.

That's an interesting point of view.

That's an interesting way of looking at it.

I like the way you had settled down.

It looks like you put a lot of work into this.

I'm very proud of the way you worked (are working).

That's certainly one way of looking at it.

Thank you for (sitting down, being quiet, helping, etc).

Groovy.

Right on.

For sure.

Sharp.

Super.

Superior work.

Exactly right.

Very interesting.

Good thinking.

Far out.

Nice going.

Out of sight.

What neat work.

You've got it now!

Cool.

That's a very good observation.

Now you've got the hang of it.

You're on the right track now.

That's quite an improvement.

My goodness, how impressive.

THIS IS JUST A BEGINNING ... I AM SURE YOU CAN THINK OF MANY MORE.

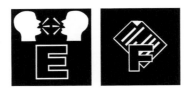

A PARENT'S PLEDGE

A parent of: _____

We sincerely and openly pledge to live our lives and take decisive action to keep our home free of drugs. Alcohol consumption will likewise be absent from our lifestyle or limited to minimal levels and occasions. To fulfill this pledge, we commit:

1. To communicate with our child/children. That means not only transmitting but receiving. Truly listening. We pledge to respect their ideas and opinions even when they differ from ours. If we disagree, we will explain why and calmly try to guide them to the best of our abilities.

2. To respond to our child/children's problems, rather than reacting to them.

3. To educate ourselves about drugs and their dangers so that we can, in turn, effectively impress upon our children why substances are bad for them.

4. To monitor our child/children's moods, habits, attitudes, and friendships, which will better enable us to recognize potential substance abuse and prevent it.

5. To help build our child/children's self-esteem; providing and promoting alternatives to chemicals; helping them feel grown up in ways other than with drugs; teaching them how to confront problems instead of seeking escape through substances.

6. To confront any youthful drug or alcohol crisis quickly and calmly so that we can make informed, rational decisions that are in our child/children's best interest.

7. To get counseling for ourselves if we have difficulty handling our child/children's substance use, so that we may be better able to help them recover and be drug free.

8. To remember what it was like to be a child; never forgetting where we came from.

_____   _____
Signature of Father   Date

_____   _____
Signature of Mother   Date

Read and acknowledged by child/children _____

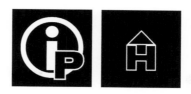

BASIC PARENTAL BEHAVIORS TO USE IN RAISING BOYS

On the following list of parental behavior patterns, rate yourself on a scale of 1 to 5, with 5 being very high and 1 being very low. Note the areas where improvement needs to be made. Note what you are doing well and keep it up. Discuss your responses with your therapist and your spouse. Also, it may be helpful, if appropriate, to discuss your answers with the entire family in a Family Council meeting.

1. Allow and encourage boys to express emotions, but only appropriately _____

2. Establish talk times _____

3. Build relationship skills by reading stories of relationships among children _____

4. Develop the "software" skills with boys, i.e., compassion, sensitivity, and caring _____

5. Use the "touch and instruct" approach when talking seriously with boys _____

6. Help boys feel how others feel when things happen, both good and bad _____

7. Allow controlled, mild physical aggression, assertiveness _____

8. Provide competition, but keep it fair and structured _____

9. Identify several male role models among the boy's peers _____

10. Identify several male role models among older men _____

11. Encourage ongoing and intimate relationships with both mom and dad _____

12. Affirm that they are boys and will soon be men _____

COMMENTS:

THE MAKING OF FAMILY RULES

The family functions best with rules and agreed procedures for handling events and the daily affairs of family life. You could try the sample below, by an unknown author, which is time-honored and has worked for many families.

House Rules

If you sleep on it – make it up
If you wear it – hang it up
If you drop it – pick it up
If you eat off it – put it in the sink
If you step on it – wipe it off
If you open it – close it
If you empty it – fill it up
If it rings – answer it
If it howls – feed it
If it cries – love it

Or you could design your own rules as a family using your individual list of desired behaviors for your children. Write a few short simple rules. Some examples might be:

- Homework must be done before supper.
- You may only get up once after going to bed.
- Instead of fighting or bickering, speak kindly and in a friendly manner.

Be sure to focus on the behaviors you *want* to occur not just those behaviors you do not want your children to engage in. The rules may be the same or different for each child. If different, make a separate list for each child and put on a separate page. Do not list too many rules; do only two or three for younger children.

Be sure to put "teeth" in it. That is, state what will happen if the rules are followed and what will happen if the rules are not followed, as agreed.

1. _____

2. _____

3. _____

4. _____

5. _____

Whatever you do, select rules that are fair, age appropriate, fun to use, and reasonable.

Exercises for Therapists to Get Children to Communicate

Section Contents

DRAWING A FACE AS A RAPPORT-BUILDING EXERCISE

MAKE A FACE

HAPPY

SAD

ANGRY

FRUSTRATED

YOU (MOST OF THE TIME)

YOU (TODAY)

DRAWING A DAD STORY FOR THE UNFORTHCOMING CHILD

Name: _____

Date: _____

The dog is dreaming. Tell a story about the dog's dream.

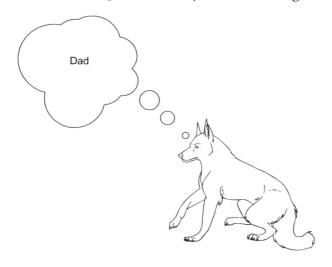

DRAWING A MOM STORY FOR THE UNFORTHCOMING CHILD

Name: _____

Date: _____

The dog is dreaming. Tell a story about the dog's dream.

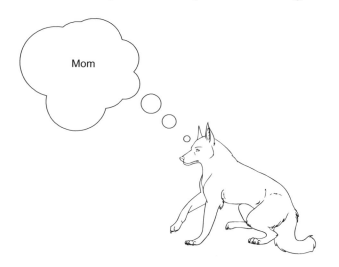

Mom

STORY TELLING FOR THE UNFORTHCOMING CHILD

Name: _____

Date: _____

It is time for the horse to come in. Draw a line to where it will go.

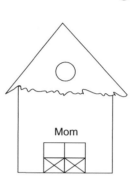

Mom

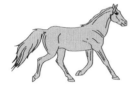

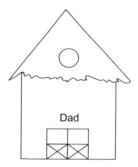

Dad

Drug Use and Eating Disorders

Section Contents

PARENTS AND TEACHERS COMBATING ADOLESCENT DRUG USE

Throughout history, mothers have generally been identified as the parent most responsible for their children's development and their behavior outside the home. Thus, mothers are the ones generally blamed for the problems their children create. However, if their children develop a respectable and admirable lifestyle, both parents are quick to share in the pride and glory of their children's accomplishments. Similarly, teachers are commonly criticized for what they do or do not do for a particular child. They are rarely affirmed or appreciated for their contribution to the successes and achievements of their students. It seems unfair doesn't it?

Recent psychological research indicates that the father plays a very significant role in the development of his children's behavior patterns, especially their level of achievement. Further, recent psychological research underscores the importance of the parenting style utilized in the home in rearing the children as compared to the mere presence of the mother or father in the home. It has also been found that children suffer and are placed at risk when the parents work outside the home a combined total of 60 or more hours per week.

Several years ago, a study was conducted among 443 youths, ages 7 through 17, relative to their drug use and the parenting style used in the home. Interpersonal and attitudinal factors were measured, along with parental relationships, parenting style, and the drug use among these young people. The findings of this research indicated that youths who abstained or used drugs infrequently came from homes where the following factors were present:

1. There was a feeling of closeness to one or both parents.
2. There was an emphasis in the home on getting along with the parents.
3. There was a desire on the part of the youth to be like one or both of the parents.
4. There was a perceived attitude of trust in the youth on the part of the mother.
5. There was regular encouragement and praise from one or both parents.
6. There was an ability and freedom to talk about personal problems with the father.

The research study also found that non-drug users or those who used drugs infrequently came from homes in which there was parental strictness or firmness, parental limit setting, and parental involvement in the decisions made by their children at all age levels. Parental lifestyle and child management style appear to be significant factors in the subsequent drug use of their teens.

Contrary to common thought, substance use by adolescents was not related to the rules set forth by parents regarding the prohibition of drug use. Further, rules about homework and television use were significantly related to teen substance usage. Parents of non-drug users were generally considered less permissive and did operate the home with rules of conduct in place and being followed. Parents of non-drug-using teens were not particularly punitive in their management of their children either.

The research results strongly indicate that drug usage is a family matter. Drug usage can be prevented and combated by the way families live together and relate to each other. Is there a role for the classroom teacher? Indeed, children spend 5 hours a day under the influence of one or more teachers. Consider the following:

1. Teachers are in an excellent position to encourage and support parents in their management of the children in the home.
2. Teachers are in an excellent position to be a consultant or coach to parents at critical times in the life of a family.
3. Teachers are in an excellent position to encourage children to talk with their parents about personal problems.
4. Teachers are in an excellent position to encourage children to seek out and solicit appropriate praise and affirmation from their parents when earned and deserved by their academic achievement.
5. Teachers can encourage children to form close relationships with their parents by involving them in the academic community and process.
6. Teachers can encourage their children to get along with their parents and can teach them to live and prevail with unity and cooperation within the home.

Parents and teachers must form a bond and commit to academic success and achievement with every child. With some parents, teachers must be creative and wise in building the bond between them. And both parents and teachers must form a bond to raise together children who will learn to live life with integrity, productivity, servitude, and with a living and expressed faith.

RECOMMENDATIONS FOR FAMILY MEMBERS OF ANOREXIC INDIVIDUALS

1. With child/adolescent anorexics, demand less decision making from the anorexic. Offer fewer choices, less responsibility. For example, they should not decide what the family eats for dinner or where to go for vacation.
2. With child/adolescent anorexics, in conflicts about decisions, parents should not withdraw out of fear that their child/adolescent will become increasingly ill.
3. Seek to maintain a supportive, confident posture that is calming yet assertive. Do not be controlling.
4. Express honest affection, both verbally and physically.
5. Develop communication/discussion on personal issues rather than on food and weight.
6. Do not demand weight gain or put down the individual for having anorexia.
7. Do not blame. Avoid statements like "Your illness is ruining the family." This person is not responsible for family functioning.
8. Do not emotionally abandon or avoid the anorexic family member. Remain emotionally available and supportive. Utilize clear boundaries.
9. Once the individual is involved in treatment, do not become directly involved with the weight issues. If you see a change in the individual's appearance, contact the therapist or other pertinent professional such as the person's physician and dietician.
10. Do not demand that the person eat with you, and do not allow their eating problem to dominate the family's eating schedule or use of the kitchen. Be consistent.
11. For child/adolescent anorexics, do not allow them to shop or to cook for the family. This puts them in a nurturing role and allows them to deny their own needs for food by feeding others.
12. Increase giving and receiving of both caring and support within the family. Develop clear boundaries, and allow each person to be responsible for themselves and setting their own goals.

Therapist's Guide to Clinical Intervention, Second Edition by Sharon L. Johnson (© 2003 Elsevier Inc.)

EATING DISORDER EVALUATION: BULIMIA

1. Psychological evaluation
   - Eating behaviors
   - Weight
   - Emotional symptoms
   - Stressful life events
   - Stressful life circumstances
   - Parental verbal abuse
   - History of mental/emotional illness
   - Mental status
   - Strengths/weaknesses
   - Motivation for treatment
   - Prior treatment experiences and outcome
   - Collateral contacts with family members/other treating professionals

2. Review diagnostic criteria
   - Episodic binge eating (eating an extremely large amount of food within a specified period of time while feeling out of control; binge eating disorder lacks purging behaviors)
   - Episodic purging behavior, which includes vomiting, laxative use, diuretic use, enema use, fasting, or excessive exercise to prevent weight gain
   - Overconcern with body weight and shape
   - History of other compulsive behaviors, such as shoplifting or substance abuse
   - Coexisting disorders (depression, anxiety disorders, PTSD, OCD, substance abuse)

3. Physical symptoms and signs
   - Dental enamel erosion and cavities
   - Swelling of cheeks, hands, and feet
   - Abdominal fullness, constipation, diarrhea
   - Abrasions on knuckles
   - Headaches
   - Fatigue
   - Hair loss

4. Medical complications (physician review). Note: This is not an exhaustive list.
   - Electrolyte and fluid abnormalities (low serum potassium values)
   - Dehydration
   - Enlarged parotid glands (glands in the cheeks associated with salivation)
   - Dental enamel erosion and cavities
   - Bowel abnormalities

Therapist's Guide to Clinical Intervention, Second Edition by Sharon L. Johnson (© 2003 Elsevier Inc.)

5. Referral
   - Physician-medical evaluation
   - Registered dietician
   - Family therapy
   - Group therapy
   - Specific eating disorder program
   - Dentist

6. Treatment recommendations
   - Psychotherapy (cognitive behavioral, interpersonal, psychodynamic)
   - Individual, family, conjoint, group
   - Antidepressant medication
   - Medical evaluation and possibly monitoring
   - Nutritional counselling
   - Self-help groups

Custody/Visitations

Section Contents

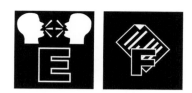

GUIDELINES FOR CHILDREN LIVING IN TWO FAMILY HOMES

The Visitation Conundrum

As parents are different from each other and have different expectations for their children, it may be helpful to write down the expectations when the child is living in the home of the mother and when the child is living in the home of the father. Expectations include both what a child may do and what a child may not do.

To complete the form and arrange for a clear understanding on the part of the children and parents, it may be helpful to hold a Family Council with the children and come to an agreeable set of behaviors in each home. Each parent is then responsible to see that the children honor the agreement and live accordingly.

A Memo of Understanding

Home of the Mother: What I *may* do

1.

2.

3.

4.

5.

Home of the Father: What I *may* do

1.

2.

3.

4.

5.

Home of the Mother: What I *may not* do

1.

2.

3.

4.

5.

Home of the Father: What I *may not* do

1.

2.

3.

4.

5.

Other Comments or Agreements:

CONFIDENTIAL COMMUNICATION

Parent to Parent Communication Form

Parents need to communicate with each other, apart from with the children. This form is designed to facilitate a flow of communication between parents about their children. It will also help parents make plans for their time with the children in a confidential manner. Send messages by mail, e-mail, hand delivery or at an agreed drop off box. Parent #1 is the parent that starts the communication; #2 is the one that responds.

The issue to be considered is: _____

MESSAGE FROM PARENT #1:

MESSAGE FROM PARENT #2:

RETURN MESSAGE FROM PARENT #1:

RETURN MESSAGE FROM PARENT #2:

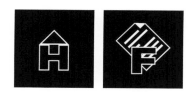

CHILD CUSTODY AND VISITATION PREFERENCES

It's all about the "Best Interest of the Children." A parent's preferences must be the advancement of the children and their best interest now and in the foreseeable future. This is the time to put aside your own desires and preferences and do what is right and best for the children. This is the most difficult and unselfish task a parent must perform at a time when it is virtually impossible to see things objectively and as child-driven. Yet, it can be done. Here is your chance.

Please complete the form prior to meeting with the Mediator of the Court or the one selected by the Court. If a private mediator is selected this form will be helpful to complete as part of the overall evaluation process.

Complete one form per child.

Name: _____ Age: _____

Grade: _____ Academic standing: _____

1. Any special needs or impairments to address?

2. Comment on the child's patterns of:

Sleeping:

Eating:

Peer play:

Educational problems:

Religious/faith development:

Sexual/social development:

Developmental milestones:

3. What is your concern for this child undergoing these significant changes in his/her life?

4. What is your best design for the child's future so that stability prevails, self-esteem is advanced, educational progress is facilitated, dependence needs met, and a positive relationship with both parents can be experienced? Briefly state your best answers below:

Custody arrangements?

Parenting plan and arrangements for sharing child:

5. Tell your story as it pertains to your parenting:

Training in child management/development:

Any arrests or jail time:

Alcohol and drug use:

Religious/spiritual commitments:

Educational history:

History of abuse; any CPS involvement:

Parenting skills:

Are you a person that praises and affirms frequently?

Do you set up and administer a behavioral modification program?

6. Tell us anything you feel should be given consideration for your child's best interest in the future:

New Drivers

Section Contents

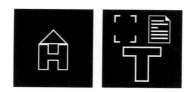

THE NEW DRIVER'S LEARNING PLAN

The following outlines the driving education plan for new drivers, which encourages safe driving for themselves as well as others. A gradual plan towards independent driving is preferred.

1. Take driver's education at school or with a private company.
2. Take driver's training at school or with a private company.
3. Pass the written driver's test and get a permit.
4. Practice driving with a parent or designated "supervisor" for a total of not less than 1,800 miles.
5. Pass driving test after turning 16 years of age.
6. Drive with parents or family members for no less than 1,000 miles.
7. Drive alone or with friends who have been preselected by the parents for no less than 1,000 miles.
8. Drive "relatively freely" as per the following parental guidelines:

_____

_____

_____

The above is agreed upon:

New Driver: _____ Date: _____

Mother: _____ Date: _____

Father: _____ Date: _____

Guardian: _____ Date: _____

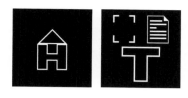

NEW DRIVER'S CONTRACT

Good communication brings about clear understanding. Develop, discuss, and sign a family contract before handing over the car keys. Different families have different ideas and rules, but a clear contract spells out exactly what is expected of your new driver, both on and off the road. Here is a suggested contract to help you.

- I will pay for my insurance and keep it current. Since I am a careful driver, I will pay weekly installments for only ___% of the cost for adding me to the family policy. This includes the driver's-training discount and the good-student discount. Should I not keep a "B" average, I will pay the increased cost or a portion of it. If I buy my own car I will pay all of my insurance.
- Driving the family car is not a right. Driving is not a contest with other drivers. I will always drive defensively.
- I will keep the car clean, help you keep the car in good running order and never leave the gas tank on empty.
- I will have no more than three passengers at any time unless I first consult you as my parent(s)/guardian.
- I will tell you where I will be and when I will be home, and will abide by the agreed plan.
- If I'm ever in a situation involving driving and any drugs or alcohol, I will call you for transportation day or night with no questions asked at the time. We will discuss the situation later.
- I will pay for any tickets I receive. If I get a traffic ticket (not parking) I will forfeit the use of the car for one day for each dollar of the fine. I will also go to traffic school and pay all costs.
- If I am involved in an accident that increases our insurance, I will immediately start to pay ___% of my portion of the damages, plus ___% of any increased cost to the family insurance policy.
- Except for a genuine emergency, I will not drive another vehicle nor permit anyone to drive our vehicles, unless I first get your permission.
- If I ever drive under the influence of a drug or alcohol, I will forfeit driving privileges until I am ___ years old and demonstrate a period of responsible living.
- Other _____

_____

The above is agreed upon:

New Driver: _____ Date: _____

Mother: _____ Date: _____

Father: _____ Date: _____

Guardian: _____ Date: _____

Other Parenting Management Strategies

Section Contents

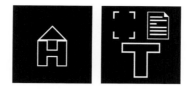

PARENT–CHILD CONTINGENCY BEHAVIORAL CONTRACT

_____

Effective dates: _____

GOAL _____

Terms to be met are as follows:

I, _____ , agree to do the following desired behavior _____
_____ for _____ minutes each day, Sunday through Saturday, with only one reminder from
_____ .

I _____ , the parent, agree to provide my child or teenager _____ so he/she can _____
_____ on Saturday if he/she fulfills the terms of this contract in according with the
conditions stated above.

Signature of child: _____

Signature of parent: _____

This contract will be reviewed on the ending date of agreement _____ .

COMMENTS:

TIME OUT AS A DISCIPLINE MEASURE

You may need or want to send your child to "Time Out" after giving an instruction that was rejected or if the child's behavior was out of control in some way. Usually Time Out is used when either: (a) a particularly flagrant rule violation occurs; (b) a tantrum period follows a request being given; or (c) you and the child need a few minutes away from each other to cool down.

The purpose of using Time Out is to make a definite statement that certain expressed attitudes or behaviors are not acceptable and the child needs time to settle down and regain composure. It is also a great alternative to criticizing, lecturing or screaming at a child. It also preserves the self-esteem of both parent and the child while motivating a child to begin a change in attitude and behavior.

The child's room may be used for the Time Out place as it is safe and comfortable. Don't worry that it may also be a fun place. The point of using Time Out is to create a time during which the requested behavior change can be initiated.

While there is no set length for a period of Time Out it is recommended that at least 10 minutes is used for 4- to 8-year-olds and 30 minutes for 9- to 14-year-olds. It is essential that the behavior of the child changes during the Time Out and that a demonstrated change is the basis for Time Out to come to an end. The child should be ready to resume proper play or do what was asked of him/her before being released and allowed to rejoin the family or activities in progress. For the younger group, you may want to set a timer and then determine if the child is ready to come out when the timer goes off.

Please note: Some children are particularly resistant to the use of Time Out periods, as well as other attempts to change a child's inappropriate behavior patterns. If this is the case with your child, you may wish to consult a professional for alternatives.

COMMENTS OR A RECORD OF TIME OUT USE:

PARENTING EVENTS TO LEARN FROM

Parenting is learned behavior. We all learn to be parents from our own parents and those other parents to whom we have been exposed. We learn to improve our parenting skill in a likewise manner, from others and from our reading. Some of us do better than others. Good parents have good kids. Yet we all do the best we can under the circumstances in which we live our lives.

- **My parenting event of which I am pleased:**

  As you look over your life, what moment are you most proud of as a parent. Tell the story of the time you did it right and are pleased with how you handled a situation.

- **My parenting event about which I am not pleased:**

  While parenting brings many good memories, there were painful ones as well. Yet, we can learn from our mistakes. Others can learn from our mistakes also, if they are shared with others openly. What was your parenting moment about which you are not pleased?

- **My parenting experiences and events that can be lessons for others:**

	Experiences or events	Lessons to pass along
1.		
2.		
3.		
4.		

26-DAY REPORT CARD ON BED WETTING

Name: _____ Age: _____

Bed Wetting Control Strategy:

(1) Rewards for being dry. (2) Mid-night awakenings. (3) No fluids before bed.

(4) Parental pep-talk at bedtime. (5) Special sleep clothing. (6) Other _____

Date	Time to bed	Size of spot				Wetting time	Comments	Strategy followed? Yes/No
		L	M	S	None			

COMMENTS, PATTERNS, AND INSTRUCTIONS:

Chapter 34

Dealing with Geriatric Patients

Chapter Contents

Dementia, within the general field of geriatrics, is a medical condition that profoundly disrupts the way the brain normally functions. All of a person's intellectual capacity becomes progressively impaired. Dementia is common but not a part of normal aging. Dementia erases treasured memories, but leaves the body intact. Dementia is the gradual loss of intellectual functioning with particular loss of short-term memory. That is, the most recent information and memories in are the first memories and information to go out. The ability to concentrate, engage in judgment and decision making, and engage in the processing of abstract thought is also impaired. And so is personality. Likewise, mood changes are likely, such as depression, anxiety, elation, and anger. Impulse control is also impaired. Grandiose and persecutory delusions are fairly common, especially in the advanced stages of dementia. For some, Alzheimer's disease becomes the next step in the breakdown of the brain's functioning.

Dementia is a physical illness also. It progressively shuts down the body as it attacks the brain. It can last for years, but in the advanced stages, life expectancy is the same as for a person with advanced terminal cancer. Alzheimer's and cancer are the most feared diseases we face.

In this chapter we have included forms, templates, information sheets, guidelines, and other tools to help the therapist address the problems of this ever-increasing segment of our population.

Assessment Scales and Checklists

Section Contents

SYMPTOMS AND DIAGNOSTIC IMPRESSIONS FOR MEDICATION USE WITH ELDERLY PATIENTS

To: MD: _____   Date: _____

Resident: _____   DOB: _____

This resident has a current psychotropic medication order. Specific diagnosis and supportive signs are needed. Current guidelines require a specific diagnosis for the use of the following medications: _____

THE MOST APPROPRIATE DIAGNOSIS

☐ Alzheimer's (331.0)

☐ Anxiety—Phobia (300.29)

☐ Dementia w/depression (290.13)

☐ Dementia w/delusion (290.12)

☐ Depression, NOS (311)

☐ Pain disorder, Psych/medical condition (307.89)

☐ Dementia, head trauma (294.1)

☐ Psychotic disorder, NOS (298.9)

☐ Bipolar disorder-mixed (296.62)

☐ Major depression (296.33)

☐ Psychotic/paranoia (295.30)

☐ Obsessive/Compulsive (300.3)

☐ Schizo-affective disorder (295.70)

☐ Schizophrenia (295.90)

☐ General anxiety (300.02)

☐ Brief psychotic disorder (298.8)

☐ Dysthymia (300.40)

☐ Mood disorder, NOS (296.90)

☐ Alcohol dependence (303.90)

☐ Psych factors affecting medical conditions (316)

☐ Adjustment reaction with mixed emotions (309.28)

☐ Anxiety—Panic (300.01)

☐ Delusional disorder (297.1)

☐ Huntington's chorea (333.4)

☐ Insomnia (307.42)

☐ Somatoform disorder (300.81)

☐ Vascular dementia with depression (290.43)

☐ Other _____

BEHAVIORS THE RESIDENT IS EXHIBITING:

☐ Paranoid talking

☐ Suicide remarks

☐ Hitting self, patients, and staff

☐ Purposefully falling/ sliding to the floor

☐ Yelling constantly

☐ Difficulty falling asleep >2 hrs or stay asleep > 4 hours

☐ Severe agitation

☐ Isolation, withdrawal

☐ Self-destructive behavior, i.e., pulling out Foley/NG tube, etc.

☐ Uncontrollable anger, verbal behavior

☐ Sexualized behavior

☐ Excessive day sleeping

☐ Irrational delusional talk

☐ Swearing, cussing

☐ Refusing care/meds > 50% per day on a routine basis

☐ Threatening other patients and staff

☐ Exaggerated pain complaints

☐ Excessive pain behavior

☐ Fearful behavior

☐ Statements of impending death

☐ Picking, scratching, biting, and drooling

☐ Play with excrement

☐ Refusal to eat, eats little

☐ Other _____

_____

_____

_____   _____   _____
MD signature   PhD signature   RN/LVN signature

_____   _____   _____
Date   Date   Date

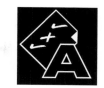

GERIATRIC DEPRESSION SCALE (SHORT FORM)

Name: _____ DOB: _____ Date: _____

Interviewer should ask the questions and record the answers.

1. Are you basically satisfied with your life? — Yes/**No**
2. Have you dropped many of your activities and interests? — **Yes**/No
3. Do you feel your life is empty? — **Yes**/No
4. Do you often get bored? — **Yes**/No
5. Are you in good spirits most of the time? — Yes/**No**
6. Are you afraid something bad is going to happen to you? — **Yes**/No
7. Do you feel happy most of the time? — Yes/**No**
8. Do you often feel helpless? — **Yes**/No/A little
9. Do you prefer to stay at home, rather than going out and doing new things? — **Yes**/No
10. Do you feel you have more problems with memory than most? — **Yes**/No
11. Do you think it is wonderful to be alive now? — Yes/**No**
12. Do you feel pretty worthless the way you are now? — **Yes**/No
13. Do you feel full of energy? — Yes/**No**
14. Do you feel your situation is hopeless? — **Yes**/No
15. Do you think that most people are better off than you are? — **Yes**/No/Some

Total number of **BOLD** answers: _____ Interviewer: _____

Answers in **BOLD** are indicative of depression. Although differing sensitivities and specificities have been obtained across studies, for clinical purposes a score over 5 is suggestive of depression and should warrant a follow-up interview by a licensed health professional. Scores over 10 almost always represent depression.

Persons scoring above 5 depressive answers should have a care plan developed to address specific mood issues.

Adapted from Cheryl Lacy, MA, *Concerns of the Heart* 2000.

THE GERIATRIC HYPOCHONDRIASIS SCALE

Name: _____ DOB: _____ Date: _____

1. Are you satisfied with your health most of the time?   Yes ☐   No ☐
2. Do you ever feel completely well?   Yes ☐   No ☐
3. Are you tired most of the time?   Yes ☐   No ☐
4. Do you feel your best in the morning?   Yes ☐   No ☐
5. Do you frequently have strange aches and pains that you cannot identify?   Yes ☐   No ☐
6. Is it hard for you to believe it when the doctor tells you that there is nothing physically wrong with you?   Yes ☐   No ☐

ADMINISTRATION: These items may be administered in oral or written format, but the former is preferred. The examiner may have to repeat a question in order to get a response that is clearly Yes or No.

SCORING: Count one point for each hypochondriacal answer. In both the institutional and community elder populations, the modal score is 0, the median 1. This test is a measure of hypochondriacal attitudes, rather than hypochondriacal behavior. It is possible for a patient to score high (e.g., 4–6) and yet manifest no somatic complaints. Any patient who has numerous somatic complaints and scores high is probably suffering from delusional illness. Any score under 3 is definitely not hypochondriacal, and so the patient's complaints should be taken seriously.

GERIATRIC DEPRESSION SCALE (LONG FORM)

Name: _____ DOB: _____ Date: _____

1.	Are you basically satisfied with your life?	Yes ☐	No ☐
2.	Have you dropped many of your activities and interests?	Yes ☐	No ☐
3.	Do you feel that your life is empty?	Yes ☐	No ☐
4.	Do you often get bored?	Yes ☐	No ☐
5.	Are you hopeful about the future?	Yes ☐	No ☐
6.	Are you bothered by thoughts that you just cannot get out of your head?	Yes ☐	No ☐
7.	Are you in good spirits most of the time?	Yes ☐	No ☐
8.	Are you afraid that something bad is going to happen to you?	Yes ☐	No ☐
9.	Do you feel happy most of the time?	Yes ☐	No ☐
10.	Do you often feel helpless?	Yes ☐	No ☐
11.	Do you often get restless and fidgety?	Yes ☐	No ☐
12.	Do you prefer to stay home at night, rather than go out and do new things?	Yes ☐	No ☐
13.	Do you frequently worry about the future?	Yes ☐	No ☐
14.	Do you feel that you have more problems with memory than most?	Yes ☐	No ☐
15.	Do you think it is wonderful to be alive now?	Yes ☐	No ☐
16.	Do you often feel downhearted and blue?	Yes ☐	No ☐
17.	Do you feel pretty worthless the way you are now?	Yes ☐	No ☐
18.	Do you worry a lot about the past?	Yes ☐	No ☐
19.	Do you find life very exciting?	Yes ☐	No ☐
20.	Is it hard for you to get started on new projects?	Yes ☐	No ☐
21.	Do you feel full of energy?	Yes ☐	No ☐
22.	Do you feel that your situation is hopeless?	Yes ☐	No ☐
23.	Do you think that most people are better off than you are?	Yes ☐	No ☐
24.	Do you frequently get upset over little things?	Yes ☐	No ☐
25.	Do you frequently feel like crying?	Yes ☐	No ☐
26.	Do you have trouble concentrating?	Yes ☐	No ☐
27.	Do you enjoy getting up in the morning?	Yes ☐	No ☐
28.	Do you prefer to avoid social gatherings?	Yes ☐	No ☐
29.	Is it easy for you to make decisions?	Yes ☐	No ☐
30.	Is your mind as clear as it used to be?	Yes ☐	No ☐

ADMINISTRATION: With frail elders, oral format is preferred. The examiner may have to repeat the question in order to get a response that is clearly a Yes or No. The GDS loses validity as dementia increases. The GDS seems to work well with other age groups, and may be very appropriate for patients with many physical problems.

SCORING: Count 2 point for each depressive answer. 0–10 = normal; 11–20 = mild depression; 21–30 = moderate or severe depression.

ADULT BRAIN SYSTEM CHECKLIST

Name: _____ DOB: _____ Date: _____

Please rate yourself on each of the symptoms listed below using the following scale. If possible, to give us the most complete picture, have another person who knows you well (spouse/family member/care provider/other) rate you as well. List Other: _____

Never (0)   Rarely (1)   Occasionally (2)   Frequently (3)   Very Frequently (4)   Not Applicable/Not Known (N)

Other   Self
_____   _____   1. Fails to give close attention to details or makes careless mistakes
_____   _____   2. Trouble sustaining attention in routine situations (i.e., chores, paperwork)
_____   _____   3. Trouble listening
_____   _____   4. Fails to finish things
_____   _____   5. Poor organization for time or space (such as room, desk, paperwork)
_____   _____   6. Avoids, dislikes, or is reluctant to engage in tasks that require sustained mental effort
_____   _____   7. Loses things
_____   _____   8. Easily distracted
_____   _____   9. Forgetful
_____   _____   10. Poor planning skills
_____   _____   11. Lacks clear goals or forward thinking
_____   _____   12. Difficulty expressing feelings
_____   _____   13. Difficulty expressing empathy for others
_____   _____   14. Excessive daydreaming
_____   _____   15. Feeling bored
_____   _____   16. Feeling apathetic or unmotivated
_____   _____   17. Feeling tired, sluggish or slow-moving
_____   _____   18. Feeling spacey or "in a fog"
                    SUBTOTAL _____
_____   _____   19. Fidgety, restless or trouble sitting still
_____   _____   20. Difficulty remaining seated in situations where remaining seated is expected
_____   _____   21. "On the go" or acts as if "driven by a motor"
_____   _____   22. Talks excessively
_____   _____   23. Blurts out answers before questions have been completed
_____   _____   24. Difficulty awaiting turn
_____   _____   25. Interrupts or intrudes on others (e.g., butts into conversations)
_____   _____   26. Impulsive (saying or doing things without thinking first)
                    SUBTOTAL _____
_____   _____   27. Excessive or senseless worrying
_____   _____   28. Upset when things do not go your way
_____   _____   29. Upset when things are out of place
_____   _____   30. Tendency to be oppositional or argumentative
_____   _____   31. Tendency to have repetitive negative thoughts
_____   _____   32. Tendency toward compulsive behaviors
_____   _____   33. Intense dislike for change
_____   _____   34. Tendency to hold grudges
_____   _____   35. Trouble shifting attention from subject to subject
_____   _____   36. Trouble shifting behavior from task to task
_____   _____   37. Difficulties seeing options in situations
_____   _____   38. Tendency to hold on to own opinion and not listen to others
_____   _____   39. Tendency to get locked into a course of action, whether or not it is good
_____   _____   40. Needing to have things done a certain way or you become very upset

_____ _____ 41. Others complain that you worry too much
_____ _____ 42. Tend to say no without first thinking about question
_____ _____ 43. Tendency to predict fear

SUBTOTAL _____

_____ _____ 44. Frequent feelings of sadness
_____ _____ 45. Moodiness
_____ _____ 46. Negativity
_____ _____ 47. Low energy
_____ _____ 48. Irritability
_____ _____ 49. Decreased interest in others
_____ _____ 50. Decreased interest in things that are usually fun or pleasurable
_____ _____ 51. Feelings of hopelessness about the future
_____ _____ 52. Feelings of helplessness or powerlessness
_____ _____ 53. Feeling dissatisfied or bored
_____ _____ 54. Excessive guilt
_____ _____ 55. Suicidal feelings
_____ _____ 56. Crying spells
_____ _____ 57. Sleep changes (too much or too little)
_____ _____ 58. Appetite changes (too much or too little)
_____ _____ 59. Chronic low self-esteem

SUBTOTAL _____

_____ _____ 60. Negative sensitivity to smells/odors
_____ _____ 61. Frequent feelings of nervousness or anxiety
_____ _____ 62. Panic attacks
_____ _____ 63. Symptoms of heightened muscle tension (headaches, sore muscles, hand tremor)
_____ _____ 64. Periods of heart pounding, rapid heart rate or chest pain
_____ _____ 65. Periods of trouble breathing or feeling smothered
_____ _____ 66. Periods of feeling dizzy, faint or unsteady on your feet
_____ _____ 67. Periods of nausea or abdominal upset
_____ _____ 68. Periods of sweating, hot or cold flashes
_____ _____ 69. Tendency to predict the worst
_____ _____ 70. Fear of dying or doing something crazy
_____ _____ 72. Avoid places for fear of having an anxiety attack
_____ _____ 73. Conflict avoidance
_____ _____ 74. Excessive fear of being judged or scrutinized by others
_____ _____ 75. Persistent phobias
_____ _____ 76. Low motivation
_____ _____ 77. Excessive motivation
_____ _____ 78. Tics (motor or vocal)
_____ _____ 79. Poor handwriting
_____ _____ 80. Quick startle
_____ _____ 81. Tendency to freeze in anxiety-provoking situations
_____ _____ 82. Lack confidence in abilities
_____ _____ 83. Seems shy or timid
_____ _____ 84. Easily embarrassed
_____ _____ 85. Sensitive to criticism

SUBTOTAL _____

_____ _____ 86. Bites fingernails or picks skin
_____ _____ 87. Short fuse or periods of extreme irritability
_____ _____ 88. Periods of rage with little provocation
_____ _____ 89. Often misinterprets comments as negative when they are not
_____ _____ 90. Irritability tends to build, then explodes, then recedes, often tired after a rage
_____ _____ 91. Periods of spaciness or confusion
_____ _____ 92. Periods of panic and/or fear for no specific reason
_____ _____ 93. Visual or auditory changes, such as seeing shadows or hearing muffled sounds
_____ _____ 94. Frequent periods of déjà vu (feelings of being somewhere you have never been)
_____ _____ 95. Sensitivity or mild paranoia
_____ _____ 96. Headaches or abdominal pain of uncertain origin
_____ _____ 97. History of a head injury or family history of violence or explosiveness

Cont.

_____ _____ 98. Dark thoughts, may involve suicidal or homicidal thoughts
_____ _____ 99. Periods of forgetfulness or memory problems
SUBTOTAL _____

SCORING KEY: Attention problems: Items 1–18
                   Hyperactivity and impulsivity: Items 19–26
                   Obsessive-compulsive behaviors: Items 27–43 (Anterior Cingulate Gyrus)
                   Depressive behaviors and disorders: Items 44–59 (Deep Limbic System)
                   Generalized anxiety behaviors and disorders: Items 60–85 (Basal Ganglia)
                   Explosive behaviors and disorders: Items 86–99 (Temporal Lobe)

INTERPRETATION: To obtain a meaningful score, add up the 3 and 4 ratings (all items scored as Frequently and Very Frequently). While there are no specific cutoff points, the higher the Score in each subcategory, the greater the probability the person is having a significant problem needing therapeutic intervention. The Checklist can also be used to assess change or improvement over time, such as after a therapeutic intervention has been attempted.

Adapted with permission from Dr Daniel Amen and Dr Bradley Schuyler, 2009.

THE GRAVELY DISABLED AND THE CARING PROCESS

The gravely disabled individual is unable to provide for their basic necessities of food, clothing, and shelter. The gravely disabled state may be due to:

1. Confusion
2. Hallucinations
3. Delusional thinking
4. Impaired reality testing
5. Psychomotor agitation
6. Lack of motivation
7. Memory impairment
8. Impaired judgment
9. Undersocialization

Some behavioral indicators of being gravely disabled include:

1. Unable to dress self
2. Incontinent (without responsibly dealing with it)
3. Not eating/drinking
4. Deterioration of hygiene
5. Inability to maintain medical regime
6. Unable to provide residence for self

TREATMENT FOCUS AND OBJECTIVES

1. Inadequate hygiene (Teach basic hygiene and activities of daily living [ADL])
   A. Person to seek assistance with bowel/bladder function
   B. Person will bathe/shower on their own
   C. Person will brush teeth, comb hair, shave, and dress appropriately daily
2. Uncooperative
   A. Person will be able to verbalize/demonstrate acceptance of daily assistance
   B. Person will comply with medication/medical regimen
   C. Person will accept assistance with living arrangement
   D. Person will accept long-term assistance
3. Inadequate nutrition/fluids
   A. Person will drink an adequate intake of fluids to maintain hydration
   B. Person will eat a balanced diet
4. Family nonsupportive or lacks understanding intervention
   A. Family education regarding person's prognosis and necessary support/structure
   B. Community support group

Therapist's Guide to Clinical Intervention, Second Edition by Sharon L. Johnson (© 2003 Elsevier Inc.)

5. Inadequate coping
    A. Consequences of noncompliance with medication
    B. Self-care management
    C. Facilitate problem solving and conflict resolution for practical situations that the person is likely to encounter
    D. Facilitate development of adequate social skills
        1. provide opportunities for social interaction
        2. model and role play appropriate social behaviors
    E. Facilitate development of management of anger and frustration
    F. Teach relaxation training
    G. Identify leisure skills
6. Improve inability to manage and improve judgment
    A. Evaluate for conservatorship
7. Inadequate/inappropriate living arrangement
    A. Consider placement
        1. Board and care facility
        2. Planned senior citizen community with therapeutic and medical care
            a. must ask permission of spouse for participation in appropriate adult activities
            b. social isolation
            c. reluctance of a spouse (offender) to allow spouse to be seen alone
            d. history of child abuse
            e. behavior problems in childhood

Successful Aging

Section Contents

AGING WITH RESILIENCY AND LONGEVITY

Everyone admires the centenarian. Living to a 100 is a remarkable feat. We all wonder how it is done by those who have achieved such a status in life. While longevity catches our attention, more important is longevity with resiliency. Even more we appreciate and admire the person who lives a 100 years and has a positive quality of life and a behavioral pattern of activity, engagement, and positive interaction. Resiliency is essentially the resistance to stress, disappointment, and the sting of defeat.

In a recent research study by M. Pipher and the aging and longevity research study conducted at Boston University, the following characteristics were associated with resiliency and longevity. The following characteristics were identified in these two research studies as being the primary factors in people who live a resilient lifestyle and had a life pattern of longevity. These identified individuals were known for the following:

1. Carried on in spite of personal losses.
2. Discovered pleasure in small moments of time and events.
3. Discovered that acceptance and gratitude were the keys to a good life.
4. Balanced sorrow with humor.
5. Had reasonable expectations.
6. Assumed responsibility for their lives.
7. Worked hard and has a sense or pride and accomplishment.
8. Played hard in their leisure time activities.
9. Minded their own business.
10. Responded to suffering with compassion rather than with anger and despair.
11. Had a strong personal and spiritual belief system that was very personal to them.
12. Clear about who they truly were … and were known for speaking out truthfully.
13. Unwilling to jeopardize and lose their own sense of personal dignity.
14. Had a sense of being connected to something meaningful in their life.
15. Known for their ability to lose weight, if needed.
16. Got adequate sleep.
17. Ate 5 servings of fruit and vegetables daily.
18. Used a seat belt.
19. Kept caffeine use below 250 mg and did not consume coffee after noon (250 mg equals two 6 oz cups of coffee, 50 6 oz cups of decaff; or seven 6 oz cups of cocoa and five 6 oz cups of tea).
20. Used vitamin supplements such as calcium, foliate, and vitamin E.
21. Flossed their teeth.
22. Consumed moderate amounts of alcohol, if they consumed alcohol at all.
23. Took a small aspirin daily.
24. Avoided falls and other forms of physical injury.

While the above list of items may characterize people who live a resilient and long life, there is no guarantee that any one or any combination of these items will produce a similar result for any particular person. The list, however, is offered as a guideline for living a generally healthy life.

LIVE TO 100 YEARS OF AGE GRACEFULLY AND SUCCESSFULLY

THE CENTENARIAN GENERATION

- There are estimated to be 70,000 centenarian elders now living, and their numbers are growing. They are 8:1 females to males; 50% live independently.
- There are 300 "super-centenarians" now living, people 110 years of age or more.
- The oldest known person, Frenchwoman Jeanne Calment, died in the 1997, aged 122.
- Life spectrum from birth to death is strongly influenced by our historic life style.

THE CENTENARIAN RECIPE

- Keep blood sugar levels low
- Keep blood pressure low, normal range
- Keep cholesterol level low
- No smoking, or stop if you do
- No alcohol, or drink little if you do
- Keep weight low and steady
- Keep calories moderate, between 1500 and 2000
- Eat extra amounts of fruits, vegetables, nuts, beans, fish, chicken, and whole grains
- Take multi-vitamins, A, C, E, and B complex; aspirin (81 mg) or low mg ibuprofen
- Exercise regularly, especially coordination exercises as in dance, knitting, biking
- Sleep well for 6–7 hours
- Challenge your mind daily with mind exercises
- Protect the brain from injury
- Keep a positive social calendar
- Clean your teeth and floss regularly
- No chronic stress; develop a "Teflon personality"
- Maintain a positive attitude and be optimistic
- Keep a diet high on antioxidants, omega-3 fatty acids (or wild fish), and folic acid
- Read widely, learn new information
- Seek consultation about the use of cholinesterase inhibitors such as Aricept, Namanda, anti-depressants, etc.

THE CENTENARIAN SUPPORT SYSTEM

- Physician(s)
- Psychologist
- Nutritionist
- Family and extended family
- Network of friendships
- Dentist
- CPA
- Lawyer
- Financial Planner, insurance agent, stock broker
- Mortician
- Minister/Priest/Rabbi/Leader of your Faith
- Others as needed

TIPS FOR RETIRING SENIORS (BOOMERS)

The primary question to discuss with a retiring senior is not financial adequacy, but how they want to live the rest of their lives. The time to think of this question is 5–8 years before the actual retirement time. Here are a few tips to make the process go well.

1. Keep your mind sharp by replacing the stimulation of work with social and intellectual activities.
2. Retirement is to be a shared experience with your spouse and family, both during the planning phase as well as the activation phase.
3. A purpose is to be sought and claimed prior to retirement with a plan on how to live it out in day-to-day experiences.
4. Live out a life plan based on your purpose during retirement.
5. Know that there is more to life than money and plan ahead for financial stability.
6. Financial stability is to be planned for and lived out in confidence.
7. Maintaining a healthy lifestyle is basic to productive living.
8. Volunteer to be of help to those in need and use it as an opportunity to meet someone.
9. Keep on meeting and getting to know new people from whom you can learn new ideas and have new experiences.
10. Consult others on how to make retirement the most wonderful time of your life.

MY RETIREMENT PORTFOLIO

To assess the breadth and meaningfulness of your retirement lifestyle, please indicate in each of the 10 ACTIVITY AREAS noted below the number of hours you devote to each activity area in a typical 40–50 hour week. For example, if you devote 6 hours to social involvement in a typical week put a check mark in the 6–10 hour designation. Consider what your typical time allocation is per week. Your total hours should approximate 40–50 hours in any given week. This could vary over time, but take your average hours per week. You need not put a mark in each ACTIVITY AREA, just the ones representing how and where you spend your time during a typical week.

ACTIVITY AREA   **ACTIVITY EXAMPLES**

Part-Time Work   Consulting – Continue in former job – New job – Odd jobs

1–6 hrs _____   7–12 hrs _____   13–18 hrs _____   19–24 hrs _____   25–30 hrs _____   31–36 hrs _____   37+ hrs _____

Family and Marriage   Family events – Grandchildren play – Dinner together

1–6 hrs _____   7–12 hrs _____   13–18 hrs _____   19–24 hrs _____   25–30 hrs _____   31–36 hrs _____   37+ hrs _____

Hobbies   Woodworking – Antiques – Crafts – Art – Gardening – Music

1–6 hrs _____   7–12 hrs _____   13–18 hrs _____   19–24 hrs _____   25–30 hrs _____   31–36 hrs _____   37+ hrs _____

Travel and Sightseeing   Cruises – International travel – Car trips – RV trips

1–6 hrs _____   7–12 hrs _____   13–18 hrs _____   19–24 hrs _____   25–30 hrs _____   31–36 hrs _____   37+ hrs _____

Cognitive Enrichment   Elderhostel classes – Lectures – Concerts – Reading

1–6 hrs _____   7–12 hrs _____   13–18 hrs _____   19–24 hrs _____   25–30 hrs _____   31–36 hrs _____   37+ hrs _____

Social Involvement   Visit friends – Club participation – Take friend to a game

1–6 hrs _____   7–12 hrs _____   13–18 hrs _____   19–24 hrs _____   25–30 hrs _____   31–36 hrs _____   37+ hrs _____

Religious Involvement   Church – Bible reading, prayer – Meditation – Bible study

1–6 hrs _____   7–12 hrs _____   13–18 hrs _____   19–24 hrs _____   25–30 hrs _____   31–36 hrs _____   37+ hrs _____

Volunteer Service   Hospitals – Clubs – Organizations – Church – Schools

1–6 hrs _____   7–12 hrs _____   13–18 hrs _____   19–24 hrs _____   25–30 hrs _____   31–36 hrs _____   37+ hrs _____

Health Maintenance   Jogging – Spa – Gym – Health classes, walks – Lectures

1–6 hrs _____   7–12 hrs _____   13–18 hrs _____   19–24 hrs _____   25–30 hrs _____   31–36 hrs _____   37+ hrs _____

Communicating Ideas   Letters – Phone calls – Visits – e-mailing – Letter to Editor

1–6 hrs _____   7–12 hrs _____   13–18 hrs _____   19–24 hrs _____   25–30 hrs _____   31–36 hrs _____   37+ hrs _____

NOTE: Review your profile and plan to make adjustments where needed to balance your lifestyle and maximize a meaningful pattern of living from day to day throughout your retirement years.

THE LONG PATHWAY OF AGING

The aging process involves a long and arduous journey on a pathway with many pot holes and unknowns. The journey takes some through the valley of death. Life is lived in the shadows of loneliness for others. The depths of depression and anxiety are an ever-present experience for most. Thankfully, for others, the pathway is relatively positive with many scenic points of interest, stimulation, encouragement, and support. The following guidelines may be helpful in relating to and helping an aging patient population in their journey during the last one or two decades of their life.

1. **Focus efforts on connectedness.** It is important that an aging individual remain connected with the people, things, places, and memories of their past. These are all subjects of good discussion. Efforts to re-involve a person with some aspects of their historical experience can be a source of strength and encouragement.

2. **Listen to their stories of loss and grief.** Do not feel sorry for what has happened in their past. It is important that the aging person has opportunity to share losses and grief experiences. Listen, support, express compassion, and be empathetic.

3. **Know that there is an open door for asking questions.** Older people love to talk about themselves and their experiences. Feel free to ask specific questions. Inquire. Ask what you can do to ease the stressful circumstances under which they currently live.

4. **It is acceptable to ask about their deceased spouse, children, family members, and friends.** Be sensitive to the feelings of distress and do not prolong the discussion unless the patient takes the lead and carries the discussion further.

5. **Invite the patient to engage in an activity with you.** It is acceptable to invite and nudge a patient into an activity that helps them connect with others and decreases their loneliness. They may not accept initially. Pursue it over time as they may accept your invitation eventually.

6. **Accept where they are at this point in life.** Some may have had a lifetime of dysfunctional relationships, pain, hurt, and trauma. Others may have had a lifetime of support, encouragement, and positive regard. Patterns may be set in how they handle events and situations and people.

7. **Let them know you have been thinking about them.** We all love to hear that we are in the thoughts of people who love us and are part of our world. It is even better to go beyond and specify what thoughts had been brought to your attention and what these thoughts mean to you.

8. **Do something special together.** If the options are few at least go for a walk, a drive or undertake a small errand together. Undertake an activity within a reasonable period of time. It is not how big or expensive an activity is but that the activity was undertaken.

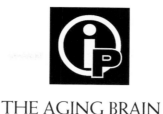

THE AGING BRAIN

Your brain is the most important and vulnerable organ of your entire body. It is like pewter, beautiful to behold, but easy to damage. The health of your brain is dependent on you to care for it, respect it, develop it, and use it wisely. Your brain was a gift to you, and you in turn may give it back as a gift to your world.

Your brain is to be appreciated. As we come together to study we can better understand and appreciate our brain. In so doing, we will also come to appreciate the entire creation process and the significance of who and what you are and for what purpose you have come to this point in your life.

Your brain is unique. Your individual approach to life is facilitated by your brain's capabilities and limitations. The unique history of experiences of your brain plays a major role in determining your future experiences in life and how you will interact with those that come into your daily world of life experiences.

Your brain is aging. You have control over the rate and nature of the changes taking place now and in the years to come. Your degree of control depends on your understanding brain structures and functions. Even a partial improvement in how you use your brain's power will yield a similar corresponding improvement in your productivity, learning and creativity.

Your brain needs to be kept healthy. To help your brain become healthy and maintain a healthy pattern of functioning, it needs the following nine events and activities on a regular bases. Then the brain will drive the body and mind functions and help you live effectively and efficiently. They are:

1. Nourishment from foods high in oxidants.
2. Protection from trauma and injury.
3. Engagement in meaningful and challenging tasks.
4. Reduced level of stress.
5. Resolution of problems before they become chronic.
6. Engagement in exercise and graduated activity.
7. Proper and needed medication and nutritional supplements.
8. Regular exposure to ideas and new information.
9. Maintain a positive pace of life without notable slowing down with age.

GUIDELINES FOR HEALTHY AND EFFECTIVE FAMILY VISITATION

Family visitation is a vitally important aspect of patient care in a skilled nursing facility. Whenever a person undergoes major life changes their family and long-term support network means much to them. The level of support provided by family and friends significantly contributes to the patient's personal adjustment and the degree to which the patient's health improves or stabilizes.

Placement in a long-term care facility such as a skilled nursing facility or an assisted living program is a major life event for all elderly people. There is a stigma associated with a skilled nursing facility which has to be addressed. There is restriction of lifestyle. There is increased loneliness and isolation. There is a fear of abandonment and being forgotten which has to be overcome. Having to face a strange environment is also a difficult issue to address alone.

The family network is the most important support system for the patient. This includes the spouse, children, grandchildren, great-grandchildren as well as other extended family members. Every patient has a historical relationship pattern of feeling closer with some family members than others. While this is not right or wrong, good or bad, it is something the family must recognize and accept. This relationship pattern is important to utilize at such critical times as making major healthcare decisions and future living arrangements.

Further, an elderly person will more likely be cooperative and participate in the decision making process when the person or persons whom they most trust guides them in their decision-making. Other family members need to play a support role and be a source of ongoing encouragement. It is important to understand that elderly people have a deep sense of love, care, and compassion for their entire family. However, there is often a greater sense of trust and confidence with certain family members. It is important for the family to recognize the fact of this special relationship and not be offended.

The following guidelines are designed to help a family know how best to utilize their time and the effort put forth to support their elderly family member who has recently become a resident of a skilled nursing facility, assisted living home, board and care home or another type of convalescent environment:

1. **Consult with nursing staff.** Be sure to understand and clarify expectations, policies, and regulations of the facility by consulting with the nursing staff. This should be done early upon admission. Every facility has certain regulations and procedures designed to facilitate healthy care, rehabilitation, and recovery throughout the patient's stay in the facility. The nursing staff can be very helpful in facilitating healthy family relationships during visitation.

2. **Brief visits are better.** Generally speaking, patients prefer brief family visits and find them more helpful than long visits. It is better to have two visits of 1 hour each or four visits of 30 minutes than one visit of 2–3 hours in length. Long daily visits may not be healthy for the patient nor for the visiting family member.

3. **Arrange prime time visits.** Quality visits can be experienced if they take place during the patient's prime hours. During certain time periods of a day, a patient may become restless, agitated or irritable. Therapy sessions are usually scheduled each day. These are not the times to visit. Better, visit at times when patients are more relaxed, rested, and more likely to be free to socialize. Select the time of the day for a visit and the duration of the visit thoughtfully and for optimum benefit. Visit accordingly.

4. **Be a positive helper.** All visits must coordinate with and advance the goals of the patient's care and treatment plan. Consider how you can help the goals being achieved.

5. **Create a change in routine.** Family visits can provide a change in the daily routine for the patient. Bringing a special or preferred food, going for a stroll, eating in a different location, and visiting in a different location in the hospital are a few examples of ways to change routine. When changing the routine, be careful to coordinate with the staff.

6. **Bring the home to the patient.** Hospitals can be very impersonal and less than homey. Bring a little of the home to the patient such as a preferred pillow, a meaningful quilt or blanket, a special knick-knack, a warm sweater or the patient's personal robe or pajamas.

7. **Help memory restoration.** When there has been evidence of memory loss, confusion or disorientation, bring photographs to review together and discuss. Remember, a picture can be more than a thousand words. Photos can bring back old memories of meaningful experiences.

8. **Praise and commend healthy and progressive behavior.** Focus on healthy talk and activity rather than discuss how the patient feels today. Praise what the patient has done recently and will be doing later in the day or tomorrow. Encourage and praise self-help behavior.

9. **Downplay pain, food, noise, and other unproductive complaining.** Be alert for positive statements and behavior to commend and encourage. Ignore or discourage complaining talk. Should you have cause for concern, tell the staff.

10. **Communicate firmly and clearly.** Support and encourage the patient to participate fully in their care plan. The patient needs to know that you as a family support the treatment plan and expect the patient to participate fully in all services rendered, such as physical, occupational, and speech therapy.

Dementia and Alzheimer's Disease

Section Contents

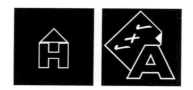

DEMENTIA AND ALZHEIMER'S TESTS

How do doctors distinguish dementia from the mental wear and tear of normal aging? Here are two tests you can give to a loved one. If the scores indicate dementia, a doctor should be consulted immediately for a full clinical exam.

PART A: ORIENTATION, MEMORY, AND CONCENTRATION TEST

INSTRUCTIONS: Score 1 point for each wrong answer, up to the maximum. Multiple the number of mistakes by the weight. Then add to get the final score.

QUESTIONS	Max no. of errors	×Weighting =	Score
1. What year is it now?	1	×4 =	_____
2. What month is it now?	1	×3 =	_____
3. Repeat this memory phrase after me: John Brown, 42 Market Street, Chicago			
4. About what time is it? (within 1 hour)	1	×3 =	_____
5. Count backwards 20 to 1.	2	×2 =	_____
6. Say the months in reverse order.	2	×2 =	_____
7. Repeat the memory phrase again.	5	×2 =	_____
		TOTAL	_____

Total score can range from 0 (no mistakes) to 28 (all wrong). A score **greater than 10** is usually consistent with dementia.

PART B: DAILY-ACTIVITIES AND SOCIAL-INDEPENDENCE TEST

EXPLANATION: This test measures how functionally dependent on others someone has become. The higher the number, the more dependent.

HOW TO SCORE: Select the answer that best describes the current situation and give the following number values:

3 points Dependent
2 points Requires assistance
1 point Does (or could do) by self but with difficulty
0 points Does (or could do) with no difficulty

SELF-HELP ACTIVITIES

	Score
1. Writing checks, paying bills, balancing checkbook	_____
2. Assembling tax records or papers, handling business affairs	_____
3. Shopping alone for clothes, household necessities or groceries	_____
4. Playing game or skill, working on hobby	_____
5. Heating water, making cup of coffee, turning off stove	_____
6. Preparing a balanced meal	_____
7. Keeping track of current events	_____
8. Paying attention to, understanding, discussing TV, book, magazine	_____
9. Remembering appointments, family occasions, holidays, medications	_____
10. Traveling out of neighborhood, driving, arranging to take bus	_____

Total score ranges from 0 (totally independent) to 30 (totally dependent). A score **higher than 9** usually indicates dementia.

Adapted from the Gerontological Society of America.

INFORMAL TESTS OF MEMORY

THE 10-WORD TEST OF MEMORY

As an informal test to assess a person's short-term auditory memory, present the following list of 10 words. After a brief delay of 10 seconds, ask that the words be recalled independent of the order in which they were originally presented. A person's memory would be considered good to excellent if at least 8 words are recalled. A person's memory would be considered fairly good if only 4–6 words are recalled. A person's memory would be considered troublesome if less than 4 items are recalled. The lower the score, the more a person's memory needs to be considered as part of the diagnostic profile and addressed as part of a treatment or care plan. Present the following 10 words, one (1) second per word:

Car	Red	Face	Grass	Scissors
Pawn	Shoe	Hand	Sky	Cup

THE 10-PICTURE TEST OF MEMORY

In addition to assessing the auditory linguistic memory, take the opportunity to assess the individual's visual memory. Perform this test using pictures of items in the same way as you did above with the words. Find 10 pictures of common items in magazines and cut them out. Paste them on a 3 × 5 card so they can be easily presented to the patient.

Present 10 pictures of items or objects, each card presented to the patient one (1) second at a time. Ask for the recall of the 10 items after a few seconds have elapsed. Score the results as was done above with words. Score the number correct.

THE 10-NUMBERS TEST OF MEMORY:

As done with words and pictures, now do with numbers. Perform the test by presenting a random list of 10 numbers as was done with words and pictures. Score the number correct as was done above. The following numbers should be presented:

7	3	5	9	12
2	8	6	1	4

NOTE: If you would like to assess delayed recall, after at least 5 minutes has passed, ask the patient to repeat as best they can the list of words, pictures, or numbers, or any combination thereof. The best way to do it is to have an immediate and a delayed recall of the words, pictures, and numbers presented with a 5-minute delay. This system will not only measure the strength of memory but also the type of memory system operating in three different areas of the brain.

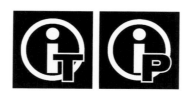

SIGNS OF ALZHEIMER'S AND ITS MANAGEMENT

SIGNS OF ALZHEIMER'S

1. Forgetting simple things more often than 6 months ago.
2. Beginning to have trouble doing simple and familiar things.
3. Putting things in odd and strange places.
4. Forgetting of common words, phrases, and even using the wrong words.
5. Having trouble and problems with complicated, yet familiar tasks and duties.
6. Beginning to experience a major change in personality.
7. Forgetting what day it is, what time it is, and where they are at any given time.
8. Losing interest in activities and people or showing a rapid loss of interest.
9. Beginning to have a sudden loss of focus or sudden changes in mood or behavior.
10. Acting in a manner that does not make any sense at all.
11. Demonstrating poor judgment in dress, personal care, and use of objects.
12. Beginning to act in a passive and unconnected manner with others and events.
13. Thinking in abstract terms is now difficult.

ACTIONS TO TAKE TO FORESTALL THE ONSET OF ALZHEIMER'S

1. Utilize one of the cholinesterase inhibitors, such as Aricept, Namanda, Excelon.
2. Stimulate the brain with thinking activities, such as crossword puzzles.
3. Maintain a physical activity level.
4. Avoid all of the addictive behaviors.
5. Protect the brain from trauma, injuries, and from chronic hurt or pain.
6. Keep a social involvement that provides stimulation and new ideas.
7. Simplify life into small sub-tasks so that success can be experienced.
8. Engage the memory in various recall and recognition activities.
9. Eat food good for the heart and brain, such as food rich in antioxidants.
10. Live a healthy life so that all the vital signs are well within the normal range.

PRECAUTIONS FOR CARE PROVIDERS

1. Live in the present, as one day can be quite different from the next.
2. Engage in relaxation exercises and activities.
3. Exercise and get plenty of activities that break the routine.
4. Manage your day by doing things in an organized and routine manner.
5. Keep in regular contact with friends and people that make you laugh and think.
6. Set daily goals and expectations that are reasonable and within your grasp.
7. Keep a daily journal and share your experiences with others.
8. Eat right and get adequate sleep.
9. Read on Alzheimer's and become an expert on the topic.

10. Engage in meditation, prayer, and time of reflection to keep a positive attitude.
11. Reset your expectations for yourself, others, and the Alzheimer's patient.
12. The use of an antidepressant may be helpful to you later in the process.
13. Don't do everything yourself, ask for help and delegate.
14. Give instructions in a simple format, use visualization strategies.
15. Be positive and use much praise, affirmation, and appreciation statements.
16. Be sure the patient is attending and listening when you are addressing them.
17. Build a strong and helpful social support system for yourself and the patient.
18. Learn to be assertive and overtly communicative.
19. Talk about the Alzheimer's patient when he/she is not present and cannot hear.
20. Speak to the Alzheimer's patient in a slow and low tone of voice.

A FEW MEASURES OF ALZHEIMER'S AND WAYS TO CHART ITS PROGRESSION:

1. Draw a key.
2. Draw a clock with the hands at ten minutes after eleven o'clock.
3. Ask the patient to write out a complete sentence.
4. Ask for a word or two to be spelled backwards, such as Watch, Grass or Window.
5. Draw a simple design; ask for it to be reproduced. Follow with a complex design.

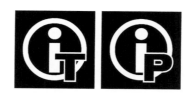

KEY SIGNS OF ALZHEIMER'S

A Step Beyond Dementia

What to notice so early action can be taken:

1. *Memory problems, especially of newly acquired information.* As the dementia increases, even former information is forgotten or difficult to recall without a prompt from someone.
2. *Complex tasks that require several problem solving steps and planning ahead.* Such tasks require more time, more concentration, and are usually troublesome, with mistakes being common.
3. *Poor judgment and decision making.* They are vulnerable in dealing with those that put pressure on them for a decision, give money, sign a document, or make a donation to some cause. They also use poor judgment in dress, appearance, and personal care habits.
4. *Misplacing personal things, putting things in unusual places, and accusing others of stealing their belongings.* As the dementia progresses, these behaviors are more common. False accusations and paranoia become increasingly common in the later stages of the disease.
5. *Perception is gone astray with much confusion and disorientation.* Reading, judging distance, determining color and mirror images are more difficult and perplexing. Seeing themselves in a mirror may give the impression that someone else is in the room.
6. *Time, date, and place are more difficult to keep track of and act in a timely manner.* They may only be able to follow something if it is happening now. Delay is not possible to process.
7. *Conversation is almost impossible to follow and enter into.* They tend to get lost and confused about the flow of ideas. Finding the right word or name of an object or person is often difficult.
8. *Daily tasks and routines become difficult and frustrating.* Even walking to a familiar location or paying routine bills become unmanageable.
9. *Mood and personality changes are noticeable.* The most likely changes are depression, anxiety, fear, paranoia, irritability, sadness, and tiredness. Intolerance for new environments, new people, and new experiences are also notable.
10. *Social isolation and withdrawal is preferred over social engagement.* They do not engage in social events very well and can't keep pace, so may prefer to avoid and isolate from others and from previously enjoyed activities.

Simple tasks to assess a person's current cognitive functioning:

1. Ask the person to draw a key, a car, or a clock with the time being ten minutes after eleven o'clock.
2. Give a series of words, numbers or letters and ask the person to repeat them right after you say them. Then gradually increase the length of the list.
3. Ask the person to tell a story using 3, 4 or 5 key items or words in the story.

Action steps:

1. Bring these observations and results to the patient's physician and psychologist for review and intervention using medication and self management strategies.
2. Consider the use of one of the phosphatidylserine supplements.
3. Utilize local professional resources and programs and read on the topic for ideas.
4. Get a case management and care plan together to follow in the home and in the community.

Truisms to be reconsidered:

1. What is good advice for the heart is also good advice for the brain. Treat your heart well and you will also be treating your brain well.
2. Good sleep is essential for clear thinking and processing of information.
3. Exercise your brain with mental activities as you would exercise your body.
4. Eat brain food, berries, walnuts, fish, and avocados, and not fast foods or a lot of diet sodas or caffeine based foods.
5. Fish oil and a good multi-vitamin are good supplements to build and maintain the brain.

Myths to be dispelled:

1. There is no cure for Alzheimer's and thus no treatment to offer.
2. Current treatment does not reverse the progressive memory loss, so why treat?
3. We just have to accept and tolerate the general decline in cognitive skills.
4. It is best not to know one has Alzheimer's; the less known the better.
5. The only basis of Alzheimer's is genetic or exposure to toxic chemicals.
6. Alzheimer's only affects those older than 80 years of age.
7. Early detection allows Alzheimer's to be reversed and effectively treated.
8. Alzheimer's cannot be fully diagnosed until death and only then with an autopsy.

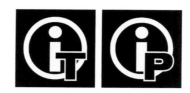

A COGNITIVE FRIENDLY UNIT FOR ALZHEIMER'S PATIENTS

Alzheimer's patients display a series of symptomatic behavior patterns that are best managed in a specialized unit with trained and experienced staff. A compassionate, supportive, and encouraging staff is also essential.

As Alzheimer's patients are very reactive to environmental stress and change, they are best managed in an environment that has an ambience conducive to calmness, quietness, relaxation, and stress reduction. Routine, regularity, and a slow pace is also needed for effective living. The goal of treatment is to preserve independence, foster meaningful relationships, and delay the advancement of the Alzheimer's process.

The following 10 components make up a positive living atmosphere conducive to the management of Alzheimer's patients with their associated impaired cognition and disturbed behavioral patterns:

1. Food served rich in antioxidants, such as multiple vegetables, fish, berries, and other such food known to enrich brain functioning.

2. Regular medication monitoring to assure that medications utilized are effective and that any risk is outweighed by the benefits.

3. A full and systematic activity program designed to stimulate brain functions and cognitive processing of information.

4. A physical activity program designed to foster daily light to moderate physical exercise, including but not limited to, walking, stretching, lifting, and cross-body coordination movements and simple reactive tasks.

5. A socialization program designed to foster social interaction, friendship building, and interpersonal support.

6. A mealtime environment that is quiet, relaxed, unhurried, and free of unrelated noise.

7. A night-time environment that facilitates sleeping. Daytime napping limited to 1 hour once or twice daily.

8. Daytime seating areas for relaxation and quietness which also provide bright light exposure during the day.

9. A unit ambiance with soft but distinct colors clearly demarcating separate living and activity areas within the unit, as well as individual rooms.

10. A systematic professional development training program for the staff of no less than 20 hours annually. Training should focus on the understanding of brain functions, conflict resolution, as well as behavioral engineering and management.

Caregivers and Caregiving

Section Contents

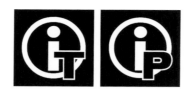

ADVANTAGES AND BENEFITS IN SERVING OLDER PEOPLE

Serving the elderly is a privilege. It is the honorable thing to do. It is the right thing to do.

We live in a world that is self-centered, self-absorbed, and narcissistic. We have been taught to look out for our self first and foremost. We have been taught to live in a self-protective and defensive mode. We have been taught the philosophy, "get the other person first before he gets you."

Servanthood is a vocabulary word we seemed to have erased from the dictionary. We certainly have erased it from our speaking dictionary. Yet, servanthood is what makes a person great. It makes a family great. It makes a country great. Why serve others, especially those who are elderly?

1. Serving gives life a new perspective

The older you are the more life seems to move at a snail's pace. The younger you are the more life seems to move like a rapid heart rate. A perspective of time comes from serving the elderly of our country, our family, and our heritage. Perspective allows us to project what life will be like 50 years in the future. What will we accomplish in the next 50 years in comparison to what we have accomplished in the past 50 years? We ask, "How will I contribute to the changes that will be occurring in the future?" A positive perspective of time promotes wonder, creative thinking, and hope.

2. Serving provides opportunity to develop special relationships

Serving brings people together. Serving bonds people together. Serving allows people to become more intimate and personal with each other than otherwise would be the case. Serving allows for time to be devoted to getting to know each other, learning from each other, and growing into a personal, deeper, and meaningful relationship. Such relationships provide strength and personal well-being for both the one who serves and the one who is served.

3. Serving provides opportunity to learn about history

History is learned from the textbooks, to be sure. However, the historical perspective of life through the eyes of a family member and close friend is priceless. Taking time to be of service to the elderly provides opportunity to sit at the feet of one who has lived a historical journey.

4. Serving teaches the importance of being flexible

Flexibility is a key trait of maturity and personal effectiveness. Flexibility is a key trait for all relationships to flourish. Older people are slow. They have their routines. They change their mind and their moods. They often make unreasonable demands on others. All this requires flexibility in providing care and serving the elderly. As a person learns to be flexible, he/she is in a stronger position to cope with any life event and unusual life circumstances in the future.

5. Serving puts faithfulness and persistence to a test

The path of least resistance is to quit. Giving up when the going gets tough is all too common. No one has ever said that serving others is a cake walk. Serving requires faithful, persistent, and determined effort. Doing the right thing when no one else is paying attention is a mark of integrity. People of integrity faithfully and persistently serve to meet the needs of dependent elderly persons. To achieve this purpose and bring meaning to the life of the entire family, faithful and persistent service is required.

6. Serving provides personal satisfaction in return for helping the helpless

There is no greater satisfaction than to know that your efforts have made a difference in the life of someone else, particularly one who is a helpless person. Feelings of satisfaction generate a corresponding sense of contentment and peace. Serving others gives a sense of empowerment and being a resource of strength for someone else. Hearing words of appreciation and gratitude is the beginning point for feelings of personal satisfaction. For a caregiver, the words, "thank you," are golden.

7. Serving teaches the essence of compassionate caregiving

Life experiences teach character and skill development. Serving others, particularly the elderly, is a primary life experience in which the character trait of compassion is learned. It is out of our sense of compassion for others that effective and positive caregiving comes forth. As we learn to be compassionate, we are sensitive to and desire to serve the needs of others. Serving others is not just the act of giving or providing a benefit for someone else. It is, indeed, one primary way we learn about ourselves to develop new character traits and become a much better and caring person. It is through the act of serving others that we become a person of quality and a person others respect and admire.

8. Serving prevents selfishness from being a prevailing attitude

Serving other people creates a sense of caring and compassion as well as an attitude of humility. Serving others prevents selfishness from prevailing as a general attitude. It is a contradiction to provide a compassionate service to someone while at the same time being self-centered and selfish. It can't be done. Wholesome living is when we live with a sense of balance and harmony between how we behave and how we think and feel

9. Serving allows opportunity to give back to a generation that has given much

Older people know how to give. Indeed, they have given. They have given to their family, to their community, to their churches and charity, to their clubs and organizations and to the general society. They gave without demanding a return on their investment. Serving this population is a small token of appreciation for all they have given. As one gives to someone who has given, we experience the adage, "what goes around, comes around." Tit for tat or reciprocation is an important element in all relationships. We learn this attitude in serving the elderly. We are then in a stronger position to act that way towards others in all arenas of life. Serving is an example of wholesome living.

10. Serving symbolizes the appreciation for what senior citizens have contributed

Older people have contributed much to their family and community. By giving of their time, they have given the best to their children, to their grandchildren, their great-grandchildren, and their friends. Nothing could be a greater contribution to another individual than to share time with them. Likewise, the older people have given of themselves in wisdom in the decision making process while guiding those younger than themselves. The older generation has given money to churches, charities, foundations, and a variety of entities to provide help to the younger generation through scholarships, grants, rehabilitation services, and countless learning and personal growth experiences. Our appreciation is expressed by providing a needed service to an older person who now has a similar need as they graciously provided others who were in need over the years.

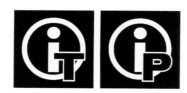

MAKING THE CARETAKING EXPERIENCE REWARDING

More than 22 million American households are involved in an act of caring for an ill, aged, or disabled family member. Caregiving is an intentional act where time and energy is given for the purpose of meeting the needs of a loved one. They are often involved in around the clock, after work, and weekend duty. While the rewards of caregiving are many, caregivers often find themselves facing physical, emotional and financial difficulties due to taking on the caregiving role in the family.

Caregiving is one phase in the long process of convalescence and aging. Home care is provided at a strategic time in the life of a loved one. There comes a time when caregiving in the home needs to give way to one of the alternative care placement facilities available in the community.

Too often, caregivers carry out their role of caregiving in a self-defeating and self-destructive manner. This need not be the case. Caretaking can be an experience that can be pleasant and satisfying for the caregiver as well as the care receiver. It takes teamwork to accomplish this, however. It takes a positive approach. It takes a long-term perspective. The following guidelines can turn the tables on a negative care taking situation and provide the caregiver with a meaningful and rewarding experience.

1. **Accept the diagnosis that has been professionally offered.** Maintain a realistic and positive expectation consistent with the future progress of the diagnosed condition. If further understanding is desired, ask the Attending Physician and professional staff.

2. **Be glad your loved one is still with you.** Enjoy each day you are able to continue to have a relationship with your loved one. Find ways to make each day meaningful for the entire family.

3. **Maintain your own support system.** We all benefit from a support system and the cheerleaders in our life. As you provide help, and care for your loved one, maintain a relationship with the people in your life who provide you with support and encouragement. Don't go it alone.

4. **Be at peace and be anxious for nothing.** The future course of your loved one does not totally depend on you. The course of any disease or disabling condition requires the involvement of a variety of caregiving resources. Utilize them cheerfully and thankfully. Ask for help, as needed.

5. **Know your own limitations.** Caregiving is usually a long-term commitment. Working night and day does not benefit anyone. Pace yourself. Conserve energy. Be sure you have the energy needed at the end states of a disabling condition and not just during the early stages. Let others help develop a teamwork approach.

6. **Sleep well.** The extra stress and strain requires rest and a healthy sleep pattern. Remember, in the middle of the night little can be accomplished. A mid-afternoon power nap can be very beneficial. Using an alarm system in the home provides extra security to allow for sound and restful sleep.

7. **Keep your emotions healthy.** Talk out and express your emotional feelings and experiences with those close to you. Take stress breaks, particularly when you feel the onset of irritability, agitation, and general restlessness. Confront and resolve conflicts and differences. The emotions of the caregiver are just as important as the emotions of the person being cared for by the family.

8. **Think straight and concentrate.** Caregiving requires positive planning and strategic thinking. There will be choice points where critical decision making is required. At such times, consult your professional and trusted resources with positive and constructive action in the best interest of all concerned.

9. **Healthy caregivers provide healthy care.** It is vital that your own health be maintained. Be sure to engage in a positive healthy living pattern so you are capable of providing the level of care needed by your loved one.

10. **Make caregiving a spiritual experience.** Caring, "for the least of these," is an expressive act of faith. Caring for others gives life meaning and brings into focus the essence of life and death.

11. **Learn to delegate.** While caregivers provide care on a person-to-person level, they also need to engage others in the caregiving process through delegation. Ask for help. Other family members may be able to play a specific role if asked. There are many support and assistance programs available in the community. Tap all the resources available to you. You need not go it alone. There are many people and services available for specific functions or for specific and designated periods of time. They are generally available for the asking.

12. **Consult professional and non-profit organizations devoted to the particular illness or disease of your loved one.** There are a number of non-profit organizations that provide information and support and could be helpful as you provide needed care. Draw upon these resources for encouragement, guidance, education, and general information.

13. **Capitalize on the opportunity to learn lessons about family history.** Spending lengthy hours caregiving also gives opportunity to discuss the history of the family and the unique experiences of various family members. This may be your best opportunity to put the family history in perspective, learn from the past, and determine how you shall live in the future. Conduct interview sessions and record them on audio or video tape. Talk about the past and enjoy the events and experiences that have happened within the family.

14. **Take every opportunity to teach independent living skills and new information.** Whether your loved one is aging or disabled, they can still learn independent living skills. Information and new ideas are still worthy of being presented and taught. Assume the role of a teacher as you provide care. People are never too old to learn. Be realistic, however. Learning something new gives encouragement and personal satisfaction. It reduces dependency.

A WORD FOR THE CARE PROVIDERS

To prevent burnout, the following suggestions are set forth. Add your own ideas as to how you successfully keep yourself from burnout. From the list below, note the four items that are most important to you (mark with *) and the four items that you need to work on and do better over the next month (mark with !).

Facilitate as much independent living and self-help skills as possible.

Friends make good medicine; be sure to have several friends with whom you spend time each week.

Home needs to be fall-proof so be on guard for ways a fall could occur.

Travel now as things could change rapidly and your future chances of travel may be limited.

Build a "War Chest" as out of pocket costs for things and services are always greater than you planned.

Velcro fastenings will make your job of caring for your loved one easier and facilitate self-help.

Keep a journal or diary of the major happening each day as looking back on this experience may be filled with lessons to pass along to others.

Know the Heimlich maneuver; you may need to use it.

Build a provider support network as you need guidance and support as much as you give support to your loved one.

Educate yourself on the problems and the disease of your loved one; knowledge helps you face the "demons."

Be positive, optimistic, and hopeful, but be realistic at the same time.

Re-shape your Box of Reality; life is not always the way you planned it or thought it was supposed to be.

Relax and enjoy the journey; don't take life so seriously.

COMING TO TERMS WITH ELDER ABUSE

A Therapist's Guide

It is generally agreed that 4% of the population will experience abuse or significant neglect sometime during their elder years. Elder abuse is defined as the subjection of persons 60 years of age and over to some type of physical and material abuse and neglect by another person, including possibly themselves. Physical abuse is the willful confinement. Material abuse involves the misuse of the older person's property or financial resources. Neglect constitutes a significant danger to physical or mental health because the family member or guardian is unable, or fails, to provide adequate food, shelter, clothing, medical, dental, or mental health care.

It is most important to understand that elder abuse can be prevented by the elderly person and/or by a family member, guardian, or friend. The essential ingredients of abuse prevention revolve around regular contact, communication, understanding, and empathy. Let's take a closer look.

WHAT THE OLDER PERSON CAN DO TO PREVENT ABUSE?

1. Stay sociable and keep in contact with friends and relatives.
2. Encourage visitors to stop by when you are unable to get out and visit others.
3. Stay organized and keep records, and know your belongings and where they are kept.
4. Take care of your own mail. Checks should be directly deposited.
5. Get legal advice before making major decisions, especially if large sums of money are to be spent.
6. Utilize various resources within the family and within the community, and ask for help when it is needed.

WHAT FAMILY, FRIENDS, AND GUARDIANS CAN DO TO PREVENT ABUSE?

1. Keep in personal and telephone contact with the older adult(s) in your family.
2. Discuss the wishes of the elder family member and respect them unless they are unreasonable.
3. Examine your ability as a family to provide long-term care, as well as the alternatives available to you.
4. Seek sources of help in the community and utilize them regularly.
5. Develop a plan as to how your needs can be met while also attempting to maintain contact and involvement with the older person(s) in your family.

Elder abuse is an unfortunate reality in our country. However, its occurrence need not result in fear or feelings of helplessness in the lives of the elder and his/her family. By taking the preventive steps outlined above, not only is the likelihood of abuse greatly decreased, but feelings of support, security, and well-being are fostered as well.

Chapter 35

Couples Therapy and Relationship Assessements and Exercises

Chapter Contents

The most common areas of difficulty and basis of referral for counseling services are marital and relationship problems. Therapists are continually being asked to assist in the strengthening or rebuilding of a patient's primary relationships. These include, but are not limited to, the following types of relationship: marital, parent–child, extended family, work colleague, and neighbors. This area of therapeutic demand speaks to the high level of value we place on our relationships, as well as the fact that we are significantly inadequate in our social relationship skills. To benefit fully from such relationships patients need to learn a variety of relationship skills. Therapy is one place such skills are acquired and implemented.

The forms in this chapter have been selected to assist therapists in helping patients build warm and effective relationships, rebuild the relationships that have been broken and make good relationships better. Templates, questionnaires, worksheets, homework exercises, guidelines, and therapy exercises have been included for the therapist's working benefit.

A "PERFECT" MARRIAGE WISH LIST

_____

Husband ☐ **Wife** ☐

List what <u>you</u> would consider to be ideal for your marriage in each of the behavior areas below. Be selfish and note what you would like if it were at all possible. Yet be realistic.

Household responsibilities: _____

_____

Rearing of children: _____

_____

Social activities: _____

_____

Money: _____

_____

Communication: _____

_____

Sex: _____

_____

Occupational progress: _____

_____

Personal independence: _____

_____

Spouse independence: _____

_____

General happiness: _____

_____

Other: _____

Name: _____ Date: _____

MARITAL HAPPINESS SCALE

This scale is intended to estimate <u>your current happiness</u> with your marriage on each of the 10 dimensions listed. You are to circle one of the numbers (1 – 10) beside each marriage area. Numbers toward the left end of the 10-unit scale indicate some degree of unhappiness and checks toward the right end of the scale reflect varying degrees of happiness. Ask yourself this question as you rate <u>each marriage area</u>: "If my partner continues to act in the future as he/she is acting today with respect to this marriage area, how happy will I be with this area of our marriage?" In other words, state according to the numerical scale (1 – 10) exactly how you now feel. Try to exclude all feelings of the past and concentrate only on your current feelings in each of the marital areas.

	Completely Unhappy							Completely Happy		
Household responsibilities	1	2	3	4	5	6	7	8	9	10
Rearing of children	1	2	3	4	5	6	7	8	9	10
Social activities	1	2	3	4	5	6	7	8	9	10
Money management	1	2	3	4	5	6	7	8	9	10
Communication skills	1	2	3	4	5	6	7	8	9	10
Sexual relationships	1	2	3	4	5	6	7	8	9	10
Occupational progress	1	2	3	4	5	6	7	8	9	10
My personal independence	1	2	3	4	5	6	7	8	9	10
My spouse's independence	1	2	3	4	5	6	7	8	9	10
General happiness	1	2	3	4	5	6	7	8	9	10
Other	1	2	3	4	5	6	7	8	9	10

NOTE TO THERAPIST: This form can be given before and after therapy with the results compared as a measure of change.

REQUEST FOR MARITAL BEHAVIOR CHANGE

List at least 3 specific answers to each statement.

A. I would like my spouse better if (he/she) would do <u>less</u> of the following:
   1.
   2.
   3.
   4.

B. I would like my spouse better if (he/she) would do <u>more</u> of the following:
   1.
   2.
   3.
   4.

C. I believe my spouse would like me better if I did <u>less</u> of the following:
   1.
   2.
   3.
   4.

D. I believe my spouse would like me better if I did <u>more</u> of the following:
   1.
   2.
   3.
   4.

E. My spouse and I do these things together:
   1.
   2.
   3.
   4.

F. I would like to do these new things together:

1.

2.

3.

4.

G. Other: _____

1.

2.

3.

4.

MARITAL SATISFACTION LIST

Marital Satisfaction: Wife

List 5 current satisfactions you are providing your partner and 5 satisfactions your partner is providing you within your marriage relationship. List specific behaviors, not general attitudes or feelings.

The following behaviors of mine provide satisfaction for my husband:

1. _____
2. _____
3. _____
4. _____
5. _____

I am satisfied with the following behaviors of my husband:

1. _____
2. _____
3. _____
4. _____
5. _____

How can I improve and do better this next month? _____

_____

* *

Marital Satisfaction: Husband

List 5 current satisfactions you are providing your partner and 5 satisfactions your partner is providing you within your marriage relationship. List specific behaviors, not general attitudes or feelings.

The following behaviors of mine provide satisfaction for my wife:

1. _____
2. _____
3. _____
4. _____
5. _____

I am satisfied with the following behaviors of my wife:

1. _____
2. _____
3. _____
4. _____
5. _____

How I can improve and do better this next month _____

_____

SEVEN COMPONENTS TO LOVING

Evaluate your marriage and loving relationship by putting the seven areas noted below into rank order from 1 to 7. Number 1 would represent complete satisfaction and frequent occurrence, while number 7 would indicate dissatisfaction and its infrequent occurrence in your relationship. Rank the seven areas for yourself and then as you think your spouse would answer. Plan to discuss your answers together.

	Myself	My Spouse	Components
A.			Verbal expression of non-sexual affection (I love you, you're beautiful).
B.			Self-disclosure for personal facts to the loved one (telling of hopes, dreams, plans and ambitions).
C.			Tolerance of the loved one (putting up with idiosyncrasies and mannerisms).
D.			Expressing concern and care (caring for the other's health, safety, welfare, and self-regard).
E.			Showing moral support (being interested in the other's work, hobbies, responsibilities and friendships).
F.			Affection shown by acts of helpfulness (buying gifts)
G.			Expressions of sexual affection (touching, hugging, kissing, intercourse)

COMMENTS OR POINTS I WISH TO DISCUSS:

-
-
-
-
-

COUPLES COMMUNICATION

"You" and "I" Messages

Read each situation, examine the "You" message in the second column, then write an "I" message in the third column. Depending on the nature of your relationship, feel free to substitute "partner" for husband/wife. Practice this exercise until you are using "I" messages more regularly.

SITUATION	"YOU" MESSAGE	"I" MESSAGE
1. Couple decides that wife is in charge of laundry. Husband notices that the laundry basket is overflowing.	HUSBAND: You lazy slob! Why can't you keep the laundry up to date?	HUSBAND: I see that the laundry basket is overflowing and I feel frustrated.
2. Husband promised to get his wife some information but forgot.	WIFE: You shouldn't make promises if you aren't responsible enough to keep them.	WIFE:
3. Husband gives wife some unexpected help with the dishes.	WIFE: It's about time you did something around here!	WIFE:
4. Husband is hurt because his wife has rejected his sexual advance.	HUSBAND: You sure didn't mind when we were first married … what's happened to you?	HUSBAND:
5. Wife has come home late while husband has been babysitting.	HUSBAND: Where the heck were you? A woman should be home with her family!	HUSBAND:
6. Husband has just announced that he has joined a bowling league.	WIFE: That's just great. Now you'll never be home.	WIFE:
7. Wife has spent $50 on a make-up kit, and husband has just discovered the bill.	HUSBAND: Don't you have any sense about money?	HUSBAND:

20 DIAGNOSTIC FACTORS THAT INDICATE RELATIONSHIP ANGER

Relationships can easily be changed from peaceful and compatible to painful and angry. It may only take a few words that make the difference. The tongue can speak peace or venomous anger as a spear to the heart and soul. Below are common attitudes and speaking patterns that are known to be hurtful to others and that may well sever any relationship. Look them over and identify the ones you may tend to utilize and which contribute to the build-up of anger within you. How can you change your manner of speaking and dealing with others when times are tough and stressful?

1. THE NEED TO BE RIGHT
2. NEGATIVE CRITICISM
3. PASSING JUDGMENT
4. THREATS
5. EMOTIONAL OUTBURSTS
6. INTERROGATING
7. LABELING
8. INDIFFERENCE
9. LYING
10. JEALOUSY
11. USING NEGATIVE LANGUAGE
12. COMPLAINING
13. PESSIMISTIC OUTLOOK
14. COMPARISONS
15. BLAMING
16. ATTACKING
17. MIND-READING
18. GIVING COMMANDS
19. PRETENDING
20. PUNISHING

What pattern from the list above do you need to change? How will you make the necessary changes? Who will help you in the process of making change?

1.

2.

3.

4.

5.

6.

I LOVE YOU AND WANT YOU TO KNOW IT

Expressing love is not as easy as it might seem. The popular portrayal of love making is usually physical sexual love. Yet we all have our own ways to knowing we are loved. We look for the signs that mean the most to us. A husband may be very different from his wife in expressing and receiving love messages. We need to know each other's preferred ways of being loved and assured of the love from our spouse. Below are typical ways couples express and receive love messages between them.

How To Love You?

Follow these three steps in your homework assignment: (1) Check the top 3 – 5 ways you prefer to receive love messages. (2) Check the 3 –5 ways you generally express love messages to your spouse. (3) Discuss together if you are accurate and on target in both receiving and expressing love to each other so that you both experience a high level of satisfaction and affirmation. This exercise can be applied to other areas and topics of communication.

1. I show my love to you by finding ways to do things together with you _____
2. I show my love to you by being available to help you when you need it _____
3. I show my love to you by engaging you in non-sexual types of affection _____
4. I show my love to you by engaging you in physical sexual affection_____
5. I show my love to you by doing things to help you without being asked _____
6. I show my love for you by making and buying things you would like _____
7. I show my love for you by directly telling you and telling others also_____
8. I show my love for you by living a life of respect and integrity _____
9. I show my love for you by keeping my promises _____
10. I show my love for you by keeping the home clean and orderly _____
11. I show my love for you by being ready and on time when it is time to go _____
12. I show my love for you by providing for you in meeting our basic needs, such as shelter, food, clothing, and a well-functioning and clean home _____
13. Other _____

MARITAL POINTERS

Many years ago, my attention was perked when I heard the following adage for the first time: "To feel the proper emotions, one must first go through the proper motions." That adage has stuck with me and has served a role in my life and in my counseling over the years. We all want to change emotions, to feel better. How does that happen? Well, we first of all need to point our attention and efforts in the direction of behavior. Once we develop appropriate and positive behavior patterns, we will soon begin to feel positive and have the desired emotions for healthy and effective living.

Another adage closely associated with the one stated above has also served well over the years. "Before one can do what is right, one must stop doing what is wrong." It is not a matter of just adding the new and better behavior patterns, it is essential that we terminate inappropriate and wrongful acts perpetrated upon the lives of others and upon ourselves. Old behavioral habits, attitudes, thought patterns, and emotions need to be eliminated as we seek ways to live positively, constructively, and righteously. Simply stated, righteousness is defined as doing that which is right. It is vital that we seek to do the right thing in our personal relationships, our business and career relationships, and in our intimate family relationships.

The following marital pointers give us direction, and focus our attention on certain issues. The admonition is to stop doing the wrong thing and start doing the right thing. As a result, our marital and family relationships can be strengthened. Marital relationships can be restructured and built on the foundation stones of caring, respect, and love.

1. **STOP** seeking more and new information, and **START** acting on what you already know as the right thing to do.

2. **STOP** placing emphasis upon external lifestyle symbols and appearance, and **START** shifting to an emphasis upon the internal qualities with each other of honesty, respect, considerations, and kindness.

3. **STOP** placing each other's worth and value on what has been earned or accomplished, and **START** sharing through open communication, feelings, hopes, future visions, and expectations.

4. **STOP** the process of mind-reading and speaking for the other person, and **START** the process of open, direct, and clear assertive communication.

5. **STOP** presenting yourself in a negative manner and **START** looking attractive at all times to increase your appeal and appreciation when together, whether that be privately or publicly.

6. **STOP** being passive, withdrawn, and discouraged, and **START** initiating activities in the life of the family. Manage family life for the purpose of productivity for each individual as a family unit.

We all struggle with the dilemma of knowing what is right, desiring to do what is right, yet doing that which we know we should not do. It is an age-old struggle. It is easy to do the familiar and the common, but it is hard to do that which is right. It is the struggle that those who have been raised in dysfunctional homes experience on a day-to-day basis.

The above six pointers apply to marriage, but also could apply to other situations. I urge you to look them over and propose to stop doing that which is destructive, unproductive, dysfunctional, and wrong, and do that which is right and beneficial to yourself and to those whom you love.

MARITAL PROBLEM AREA QUESTIONNAIRE

Name: _____ Date:_____

Please complete the following by answering (T) true or (F) false:

AFFECTION:
_____ Seems to care for others more than he/she cares for me.
_____ Is sometimes quite warm and other times quite cold to me.
_____ Does not show enough affection toward me.
_____ Demands a great deal of affection from me.
_____ Other (specify) _____

COMMUNICATION:
_____ Does not let me know I'm important to him/her.
_____ Does not listen to what I have to say.
_____ Holds things inside until he/she eventually "blows up."
_____ Does not take the time to talk to me.
_____ Only criticizes me for what I do wrong; few compliments.
_____ Other (specify) _____

FINANCES:
_____ Spends money on himself/herself but not on me.
_____ Refuses even to spend money on necessities.
_____ Wants to control the finances without consulting me.
_____ Spends money foolishly.
_____ Other (specify) _____

RESPONSIBILITY:
_____ Will do things for others before doing things for me.
_____ Does not take good care of our home.
_____ Does not finish what he/she started.
_____ Does not take part in decisions affecting our family.
_____ Other (specify) _____

SEX:
_____ Does not seem concerned about my sexual satisfaction.
_____ Is sexually attracted to others.
_____ Is too demanding of me sexually.
_____ Seems to dislike sexual relations with me.
_____ Other (specify) _____

UNDERSTANDING:
_____ Does not seem to care about my feelings.
_____ Burdens me with his/her problems.
_____ Does not try to help me understand how he/she feels.
_____ Does not seem to realize the effect his/her behavior has on me.
_____ Other (specify) _____

CHILD REARING:
_____ Does not pay attention to the children.
_____ Does not participate in decisions about the children.
_____ Does not discipline the children appropriately.
_____ Expects too much from the children.
_____ Other (specify) _____

RELATIVES:
_____ Does not get along with my side of the family.
_____ Spends too much time with his/her side of the family.
_____ Belittles my relatives.
_____ Avoids being with my relatives.
_____ Other (specify) _____

Marital Problem Area Questionnaire *(Continued)*

ALCOHOL:

_____ He/she really wants to stop drinking alcohol.
_____ Has caused major problems between us.
_____ He/she is physically and psychologically addicted.
_____ If he/she stops drinking, so will I.
_____ All alcohol has been removed from our home.
_____ Other (specify) _____

Answer by indicating the percentage number:

1. I feel _____% satisfied in my marriage.

2. I feel _____% committed to remaining married to my spouse.

Indicate which 3 problems you would like to address and change first:

1.

2.

3.

What are you willing to do to start the process of making a change in your marriage relationship?

PRE-MARITAL QUESTIONNAIRE

Male partner ☐   Female partner ☐

Please complete the questions listed below and bring them to the next session for our mutual discussion. We may need to spend two or three sessions discussing your answers.

1. Please define marriage:

2. Please define love:

3. How were you reared in the home of your parents regarding examples of love, intimacy, tenderness, communication, etc.?

4. How would you like your marriage to be similar to your parents' marriage? How do you think it should be different from your parents?

5. As you anticipate marriage, what fears and concerns do you have?

6. List several reasons you feel this is the person to marry at this time:

   a.

   b.

   c.

   d.

   e.

7. What is it about your relationship with your intended spouse that indicates that this marriage is the right thing for the two of you?

8. What is it about your intended marriage that you want to be known for or to achieve together?

9. Other areas you would like to discuss with your intended spouse?

   a.

   b.

THE SCOPE OF INTIMACY IN MARRIAGE

Review the full scope of intimacy with a couple in the early stages of marital counseling. Note the dimensions that are problematic and then plan to address these areas during subsequent sessions. This is an important task during the rebuilding process.

DIMENSIONS OF INTIMACY

1. Emotional intimacy – ability to share feelings and emotions.
2. Intellectual intimacy – ability to discuss ideas and thought events.
3. Sexual intimacy – ability to share physical closeness, sexually and nonsexually.
4. Creative intimacy – ability to create something new and different.
5. Aesthetic intimacy – ability to share acts of beauty and artistic events.
6. Recreational intimacy – ability to play and have fun together.
7. Work intimacy – ability to engage in tasks and projects together.
8. Conflict intimacy – ability to face and solve problems together.
9. Crisis intimacy – ability to face painful and hurtful events together.
10. Spiritual intimacy – ability to share in spiritual events and pray together.
11. Communication intimacy – ability to talk openly and freely together.
12. Commitment intimacy – ability to trust each other for the long term.

AREAS TO BE FURTHER EXPLORED:

NAVIGATING THE CONFRONTATIONS OF A DISCOVERED AFFAIR

The discovery of an affair or other moral or marital departures comes with hardship and pain. As a couple in the midst of such suffering, the following checklist may help the recovery process, ease the pain of healing, and bring restoration. Research has shown that couples that stick it out are glad they did after 5 years. Discuss the following issues together in therapy or at home, if possible.

DISADVANTAGEOUS	ADVANTAGEOUS
1. Persist in demanding to know why.	Accept the fact that there were reasons and focus on them.
2. Concentrate on the details of the affair.	Consider the overall factors that brought it about.
3. Withdraw from others and events.	Realize you are not alone; communicate all the more.
4. Decide that you have reached the limits of your endurance	Know that your limits are beyond your current inner resources
5. Be impatient, demanding, and panicky	Be sensitive and seize the right time to talk and take action.
6. Give up in despair and frustration.	Wait and see; be alert to the cues of encouragement and hope.
7. Seek out your own remedies, and solutions.	Trust in and seek the guidance of professionals and others.
8. Indulge yourself and seek self pleasure.	Stay focused on the long run and act responsibly. View the future as what is best for all.
9. Delude yourself; deny the reality.	Seek the truth; check out the facts and act wisely.
10. Become angry, hostile, and retaliatory.	Master the management of your acute moods and feelings.
11. Let discouragement, depression, and helplessness win.	Keep the faith utmost; focus on hope and see the humor in it.

THE PATHWAY TO RECONCILIATION

When hurt occurs between two or more people, a reconciliation process may need to be implemented. This is more so in close relationships and when it can affect a large group of people, as in a church or club, office or organization. The following steps generally resolve most disputes and hurts between people. The steps to forgiveness follow those formulated by psychologist Dr Frederic Luskin.

THE STEPS TO RECONCILIATION:

1. Overlook the minor offenses by accommodation, compromise, or just giving up a personal right or privilege. Learn to forgive and move forward without malice.
2. Seek out a private opportunity to speak on the issue with the other party. Should you become aware of a wrong, it may be appropriate to go to the person and discuss your observations of the wrong and what can be done to set it right.
3. Take one or two people with you to address the other party. If the attempt fails as is set forth in point 2, go with a witness or two or three who may act as intermediaries or mediators.
4. If no reconciliation occurs, you are free to bring the issue before some body of authority such as the person's pastor, priest or rabbi, employer, or family, for their intervention and assistance. Accountability is the purpose of this higher-level involvement.
5. Cut off or greatly reduce the relationship or contact with the person who refuses to reconcile after positive steps have been undertaken.
6. If the conflict or dispute or hurt is deep and irresolvable and involves the loss of funds, functions or possessions, a higher level of resolution may be sought, such as mediation services, arbitration or filing for a Court hearing of the principal matter. It is advisable to seek much consultation and guidance before litigation is pursued.
7. Finally, at all steps along the way to reconciliation, seek the advice of wise friends and professionals. Look into the short-term and long-term consequences of any actions considered. This is a delicate area of relationships and one needs to be thoughtful and not act hastily.

THE STEPS TO FORGIVENESS

1. Breathe deeply for a few minutes and relax while visualizing a time when you felt cared for and loved. Think of the situation that did not go as you had wished and what you had hoped for. What would you have preferred to have happened?
2. Look at the world around you. Have others experienced what you just went through? Try to look at it less personally.
3. Realize that you should not give up trying to have your needs met even if you did not get from a situation what you wanted. Feel the part of you that's lost when you were hurt. Your intentions are still valid so reclaim your power from the one who hurt you. Your future can be clearer and yet attain what is important to you.
4. Pledge to practice letting go of grudges forever. The cycle can be broken as you breathe deeply and relax and then visualize something positive and wonderful in your life.

THE FINAL THOUGHT

Hurts and grudges can be long term and follow us for years. They take a toll on our spirits and mind and body. Learning to forgive and reconcile is the only way to release a burden. Even small burdens get heavy after a long period of time of carrying them all alone. "Burden release" is a prescription for improved mental and physical health.

MARITAL ACTION STEPS FOR THE LONG RUN

Marital relationships like any other relationship must be developed into a primary and strong bond between husband and wife. How to build that relationship is learned. We learn it from our primary parents, the marital relationships of our parents' friends, from our friends who are married, and from a variety of other sources, such as books and magazine articles, movies, and general observations made in public places.

Marital bonds result from intentional efforts on the part of a couple to build and strengthen and expand their relationship. A strong marriage is not a private relationship but one that has a public face and is inclusive of others.

There are eight acts of marital relationship-building. They are as follows:

1. **Acts of service** are a strong way to express consideration and care for your spouse. It is essentially a helping relationship that is built through service one to the other. Service represents a language of compassion and consideration and thoughtfulness. Demonstrating one's love for another through serving is one of the oldest acts in history that one can do for another.

2. **Acts of reassurance** can be expressed verbally as well as through various physical acts. Reassurance builds up, supports, and strengthens the spouse. The issuance of reassurance reduces anxiety and fear and uncertainty. Reassurance is a building block for self-esteem. Reassuring the spouse of ongoing love and care counteracts the threats, insecurities, and anxieties normally associated with any marital relationship. Uncertainty stirs up fear. Reassurance calms.

3. **Acts of focus** carry a message of importance and value when attention is placed upon the other spouse. It communicates that that person is special, valued, and worthy of intentional focused attention.

4. **Acts of appreciation** carry a message of satisfaction and acceptance. When appreciated, a person desires to continue to do those things that please and are desired by their spouse. Appreciation is a form of reward and re-enforcement for behaving in a desired manner.

5. **Acts of commitment** anchor the marital relationship. Commitment communicates security, assurance, and removes the uncertainty that prevails in any marital relationship. Commitment provides opportunity to look forward and plan the future. It allows planning to be undertaken to enhance and strengthen the relationship for the future. Someone has said that, "Marriage is a marathon and not a sprint." Commitment means that you are in it for the long haul. Pulling out is not an option. Marriage does not just begin with engagement, but lives a lifetime of engagement. Your marriage is to be celebrated and enjoyed.

6. **Acts of enjoyment** recognize that relationships need to be bathed in fun, laughter, pleasure, and even times of hilarity. Enjoyment is soothing, healthy, and lightens a personal burden otherwise carried as a load.

7. **Acts of communication** reduce isolation and separation. When we speak to each other, needs are met and distance is broken down. Closeness is achievable. Communicating with your spouse carries the message of value, importance, recognition, and acceptance.

8. **Acts of intimacy** come in two forms, sexual and non-sexual. Relationships thrive and strengthen on non-sexual acts of intimacy. Intimacy comes in the form of sharing experiences, telling of historical events, opening up and talking of hurts as well as accomplishments. The freedom to ask for support and encouragement when needed is clearly an act of intimacy. Knowing about each other in a deeper and more personal way is the ultimate act of intimacy. Intimacy requires that hurts and disappointments be settled through forgiveness.

Enjoy the journey of your relationship. Embrace the journey you have chosen with your person of choice.

INTERPERSONAL RELATIONSHIP DISTINCTIONS

Interpersonal relationships require discipline and reason as prevailing guidelines. However, they can easily get out of control and become harsh, even abusive. Below are the key words or distinctives that separate harsh and abusive relationships from healthy and well-disciplined relationships. We need to assess our relationships periodically and improve them as needed. Review the list below and identify those aspects of your interpersonal behavior that needs improvement. Make a plan to do so in the space provided below.

	Harsh, Abusive	**Healthy, Disciplined**
1.	Unfair	Fair
2.	Unexpected	Expected
3.	Degrading	Upholds dignity
4.	Extreme, strong, harsh	Held under control
5.	Torturous	No lasting scars
6.	Hatred, twisted mind	Love
7.	Creating terror	Creating respect
8.	Damaging esteem	Strengthening esteem
9.	Crushing the spirit	Shaping the will
10.	Public	Private
11.	Tongue lashing	Reproving
12.	Lack of assurance	Reassurance expressed
13.	Out of balance, lacking perspective	Staying balanced, showing moderation
14.	Undertaken late	Starting early
15.	Inconsistent	Consistent
16.	Unreasonable	Reasonable
17.	Humiliating, embarrassing	Retaining integrity

PLAN HOW YOU WILL TRY TO CHANGE IN HOW YOU TALK AND ADDRESS OTHERS:

VIOLENCE IN THE HOME: PARTNER VIOLENCE AND WHAT CAN BE DONE ABOUT IT

INTRODUCTION

Until the mid-1970s, no one talked much about abuse between adult partners. We were taught to think that criminal violence occurred on the street or in bars. Home was thought to be a safe place.

Now we know that violence in the home is very frequent. According to Drs Angela Browne and Laura S. Brown of the American Psychological Association, more than 2 million American women each year are physically attacked by their male partners; violence can also happen in same-sex relationships, and some men are beaten in heterosexual relationships, although what is most common is that women are battered by men. Some of these assaults are severe. During the first half of the 1980s, the deaths of nearly 17,000 people resulted from one partner killing another, with women twice as likely to be victims of such fatal partner violence as men. *Violence between partners happens in all groups in society. No group is immune. If your intimate partner has beaten you, you are not alone.*

HOW DO I KNOW IF I'M AT RISK?

Violence in a relationship is never OK and never justified. A "little slap" is violence. So is pushing, shoving, throwing things, threatening violence, or forcing a partner to engage in sexual activities against her or his will. All of these things, along with punching, kicking, biting, choking, burning, and injury with weapons have happened to victims of partner violence.

If violence or a threat of violence of any kind has happened more than once or twice, it is extremely likely to happen again. It may get more frequent or more severe. If this describes you and your relationship, you are at risk.

AM I OVERREACTING?

Very often abusers will tell victims that they are overreacting and causing the batterer to become violent. You are not overreacting or causing the violence. It is *normal* to feel frightened and angry when your spouse or partner is violent with you. Your reactions to earlier abuse are no excuse for someone to be violent toward you.

WHY DON'T I JUST LEAVE?

This is a common question that people ask about victims and victims ask of themselves. It is almost always more complicated than just leaving. Sometimes the batterer will not allow you to leave and may threaten to kill you or other family members if you do. These are not always idle threats. Research tells us that women are more likely to be killed by their battering mates at the time these women try to leave. You may still feel love and compassion for the abuser and worry about hurting that person's feelings. You may be afraid to be alone and on your own. You may worry about how to support yourself and your children without the batterer. You may blame yourself, wrongly, for causing the violence and feel ashamed and afraid of exposing yourself. It may be against your religious or other beliefs to end a marriage or committed relationship. It's important for you to get help in learning how to answer these questions for yourself.

WHAT CAN I DO?

If you are a victim of violence:

- Begin to think about how you can plan for your own safety and happiness. Waiting for abusers to change and trying harder to please them will not work.
- Find out what resources are available in your area for victims of partner abuse. At a safe time, when the abuser is not around, call a local battered women's shelter or domestic violence hotline. Tell them what has happened; ask them what your choices are to protect yourself and to end the violence. Think about the answers to your questions and call again if you need to know more.

- If you are considering leaving your abuser, make safety plans *before* you talk about separation. Discuss the abuser's pattern of violence with someone at a shelter or crisis line and think about what risks there might be if you talk about leaving. Try to keep enough money in a protected place to use when you need to get to safety. Some victims find it best to go to a shelter where they can be safe before they tell the abuser that they are leaving.

- If you can do this safely, encourage the abuser to go to a group for batterers. There are now many such groups for men who batter their partners. Some large cities also have groups for gay men and lesbians who batter their partners and for people from particular ethnic or religious groups. In such a group, batterers can get help from experts specially trained to treat violent people and may learn to change their beliefs and behaviors. You still may need to live apart from the batterer while that person is in the group. Changing patterns of violence can take a long time.

- If you think you are in *immediate* danger, you probably are. You are expert at sensing when things are getting really bad. Flee at once to a safe location or call the police if you can. When police arrive, ask what legal protections are available to you, and use whatever you need to be sure you are safe. Don't let the police leave you alone with the abuser once they've arrived. If you are hurt, ask for medical help. Be sure that the doctor or nurse makes a record of your injuries and notes that those injuries were the result of an assault, not falling down stairs or bumping into a door.

IF YOU ARE AN ABUSER

- Get help to end your violent behavior. Hurting the people you love will cost you their trust and respect and your own self-respect as well. You may lose your loved ones permanently. No one likes to be violent or to get hurt.

- Realize that you *can* change. Others have gone through this and found ways to stop their patterns of violence. Their lives and relationships with those they love have gotten better. Call a state or local domestic violence hotline (you don't have to give your name to get information) and ask for referrals to a batterer's group or to expert therapists in your area. Be honest with the people running the group or with an individual therapist about your history of violence. Tell the leader or therapist that your violent behaviors are the ones you want to change. Don't wait until a judge requires you to go to treatment.

IF YOU ARE A FRIEND OR FAMILY MEMBER

- You can do something. Encourage the victim to get to safety and help keep that person safe. Confront the abuser if you can do it safely (you may want to have someone else with you when you do this). Don't accept excuses for violence from people you love.

- Call the police if the victim cannot. Sometimes this can help stop or reduce the violence.

SUMMARY

Take action. Do not let the situation go on and on while being ignored and unaddressed. The sooner action is taken the more quickly the rehabilitation process can begin and the more effective it will be in the long term. The aim is to bring about healing in the abused as well as the abuser. Only then will it stop and not continue on to the next generation.

HOW TO PREDICT A POTENTIALLY VIOLENT RELATIONSHIP

At the core of any violent relationship is the use of power and control. People often express interest in how they might be able to predict if a potential partner may be someone who is emotionally, sexually, or physically abusive. Consider the following points in increasing awareness for concern.

1. **Controlling behavior.** Where the person is allowed to go; who he or she is allowed to see or talk to. How the person dresses, and how a woman does her hair and make-up. This behavior tends to escalate under the guise of trying to be protective or to prevent someone from being harmed by their own poor judgment – therefore, they need to be told what to do and how to do it.

2. **Jealousy.** Expresses jealousy as a sign of love and concern. There may be accusations of flirting or being questioned for talking to someone. The person may be isolated from their family and friends. As jealousy intensifies, they may be monitored by frequent phone calling and will not be allowed to make personal decisions. Ultimately, he or she may not be allowed to do anything without the permission of their partner.

3. **Neediness.** Insecurity is expressed as "I have never felt like this about anyone" or "I have never been able to talk to someone or trust someone like you." There is pressure to commit quickly to an exclusive relationship. There may be pressure to have sex or to move in together.

4. **Isolation.** There is an attempt to isolate the abused person from family and friends. There will likely be efforts to sabotage close relationships and accuse others of causing difficulties in the relationship. There may also be efforts to limit phone contact, use of a car, or even from going to school or work.

5. **Projecting blame onto others.** Almost anything that goes wrong will be blamed on the abused person or on other people.

6. **Unrealistic expectations.** Expectations of the perfect partner, who has nothing out of place in the home, and who will be his/her everything. The abuser may have the expectation that all their needs will be met in this relationship.

7. **Blaming others for the abuser's feelings.** The abuser does not take responsibility for his/her own emotions. Blames the abused partner or others for how they feel and may use it as a means to manipulate. Makes light of abuse through minimizing, denying, and blaming.

8. **Verbal and emotional abuse.** Saying things to be hurtful and cruel – minimizing ability, accomplishments, and overall degradation. There may be awakening during the night out of sleep to be verbally assaulted, questioned, and called names. There may be added manipulation such as threats to end the relationship, to harm themselves, to abandon the abused person or kick them out of their home. There is game playing, resulting in the abused experiencing low self-esteem and feeling crazy.

9. **Rigidly traditional roles.** Expectation of the woman being in the home, being the central caretaker, being submissive, being unable to make decisions independently and seen as inferior. This can be a part of economic abuse. The abused may become totally financially dependent on the abuser. This is also where children can be used to make the abused feel guilty for their own strivings. Or children can be used to relay messages. Using male privilege, treating her like a servant, creating the rules for men and women.

10. **Coercion and threats.** Cruelty to children or pets. Having unrealistic expectations about children's abilities. Pets may be harmed or even killed.

11. **Using force sexually.** Desires to act out fantasies during sex in which the woman is forced, bound, or hurt. There is little concern about what the woman wants or needs. There may be manipulative behavior such as withdrawal, anger, or guilt to get the partner to comply. There may be no empathy for illness, and demands may be made for sex, or sex may be initiated while the partner is sleeping.

12. **Using force during conflicts.** The use of force, such as being prevented from leaving a room, held down or restrained.

13. **History of violence in a relationship.** History of physically hurting a past partner but blaming them for what happened.

Therapist's Guide to Clinical Intervention, Second Edition by Sharon L. Johnson (© 2003 Elsevier Inc.)

14. **Threats of violence.** Making or carrying out threats of harm, threatening to leave, or harm self. Coercing someone into illegal behavior. This is meant to control. There may be excuses later, such as "I was just upset because of what you did. I wouldn't do that."

15. **Throwing or breaking things.** This behavior is threatening and is often used as a punishment and to terrorize another person into submission.

16. **Mood swings.** This is the confusing behavior where one minute the person is nice and the next minute the person is upset, angry, or out of control.

WHY VICTIMS OF DOMESTIC VIOLENCE STRUGGLE WITH LEAVING

1. **Fear in general.** Often they have been cut off from all of their resources and have lived under threat and control, not being able to rely on their own decision making.

2. **Low self-esteem.** People who have been emotionally beaten down over a period often begin to see themselves as failures at everything they do. Offenders reinforce this belief to maintain their control.

3. **Self-blame/responsibility.** Victimized people blame themselves for the abuse. This is constantly reinforced by the offenders who blame them for the abuser's violent behavior.

4. **Holding the family together.** Women are raised and socialized to see themselves as the center of family cohesiveness – for keeping their families safe and together. Women often believe they must do this at any cost to themselves, while at the same time questioning their parenting abilities.

5. **Fear of being crazy.** When you are told you are crazy often enough you begin to believe it. As a result, these victims question their ability to cope with all of the responsibilities of the outside world.

6. **Dependence.** Victims of domestic violence have likely had their worlds made very small so that they could be controlled. As a result, they lack experience in making their own decisions and acting independently.

7. **Isolation.** One of the most common things done to victims of domestic violence is to isolate them from family and friends, physically and emotionally. The more isolated they are, the less likely they will seek help or be aware of the help available in their community.

8. **Traditional values.** Traditional male–female roles are in conflict with separation and divorce and support the notion of "keeping the family together at all costs." There may also be strong religious influences and unsupportive family members that reinforce a victim's belief that he/she must stay in an abusive relationship.

9. **Learned behavior.** When you live in an isolated and abusive environment, over time the experience takes on a normalcy because there is nothing else to compare it to. When combined with a lack of belief in oneself, the victim may come to believe that the situation is impossible to change. This may be further embedded if the victim grew up in an abusive home.

10. **The honeymoon stage and promises of change.** Victims often love their partners and want a good marriage and a stable family life for their children. With the promise of change is the hope that all of these things are possible. In the hopes that the promise of change will be kept, the victims will forgive and give the relationship another chance for a new beginning.

Deal with what is, not what if. If things were going to change on their own they would have. If there is to be any chance of hope for change, for the victim and the victim's family, it is necessary to take action.

Therapist's Guide to Clinical Intervention, Second Edition by Sharon L. Johnson (© 2003 Elsevier Inc.)

Form Development and Usage for a Clinical Purpose

The development of a form for clinical use is generally thought to be easy and straightforward. All that you do is take out a piece of paper, write down some questions, and then give it to someone to complete their answers. Zippo you are done! Unfortunately, it is not quite that easy.

Form development follows a sequence of formal steps. These steps include, but are not limited to, the following: item selection, answer options, choice of wording, layout attractiveness, usability, and the design of an easy and quick scoring system.

Once the form has been designed, it requires a test run to see if its purpose, use, and design are actually fulfilled. It is important that the results from the test run are subject to analysis and interpretation. This will help determine if the questionnaire or form is useful and provides meaningful information to the decision making process of a clinician.

It is important that the form be designed with the intention that it will be included in the formal record of the patient, whether that be in a paper folder or a computerized data storage system.

The following components comprise the thought process and design procedures utilized by the clinician in developing a form or questionnaire:

1. *Purpose.* The purpose of the form should be clearly understood and be reflected in the nature of the questions and the corresponding responses or answers by the patient. Every form has a purpose and the purposes justifies its use.

2. *Item selection.* It is not uncommon to select items from a variety of sources but all items should be consistent with the purpose of the form and allow the purpose to be fulfilled. At times, items have significance in and of themselves. At other times, items lead to a more general factor comprising several items of a similar nature.

3. *Wording.* The wording should be clear and concise. All items needs to be communicated in the language and vocabulary of a person with a sixth grade reading level. Be careful not to express compound questions, or questions that could have a double meaning.

4. *Design of forms.* The simpler the design of the form, the better. It should be a form that can be completed quickly and without stress or frustration. The design should lead to a relatively easy scoring procedure and allow for interpretation to be conducted in a straightforward manner.

5. *Test run.* Any form should be submitted to a sample population not only to complete but to provide feedback as to their experience in completing the form. It should not be considered offensive, raise stress or stimulate emotional experiences for the person completing the form.

6. *Item interpretation.* Completed forms are evaluated relative to a particular theory, a particular data base, or a predetermined line of evidence.

7. *Storage of answers and responses.* Once a form has been completed, it should be readily filed and maintained in the patient's clinical file, or in the data base that is maintained on the patient. The form should be readily accessible for future reference.

8. *Confidentiality and privilege.* A complete form is considered confidential and privileged information with the patient being the holder of the privilege. The questions and answers become part of a patient's chart and must be stored in the context of the laws of confidentiality.

Forms for the Therapist

Professional Issues in Clinical Practice

CLINICAL CONSIDERATIONS

In the course of clinical practice, we have all occasionally faced situations and circumstances which raise the question of professional ethics and practice. We wonder, are we working within the guidelines of accepted standards and professional practice?

To be sure, practitioners are people of conscientiousness, integrity, and compassion. Therapists are caring individuals. Professional therapists are ethical individuals. Yet, all of us are vulnerable and fallible. As we strive to be helpful, compassionate, and cost-effective, it is easy to cut corners to the point that we may not see around the corner. That is when trouble raises its ugly head.

One of the areas of vulnerability is in the use of clinical forms. For example, forms contain confidential information and can be easily misused to a patient's detriment. A form contains information that needs to be interpreted. At times a clinician's interpretation can be less than accurate and lead to a course of action that unwittingly may not be in the best interest of a patient. Forms can also request information or pose a question for patients to complete or respond to that may produce emotional hurt and emotional re-traumatization even though this was not meant to be the case.

As the use of forms carries risk, therapists have to have foresight and think conscientiously and thoroughly about their use of forms. How the information on forms respects the privacy, dignity, and the integrity of the one who completed the form must be given careful consideration, as any other clinical data base.

When using forms, it is advisable to review the relevant code of ethics of one's profession to know the areas of sensitivity and areas of caution.

These words are said only to bring awareness and sensitivity to the issue of ethics. These words are not meant to discourage the use of forms. Clinical freedom must prevail in the interpretation and the use of information obtained through forms and questionnaires.

The main point is to be careful, considerate, thoughtful, caring, conscientious, and committed to ethical behavior in all that one does and through whatever means available. This includes form construction and use.

PROFESSIONAL CONSIDERATIONS

A clinician's ethics goes beyond what a managed care company prescribes or allows. It goes beyond what the code of conduct or code of ethics articulates for a particular professional association. It goes beyond the definition of what is legal. Ethics for the individual practitioner is acquired from a variety of sources including one's professional association, managed care companies, and the articulation of practice guidelines through books, articles, and papers written by colleagues. Indeed, it becomes a personal matter arising out of one's childhood development of a value, moral, religious, and ethical system that has been personalized over the course of professional training, educational experience, and life events.

Similarly, professional guidelines and professional standards also are operative in the development of clinical forms of various kinds. In the use of a form, helpful information is the objective as compared to being an instrument of snooping into the private life of an individual. Is the information obtained evaluated and utilized in the therapeutic context? Are the forms selected given serious consideration as to their purpose and face validity?

Information obtained on whatever form one selects for use is confidential psychological data. It must be maintained in a secure, limited access, archival system. As in other information, the patient holds the privilege; the therapist is to be confidential in dealing with such information. Release of data should be guided by strict and careful conditions and policies. Such information can be released only to proper sources and upon the execution of a formal signed release of information.

The use of forms should be conducted in the context of informed consent. It is important that the patient understand the reason for the use of forms and how they are going to be used as professional services are provided. A therapist must fully inform a patient as to the purpose and nature of an evaluative, therapeutic or educational form used in clinical practice, research, or for administrative purposes.

As in psychological testing, there are factors that must be taken into account when forms are utilized, interpreted, and incorporated as part of a clinical practice and the therapeutic strategies. Response bias is one example. Patients are known to fill out forms in the context of the bias they hold on any particular topic or issue raised by that form. For example, there are people who appear to function within the normal limits on a screening measure because they hold a particular "mind-set" as they complete the form. Some patients fill out forms to impress. Others fill out forms to indicate a cry for help. Others fill out forms from the perspective of trying to give a covert message through the therapist.

Lastly, it may be necessary to use an imperfectly designed screening device or form rather than not have any such screening device or form at all. Completed forms represent a snapshot, a photograph, of a person at one point and time in their life related to some particular issue or event taking place. Every form has historical value but may have only limited contemporary value. As a patient's circumstance changes, even as a result of therapy, the information obtained may come to have less value even though it had great value at an earlier time.

INDEX

Printed and bound by CPI Group (UK) Ltd, Croydon, CR0 4YY

10/05/2025

01866281-0001